STATE

of the

HEART

ALSO BY HAIDER WARRAICH

Auras of the Jinn

Modern Death

STATE

of the

HEART

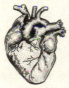

Exploring the History, Science,
and Future of Cardiac Disease

—⩘—

HAIDER WARRAICH, M.D.

ST. MARTIN'S PRESS

NEW YORK

First published in the United States by St. Martin's Press, an imprint of St. Martin's Publishing Group

www.stmartins.com

Designed by Kathryn Parise

The Library of Congress Cataloging-in-Publication Data is available upon request.

ISBN 978-1-250-16970-9 (hardcover)
ISBN 978-1-250-16971-6 (ebook)

Our books may be purchased in bulk for promotional, educational, or business use. Please contact your local bookseller or the Macmillan Corporate and Premium Sales Department at 1-800-221-7945, extension 5442, or by email at MacmillanSpecialMarkets@macmillan.com.

First Edition: July 2019

10 9 8 7 6 5 4 3 2 1

To Ammi and Abbu,
who taught me everything good I know

Contents

Acknowledgments

My grandparents were small-time farmers in Pakistan and my parents were the first generation in their families to go to school. They sat on the floor in their classrooms on mats woven from jute; instead of notebooks, they had slates which they would reuse the entire year. Education was their only way out of the village, and that idea stayed with them as they set about raising me and my two siblings.

My parents were never distracted and they were never impatient. They didn't just teach me that I should be kind, they showed me through how they treated everyone they met. They somehow found the perfect balance between providing structure and freedom. Now that I have a daughter myself, I am in awe of how they did so much, but made it look so easy. They provided me with the tools and the intellectual space to really be who I wanted to be even though I had no idea what that was.

As my medical training wraps up and I look back on five years of medical school at the Aga Khan University in Pakistan, three years of internal medicine residency at the Beth Israel Deaconess Medical Center in Boston, and three years of cardiology fellowship with a final year of training in advanced heart failure and transplantation both at Duke University Medical Center in North Carolina, I would be remiss to not acknowledge the hundreds of peers, faculty, nurses, and patients, who have helped make me the physician I am today. Being a physician is the greatest privilege of my life and that patients have provided me opportunities to be involved in some of the most vital moments of their lives is something I never take lightly. It has been an exhilarating journey and I still remember every single time a peer or faculty member gave me a few minutes of their time or more, to help me become a better doctor. I can never pay them back, but I do hope to pay it forward and keep this circle going.

As an immigrant, I am also grateful to the people of the United States who have welcomed me, my wife and our daughter. Like so many others who found a home here, we have received so much love in this country, from strangers in restaurants to our dearest friends. I couldn't have asked for a more thoughtful editor than Daniela Rapp at St. Martin's Press. This is my second book with her and she has made what can be a painful process a breeze. My agent, Don Fehr, always keeps me thinking about what is next.

And finally, no book can be written without acknowledging the love, care and support of my wife, Rabail. Between my last book and this, we had our daughter, who is the light of our life. And through my clinical training, my writing and my research, and now fatherhood, it has been Rabail who has held it all together for me, and who has allowed me to pursue my dreams. To date, the two best days of my life remain the day I first ran into her in Karachi more than a decade ago and the day that we got married. I know if I were to redo my life, I would never pick it any other way. My only hope is that I can give her back the joy she has given me, and that she would pick me again, too.

STATE

of the

HEART

1

—⩗—

DARKNESS BEFORE DAWN

The human heart has hidden treasures,
In secret kept, in silence sealed.

—Charlotte Brontë, "Evening Solace," 1846

Before I walked into my patient's room, I huddled outside with the rest of the team to make sure we were all on the same page. He had come to the hospital after he had caught a serious infection while on a cruise with his wife in the Caribbean. Tests confirmed that he had bacteria growing in his blood, which he had likely contracted from using a catheter to urinate while on the cruise. We treated his infection with antibiotics, but what we couldn't fix was his heart. He had been seeing a cardiologist regularly for his feebly beating heart, had been taking heart medications for decades, had even received a special pacemaker to help his heart beat synchronously. Despite all that had gone into trying to overcome his weakening heart, he was now fast approaching what seemed to be an imminent end. The entire medical team was convinced he didn't have long to live, maybe a few months at best. Everyone nodded in agreement one final time, like a football team about to take the field or a group of paratroopers about to leap from the back of a plane. After we filed into his room and made the customary introductions, the team settled in like a dense air freshener. As we had decided, I started talking, slowly.

"While you have recovered well from your infection, the one thing we cannot help you recover from is your heart failure."

"Wait—*what*—I have heart failure?" he asked abruptly. Startled, he looked to his wife, who started crying. "He has *heart failure?* No one told us he has heart failure! What *is* heart failure?" she wailed.

I was completely taken aback. These conversations can sometimes take their time to come to a full boil, but in this instance, it had bubbled over almost as soon as the stove was lit. The patient had been living with heart failure for almost two decades, and by all accounts, his cardiologist had been managing his heart failure diligently, yet somehow, the man had no idea what it was or what it meant, and worst of all, it appeared as if no one may have ever told him either. For some reason, the words *heart failure* had never been used around him. I had to back up, change gears immediately, and scrap the conversation about his mortality for another day. But that day never came—he died two weeks later in the intensive care unit.

More people die of heart disease than any other disease in the world, including even cancer. In fact, deaths from heart disease are on the rise around the world and in the United States as well.[1] When any heart disease becomes advanced enough, it frequently results in the development of heart failure. In the United States, heart failure is the most common reason for admission to the hospital.[2] Heart failure strikes both the abject and the affluent, the young and the old. In the past few years, both the pop singer George Michael and former first lady Barbara Bush died of heart failure. And yet, in many ways, heart failure is a disease few know about and fewer still understand. Even though the words *heart failure* are more likely to show up in common use these days than in times prior, many continue to ask the same question as my patient's wife—*what* is *heart failure?*

Heart disease, in many ways, is the overlooked affliction of our times. That seems like a curious thing to say for a disease that touches so many, young and old, man or woman, black or white, rich or poor. And even as the number of people dying from heart disease continues to rise. Many proclamations of the end of heart attacks have been made. And such pronouncements are having an effect; funding for research for heart disease and the development of new innovations for heart disease continues to lag behind other diseases such as cancer.[3] Fewer therapies are in development for heart disease today than before.[4] This is driven by many thinking of heart disease as a battle that has already been won, with funding being increasingly diverted to other conditions such as cancer, dementia, and diseases such as amyotrophic lateral sclerosis (ALS). Breast cancer, for example, receives seven times more research funding than heart disease for every death that it causes.[5] The media is far more likely to play up incremental and unproven advances in other diseases while ignoring proven and lifesaving therapies for heart disease.[6] Many people think that when people get heart disease, it is their fault and, increasingly, as treatments get better for heart disease, people acquire it in older age rather than in their younger years.[7] Even some of the leading experts in cardiovascular research are not optimistic about the future of research in heart disease. And despite the amazing reduction in the death rate from heart disease over the past few decades, the last few years have seen that progress effectively plateau and even some disconcerting reversal occur in the rate of death from heart disease.[8]

And yet, the present and future of how we can treat and prevent heart disease have truly never been more awe-inspiring. There is almost no parallel in human progress that mirrors how we have managed to change a heart attack from a death sentence to something that for the most part can be managed safely. Just over the past few years, I have seen technology become commonplace that could easily have been conflated with science fiction.

The heart, that muscular organ beating in your chest as you read, sending pulsations throughout your body, is perhaps the part of the body most associated with life at both ends of human existence. Hearing a heartbeat has become a rite of passage for anyone who becomes pregnant. When my wife got pregnant, it wasn't until our visit to the gynecologist at the eight-week mark that we heard that machine-gun-like heartbeat and the pregnancy was truly confirmed and we breathed a sigh of relief.

On the other end of existence, when someone falls to the ground unconscious, the reflex of anyone with an ounce of knowledge about the human body will be to reach for their wrist and feel for a pulse. If there is a pulse, there is life. If there is no pulse, there is no life, and hopefully someone is straightening out their elbows and locking their fingers as they get ready to perform cardiopulmonary resuscitation.

The pumping heart keeps the circulation of the body going. Blood seeping through the vine-like arterioles webbed through the lungs picks up oxygen that we breathe in. These vines then merge to form bigger vessels, which lead into the left side of the heart. The left side of the heart, the most muscular part of the heart, then pushes the blood to every part of the human body, from the kidneys, to the intestines, to the limbs, and all the way to the tips of the toes and fingers, but most importantly, to every vital nerve cell in the brain. These organs suck out oxygen from the blood like you would the last bit of that Slurpee with a spiral straw. This oxygen-deprived blood is sucked all the way back to the right side of the heart, which then squeezes this oxygen-poor blood into the vine-like arterioles lacing the lungs to fill up on oxygen.

The constant circulation of blood is like a divine, life-giving pilgrimage. When blood reaches the lungs, the temple of life, each red blood cell— all five million or so of them—squeezes into teeny-tiny alleys as opposed to the large highways it drove in from. These tiny alleys are called capillaries. It is in these capillaries that each and every red blood cell comes face-to-face with the invisible source of life—air. The air that we breathe in remains confined to tiny sacs of air called *alveoli*, which look like a bunch of grapes at the end of a stem. These alveoli are wrapped by the capillaries. So here the capillaries and alveoli come up right against each other, but they never mix, never touch the other. And yet, because of how thin the membranes that separate the two are, the red blood cells are able to absorb oxygen from the air, while unloading the carbon dioxide they are burdened with in exchange for the oxygen they have previously delivered to the tissues of the body. In essence, each and every one of the millions of red blood cells is cleansed, and their sheen so visible, so evident, that the blood actually changes color, from the dull and murky maroon of oxygen-deprived blood in the veins to the flush and vibrant crimson of oxygen-rich blood cruising through the arteries.

The heart is not the temple, but it is the stream that keeps this pilgrimage flowing uninterrupted. The heart is so essential to life that within seconds of its stopping, the body starts to undergo irreversible damage. It is a miracle that the heart, which beats more than two billion times in an average human being's lifetime, doesn't ever stop unless catastrophe happens.

The heart is one of the most complex structures in the human body, in charge of an incredibly high-stakes job. It is one of the first organs that forms in the growing human fetus. Although initially it starts off as one long tube while in the fetus, the heart folds in on itself, undergoing a dramatic but meticulous transformation, emerging as the four-chambered heart we are familiar with. The more one studies it, though, the more one is drawn into its complex yet elegant mechanisms. Every bit of the heart serves a purpose, and any small deviation can result in life-threatening consequences. This is particularly true when the heart is forming in the fetus.

How the fetus just knows what to do as it constructs itself out of a single embryonic cell into the most complex piece of organic machinery in the known universe is something that is worth pausing for. Without almost any outside guidance, within every human embryo lies all the knowledge needed to build itself. It's like an IKEA cabinet that can assemble itself just from a single piece of paper with directions on it. The worst a poorly assembled chest of drawers can do is not operate as smoothly as one would like. A poorly assembled heart with even the slightest flaw can be fatal.

Nature gets the heart right 99 percent of the time.[9] That sounds pretty great until you realize that in the United States, the 1 percent of children born with congenital heart defects amounts to forty thousand babies a year.[10] Most of these defects are not life-threatening and can be easily repaired or, in many cases, simply observed. A quarter of that 1 percent, though, almost ten thousand infants, have critical congenital heart disease, requiring major surgery within the first year of life.

The smallest aberrancy in the human heart can have devastating consequences. Recently, I took care of a woman who had a coronary artery, the teeny blood vessels that supply oxygen to the heart itself, taking a slightly different route. Instead of falling right onto the heart, it coursed between two large blood vessels. This simple rerouting meant that the lifeline to her heart could be blocked off at any given moment as the large vessels pulsated, sandwiching the coronary artery between them, and she needed to have it surgically corrected. Yet advances in surgery now mean that the vast majority of babies born with defected hearts can live into adulthood.

For the rest of the 99 percent, those without any obvious defects at birth, it is easy to think of the heart as perfect. Yet, in nature, there is no such thing as one perfect heart, for there is a different type of perfect heart for every different organism.

Just like there are many animals on the planet, there are different types of hearts.[11] A hummingbird has a heart that beats a thousand times a minute, while that of an elephant beats only about thirty times a minute. The heart of a blue whale weighs 1,300 pounds, is as big as a car, and pumps 92 gallons with every contraction, while the human heart pumps only about 70 milliliters with every squeeze. Octopuses have three hearts, two for each gill that serves as a lung, and one for the rest of the body. The Burmese python's heart can double in size within a day after it has a nice meal like a mouse or even a deer to accommodate for the sudden boost in metabolism before shrinking back to its previous dimensions. And dogs have a bigger heart relative to the size of their bodies than any other mammal, a fact that many dog owners might have already intuited.

So there is no one perfect heart, but each heart seems to be perfect for the body that it dutifully serves. But if the heart is so perfect, why is it that to this day, there are organisms that can exist just fine without one? While many readers have, at various points in their lives, been accused of being so, the truth is that when life started out, all the beasts that wandered the earth or swam in the oceans were heartless. Many of those exist as such to this day, but they are mostly tiny invertebrates. Some heartless organisms, such as sea spiders, actually move oxygen-rich blood within their bodies with the help of their pulsating guts.[12] The question—one that is starting to take on even more import as we humans advance to a stage where we can effectively replace people's hearts—is why do we even need the heart to begin with?

While many think of the heart in isolation, the truth is that the heart is in fact just the most visible part of the entire cardiovascular system. Focusing on the heart is like focusing on the air traffic control tower and ignoring the rest of the airport. Each and every blood vessel in your body, from the artery in your foot that you can feel between the webbing of your big toe and the second digit to the vessels supplying blood to your eyeball, is connected to the heart.

The heart is central to what it means to be human, yet modern medicine, having fundamentally changed how we live in so many ways, is now on the verge of unseating the heart from its throne. Over the past decade, new technology has been developed that allows people to live far beyond when their hearts fail. Heart failure, which used to be a terminal diagnosis, has been effectively transformed into a chronic disease that people live many years with. This technology effaces some of the most elemental aspects of what the heart does. Left ventricular assist devices (LVADs) are mechanical pumps that are surgically sewn into patients' hearts and take over the pumping function of the heart. If you put your fingers on the wrist of a patient with an LVAD, most of the times you will not feel a pulse. If you put your ear on an LVAD patient's chest, you will actually hear the pump humming, not the heart beating. When patients with LVADS get really sick, sometimes they don't need a doctor or a surgeon—they need a mechanic. LVADs are not only changing how patients with heart disease are being treated, they are changing what it means to be human.

Over the past century, heart disease has been the focus of intense scientific scrutiny, and the journey to rid the world of heart disease is very much reflective of the journey of medical science at large. So many issues that are relevant to science—the introduction of empirical testing, the industrialization of the scientific vocation, the epidemic of "fake news" and hype—are most apparent when it comes to heart disease. In understanding how our knowledge of the heart evolved, we inevitably trace the twisting and turning road all the way back, which allowed us to reach our present understanding of our biology and ourselves.

Just during my own training, I have seen the treatments for heart disease change in unimaginable ways. Take, for example, a condition in which the valve of the heart that connects the heart to the rest of the body, the final door the blood has to pass through as it enters the great vessel supplying the body with oxygenated blood, the aorta, becomes really tight. Aortic stenosis most commonly affects us as we get older, typically resulting in the soft and pliable aortic valve becoming hard and calcified. When it's severe, aortic stenosis can cause very high pressures the heart has to beat against, and it can limit how much blood can be ejected from the heart. Not too long ago, severe aortic stenosis was a death sentence. Then one doctor, who saw one case and was asked one simple question, changed all of that.

Eugene Braunwald is almost ninety years of age and to this day is one of the most prolific cardiology researchers around. Back in 1958, he was working at the National Institutes of Health, in Bethesda, Maryland, and a patient with aortic valve disease was seen by him and a heart surgeon.

Aortic valve surgery, which was done through the placement of an artificial heart valve after open-heart surgery, was just in its nascent stage, and the surgeon asked Braunwald, "What would you expect would be his prognosis in five to ten years if we don't operate?" Braunwald was caught off guard because no one really knew what the answer was. "What the hell are you good for?" he recalled the surgeon telling him when I spoke with Braunwald recently. "You can't fix the valve, and you can't even tell me what will happen to this patient if I don't fix it." Braunwald then launched a project to understand what happens to patients with severe aortic stenosis and found that once patients develop symptoms such as chest pain, fainting, or heart failure, they pretty much fall off a cliff and die within weeks to months, effectively defining the natural history of the disease.[13] Aortic valve surgery, the culmination of decades of technological developments that would have previously been unimaginable, was able to yank people off that ledge and provide them long and healthy lives.

Yet for many patients, aortic valve surgery was a tall task, and too many patients were too sick to be able to get this procedure. On the other side of the Atlantic, the French cardiologist Alain Cribier was planning an entirely radical treatment for severe aortic stenosis. He had devised a procedure in which, through a small incision in the leg, he would introduce a long, thin plastic catheter that would reach all the way up to the patient's heart and then blow up a balloon across the stiff aortic valve. After Cribier first performed this procedure in 1985, it spread around the world like pandemic flu, but the excitement was short-lived.[14] "The procedure appeared to provide only a temporary improvement in symptoms and, at best, a modest survival benefit," he told me in an email. Blowing a balloon open in a diseased valve was a Band-Aid at best. Cribier's eventual goal was much loftier: he wanted to transform aortic valve replacement from open-heart surgery to a minimally invasive procedure by "implanting a valve prosthesis within the diseased calcific native valve, on the beating heart, using catheter-based techniques and local anesthesia." He faced extensive challenges to be able to even imagine what this might look like, but the biggest one had nothing to do with science and technology. "The negative opinion of experts was definitely the greatest barrier," he wrote to me. "The idea was even considered the most stupid idea ever heard."

Cribier, though, was never going to take no for an answer. He developed a cylindrically shaped wire frame a few inches in length that housed a valve taken out of a pig or a cow. After a series of experiments in cadavers and animals, in April 2002, he implanted the first such valve in a fifty-seven-year-old man who was dying of severe aortic stenosis and was too high risk for surgery.[15] The procedure was so well tolerated that Cribier's team, in very French fashion, drank "champagne with him, in his room, on the same day."

Fast-forward to 2010, and I found myself standing in the operating room at Beth Israel Deaconess Medical Center in Boston, where I was doing research, and the first-of-its-kind transcatheter aortic valve similar to the one developed by Cribier was being placed in a patient. It was the first implantation of this valve in the United States as part of a large clinical trial that was just kicking off. The operating room was full of dozens of people with multiple cardiologists, surgeons, and anesthesiologists in attendance. Tension was high, but there was a sense that history was being made. Since then, hundreds of thousands of people have avoided open-heart surgery to receive this procedure that has single-handedly transformed the fate of patients with this life-limiting diagnosis.

To many, the best years of heart science are in our rearview mirror. Eugene Braunwald said, "If I were to start over today, I would choose a career in neuroscience, because the next forty or fifty years will be the golden period for discoveries in treatment of neurologic disorders, just as the last half century has been the golden period of cardiology, even though we have a long way to go." Yet, as you will find out, the golden age of cardiology is only just beginning, and it could end not by elevating the status of the heart but by entirely usurping it, effectively developing devices that can replace the human heart. Heart disease has been around for a while, but the type of heart disease people have, why they have it, and how it's treated is changing. And with treatments of heart disease altering the very definitions of human life and death, there is no better time to look at the present and future of heart disease, the doctors and nurses who treat it, the patients and caregivers who live with it, and the stories they hold close to their chests.

2

-\/\-

THE HEART—A LOVE STORY

Hearts are wild creatures,

That's why our ribs are cages.

—Elalusz

was sitting in a coffee shop with my wife and baby daughter, our table awash with sunlight, when the barista tiptoed over, delicately balancing the latte my wife had ordered. As he placed the large ceramic cup in front of her, something instantly made us smile. Beneath the reams of steam rising from the coffee, he had drawn an immaculate and whimsical heart in the foam. It made our day.

The heart is as much an organ that keeps us alive as it is a metaphor that helps define some of the most powerful, at times irrational, impulses we feel. It aids songwriters at wit's end, helping finish unwritten songs. It helps lovers put down in words what only the other can see, the other can feel. One doesn't even need to know how the heart works, how the heart comes to be formed, and all the beautiful mechanics that constitute its immaculate design to be bathed in its self-evident splendor.

The heart, though, is not just a symbol of beauty or love; the more you understand its actual function, its day-to-day existence manifest in every beat, the more its actual living beauty is actualized. Cardiologists dedicate their lives to appreciating what the heart is and then using that understanding to mend people's hearts—as much in allegory as in actuality. Between medical school and clinical training, it takes more than a decade to gather all the knowledge needed to be able to diagnose, prevent, and treat all the afflictions the heart can gather over a lifetime of hard, incessant labor.

There are many perks to being a cardiologist, but the one thing that unites us all is our fascination with the sheer, untainted beauty of the heart. Like a labyrinth that goes deeper and deeper, like a code that can never be cracked, the heart is so obvious in its magnificence that it is in its enigmatic details that its intricacy emerges. On any given day, using several different advanced imaging technologies, we get to see the hearts of many beat away, in radiographic loops that seamlessly flow in infinite cycles. At the same time, we talk to patients and their families at length about their cardiac health, the treatments they may or may not be able or willing to get. Interventional cardiologists who do invasive procedures, including inserting miniscule metal stents to open up the blood vessels supplying the heart, get even more up close and personal with the heart. And perhaps, no one is closer to the human heart, and is more aware of its maze of vessels and chambers, than the surgeon who can hold the heart of another in their hands with the human chest splayed wide open.

There are a variety of reasons behind why many choose to go down this path of training, and most of them are less romantic. During the first year of my cardiology training in the middle of the night in Durham, North Carolina, while I slept, on the very other end of the planet in Pakistan, a man in his mid-sixties started to sweat profusely early in the morning. He then felt light-headed and had to sit down to gain composure, not knowing what was going on. His wife, my mom, knew: my dad was having a heart attack. There was no one else at home. She didn't call the ambulance. She put him in the back of the car and rushed him to the nearest hospital.

About an hour after they had reached the emergency room, my mom called me. During that hour, he'd had an electrocardiogram, which was read by a cardiologist who immediately knew that he was having a heart attack—a serious one. The cardiologist activated the cardiac catheterization lab team, who swooped in and took Dad right in. Within minutes of him getting there, through a small puncture in his leg—using a long, slim, plastic-based catheter—they had made it all the way up to his heart, where they saw a blood clot completely obstructing the main blood vessel supplying it. They deployed a small metallic stent in the blocked blood vessel, restoring blood flow.

When I talked to Dad only moments after the procedure was over, he told me how everyone seemed so calm, that there was no commotion, that they just went ahead and did their jobs. In this instance, their job saved his life, and their timely response ensured that his heart was not affected in any way. All this happened while I was still asleep seven thousand miles away. In modern medicine, where chronic disease dominates, there are few moments one can look back on and truly feel like they saved a life. For those taking care of patients with heart disease, moments like these are not an exception—it is their very job. More than anything, it is for moments such as these that many embark on this journey.

Not all love stories have happy endings, though. My first memory of being in a cardiac hospital is very vivid to this day. I was around six or seven when one of my uncles was admitted to that very same hospital my mom drove my dad to after his heart attack. When I went with my parents to visit my uncle, a curious sign greeted us at the entrance: *Children are not allowed in the hospital*, it proclaimed. It was too late for us to turn around, so my parents snuck me in, something that was perhaps not so out of the ordinary back in Pakistan. I was walking down the main hallway when suddenly, I heard a loud shriek. Ahead of us, I saw a young woman wrapped in a large shawl who was running from side to side in the hallway, flailing her arms, until she collapsed to the ground. Her family rushed to her and tried to lift her off the floor, but she fought for her right to stay down. She was wailing in a way I could never have imagined would be possible. I had never heard sounds like that coming from a human being, and that traumatic sight lives with me to this day. She had not been as lucky as I would be almost two decades into the future. Her dad never called her after the heart attack—and he never would again.

With time, as our understanding of the heart's mechanics has changed, this knowledge has also changed the arc of the metaphorical heart. The heart is no longer hallowed ground, but a machine, which breaks down and needs a tune-up once in a while, with pipes that get clogged and that frequently need to be opened up by plumbers. When the heart is weak, the heart doesn't need love, it needs rocket fuel. In that way, the heart as metaphorical symbol has experienced as much of an arc as has the biological organ it represents.

For physicians and romantics alike, the heart has always been an irresistible, shimmering mirage on the horizon, forever drawing both toward it. The connection between us humans and our hearts always come down to anguish or elation, agony or exhilaration, affliction or enchantment. Never one for the fainthearted, many have trodden this path to unlock the secrets of the heart so as to conquer it, through words or verse and analysis and experiment. Walking back down these footsteps leads us all the way back to ancient Egypt, where the first records of our study of the human heart were unearthed.

Physicians and surgeons are frequently accused of having a god complex. Not too long ago, though, perhaps many did feel like they were the ultimate authority over their patients and what was best for them. If you look even further back, such as during the time of the pharaohs, physicians were very *literally* considered gods. Yet it is during that time, thousands of years ago, that we started to take baby steps into understanding the basic fundamentals of how our body works. What is intriguing is that for a long time, we were much better at understanding the universe around us, the one in which we are mere specks, than the universe that existed within.

The unassuming plant growing extensively in the Nile River delta wetlands, *Cyperus papyrus,* which was used to create the scrolls that allowed for the documentation and preservation of information, is why we can go back in time and tap into the vast wealth of knowledge that was being generated in Egyptian society, which was obsessed with medicine, chemistry, architecture, metaphysics, and the arts. What the Egyptians left behind was not just some of the first formal observations of medical science and the birth of the physicians' profession but something much greater. Sir William Osler (1849–1919), the famous physician who was one of the founding professors of Johns Hopkins, said in 1913, "In records so marvelously preserved in stone we may see, as in a glass, here clearly, there darkly, the picture of man's search after righteousness, the earliest impressions of his moral awakening, the beginnings of the strife in which he has always been engaged for social justice and for the recognition of the rights of the individual. But above all, earlier and more strongly than in any other people, was developed the faith that looked through death, to which, to this day, the noblest of their monuments bear an enduring testimony."[1]

No one is more singularly associated with the birth of medicine than Imhotep, who lived during the twenty-seventh century B.C. and was one of only two commoners ever elevated to the honor of full deification.[2] Considered the Egyptian god of medicine by the people of his time, he was outlived by temples erected in his honor, where the sick and debilitated would come for healing. These facilities were precursors to the modern hospital. Imhotep was much more than a physician: he was the chief minister to Pharaoh Djoser and was the principal designer of the step pyramid, the oldest hewn stone monument still left standing in the world. He truly was a god among men.

While no medical work is directly attributed to him, Imhotep's legacy was best documented in the Edwin Smith Papyrus, which gives us a glimpse into how medicine was practiced five thousand years ago.[3] While dated to the seventeenth century B.C., it is believed to have been copied from a document written possibly by Imhotep himself between 3000 and 2500 B.C.[4] The Edwin Smith Papyrus is a methodical analysis of forty-eight cases, ranging from infections to wounds, from the head to the feet, presented in what can now be considered a classic format. Every case has a title, followed by findings on physical examination, followed by one of three proclamations by the physician. When the ailment is one such as a chest infection (case 39), the physician "can handle it," and treatment is described. When the physician faces an ailment in which cure is not guaranteed, such as a chest tumor (case 45), the physician says that they "can fight with" or "contend with" it. Finally for ailments that just require observation, such as a rib fracture (case 44), these cases are described as those for which "nothing is done."

The Egyptians got much wrong about how the body works, and those misunderstandings would not be corrected for several thousand years, but they also got much right. The Egyptians were correct in understanding the centrality of the heart in human circulation, and the Edwin Smith Papyrus provided the first account of the human pulse linked to the heart. In poetic hieroglyphs they wrote, "It [the heart] . . . speaks in every vessel, every part of the body."[5] This might sound intuitive now, but almost a thousand years later, the Greek physician Hippocrates was still adamant that the circulation of blood started in the liver and not the heart.

But what was the heart circulating? The Egyptians thought that the heart was the central organ connected to channels spread throughout the body, transporting air, blood, bile, feces, semen, the spirits, and even the soul to every part of the body.[6] They also thought that it was air in the vessels that causes them to pulsate rather than a literal conduction of the heart's contraction through the arteries of the body. Furthermore, Egyptians, like many others to this day, had difficulty separating the fantastical from the empirical when it came to the heart. Blood, air, and all sorts of other bodily fluids were brought to the heart through a receptor vessel, likely the aorta, and were then transported to organs around the body, never to come back. The soul, while centered around the heart, also had another collection zone around the anus, which is why keeping the anus clean was an essential ritual necessary to cleanse one's soul.

Over the course of their civilization, the Egyptians continued to keep a magnifying glass on the heart, and their understanding evolved. Even how they drew the heart changed, starting from a blob with eight vessels looking like a latex glove blown up like a balloon to a more realistic jar-like shape. The heart was the seat of emotion and the spirit, a living record of one's deeds both good and bad, so essential that it was left behind in the chest when bodies were mummified. It was believed that when the deceased were ushered into the hereafter for judgment by Anubis, the canine-headed Egyptian god of the afterlife, the heart of the dead person was weighed on a scale against an ostrich feather. A heart weighed down by sin would be fed to the devourer of the dead, Ammit, the crocodile-lion-hippopotamus hybrid, and the deceased could no longer enter the afterlife and were damned to eternal restlessness. A heart devoid of debauchery, floating like a feather, would allow the deceased entry into the eternal underground, promising an unending life of peace.

Sin didn't just burden the heart in the afterlife but could actually lead to disease in the mortal life. This concept formed the basis of seminal descriptions of some of the most common heart conditions, such as heart failure, that we see and struggle to treat to this very day.[7] These diagnoses were documented in the Ebers Papyrus—one of the longest-surviving papyruses, written almost 1,500 years after the Edwin Smith Papyrus, around 1,500 B.C.—bought in 1873 by the German Egyptologist Georg Ebers from its Egyptian owner and translated by Heinrich Joachim. Many think of heart disease as a modern disease, and yet it has continued to maim men and women for as long as they have had hearts.

For many, a single degree connects them to the earliest accounts of heart disease and the most primitive ideas about how the body was assembled. For me, it is the wedding ring I have worn so long on my finger that the skin underneath it is slick and several shades fairer than the uncovered rest of my hand. What dates back even longer than my marriage is the tradition underlying why exactly so many wear wedding rings on the fourth digit on their left hands. The answer to that may lie in a roll of papyrus a hundred pages long, written in 1555 B.C. The Ebers Papyrus contains an encyclopedic amount of information, from treatments for night blindness (ox liver) to some of the first descriptions of diabetes, yet it was its description of different types of heart disease that cemented its place in human history.

To this day, there is no image more classically associated with potentially fatal heart disease than a man or woman clutching their chest in pain. The clenched fist over the breastbone, referred to as the Levine sign, is almost synonymous with *angina pectoris*. Angina, the pressure-like feeling in the chest that frequently travels down one's left arm and up the neck, occurs when there is a restriction in the blood supply of the heart, which, if it continues unabated, represents a heart attack.

It is important to understand here that even though the heart is pumping blood at all times, this blood does not actually supply the heart itself with oxygenated blood. In fact, the heart muscle is supplied with oxygenated blood from a system of blood vessels referred to as the *coronary circulation*. Derived from *crown*, the coronary arteries emerge right from where the aorta leaves the heart and descend on it like ivy embedded in the heart's wall like termite tunnels. It is these tiny vessels on the outside of the heart where blockages from cholesterol in the blood vessels can cause heart attacks and result in people feeling pain or a pressure-like sensation in their chests. For most of modern times, the discovery and initial description of angina was attributed to British physician William Heberden (1710–1801), in his very vaguely titled paper, "Some Account of Disorder of the Breast," which he presented to the Royal College of Physicians in London in 1768; it was published in 1772.[8] Heberden provided an arresting and incredibly accurate description based off an analysis of only twenty patients: "Those who are afflicted with it, are seized while they are walking with a painful and most disagreeable sensation in the breast, which seems as if it would extinguish life if it were to increase." While these patients had angina, Heberden felt their pulse and, given the lack of any abnormalities there, incorrectly determined that the pain was not from the heart but from an ulcer in the stomach, yet despite this misattribution, he knew what happened when angina went on unabated. "If . . . the disease goes on to its height, the patients all suddenly fall down, and perish almost immediately." After not finding any abnormalities in autopsies in patients suffering angina, having again missed the coronary circulation, Heberden concluded, "Since it was not due owing to any malconformation, or morbid destruction of parts necessary to life, we need not despair of finding a cure."

Heberden, though, was far from the first to describe angina. In fact, several thousand years ago, an equally compelling description of angina was noted in the Ebers Papyrus, also predicting a grim ending: "And if thou examinst a man for illness in his cardia and he has pains in his arms, in his breast, and in side of his cardia . . . it is death that threatens him."[9] In fact, the Egyptians were likely a step ahead since the left fourth digit, the very finger many people wear rings on as signs of sexual and emotional commitment, where the pain of angina frequently radiates to, was widely referred to as the "heart" finger. They believed that angina was related to the heart and not in fact the stomach or intestines as Heberden did. In fact, it was later hypothesized, and widely believed to this day, that a special vein, the so-called *vena amoris*, forms a direct connection between the heart and the fourth finger.

While angina occurs because of restricted blood flow supplying the heart muscle, the Egyptians also provided the first description of a different type of heart disease, one that is rearing its head today more than ever before—heart failure.[10,11] The papyrus describes it as a weakening of the heart muscle, which it calls in other places a "weakness or feebleness" of the heart, a "kneeling of the heart." Elsewhere, the author states "his heart is bored," although the cause of this boredom was perhaps misattributed: "This means that his heart is weak because of heat of the anus." Many patients with heart failure develop swelling of the legs and can collect fluid in their lungs, causing difficulty breathing and a wet cough, and this, too, was addressed. "His heart is flooded. This is the liquid of the mouth. His body parts are all together weak." And finally, the unknown author of the Ebers Papyrus also reported on the fatal final act of heart failure for many patients, which takes lives without announcement to this day: ventricular fibrillation. "When the heart is diseased, its work is imperfectly performed; the vessels proceeding from the heart become inactive so that you cannot feel them. . . . If the heart trembles, has little power and sinks, the disease is advancing." This trembling of the heart, which effectively leads to a stoppage of the circulation of blood, occurs when an abnormal heart rhythm originating from the pumping chambers of the heart, the ventricles, causes the heart to rapidly quiver, at times more than two hundred times a minute, and can be fatal within seconds. Patients with heart failure are at particularly high risk of developing ventricular tachycardia or fibrillation.

These breathtaking discoveries, these complex descriptions of heart disease, in all their different forms, though, would remain unknown for centuries. While much of Western medicine draws a straight line back to the Egyptians, in many ways, much of what was learned in the cradle of human civilization was lost, and many of these conditions, such as angina or heart failure, would not be "discovered" until centuries after they had already been recognized. It was our inability to comprehend their ancient language that prevented these findings from being transmitted and built upon rather than buried underneath the ruins of time.

These discoveries could still have been outside our reach were it not for one of the most serendipitous moments of human history. During Napoleon's Egyptian campaign in 1799, Pierre-François Bouchard, a French soldier, was put in charge of rebuilding Fort Julien, an old Ottoman fort near the Egyptian town of Rashid. He came across a large granite slab, which was being used as fill, but there was something quite remarkable about it. On the slab was inscribed ancient text, which was subsequently revealed to be three versions of the same royal decree. The top two texts were in ancient Egyptian scripts while the bottom one was in ancient Greek. The stone was captured by the British, who transported it to the British

Museum, and almost twenty years after it was first discovered, using his knowledge of the ancient Greek language, the texts were transliterated by the French Egyptologist Jean-François Champollion, opening up the entire Egyptian civilization and its myriad time capsules jotted on hardy papyruses to our comprehension.

By the time the Rosetta stone blew humanity's collective minds, Egyptian knowledge had gathered two millennia worth of dust, and it was the Greeks and Arabs who came to define our modern knowledge of the heart and the human circulation. A scientific theory originating in ancient Greece and popularized by the scholars Hippocrates and Galen defined not only how we thought of the human body but also the human soul. For the almost two millennia that separated the creation of the Rosetta stone to its eventual rediscovery, civilization found itself neck deep in blood, phlegm, black bile, and yellow bile—the four humors.

Before a time when we could go online and take a quiz to figure out "Which *Game of Thrones* character am I?" many looked to the concept of the four humors to explain one's temperament. While the humors were used to organize all of human existence into one theorem, at their core they were a personality test, one that persists to this day, and you can go online and take it for free. Different tests, though, gave me a different personality type, with one defining me as sanguine while another found me to be phlegmatic. The four temperaments associated with the humors form the backbone of some more widely used tests, such as the Myers-Briggs Type Indicator.

The humors centered around the number four.[12] There were four primary qualities in nature—hot, cold, dry, and wet. There were four central elements—earth, wind, fire, and water. Corresponding to these elements and qualities were the four temperaments of human nature—melancholic, sanguine, choleric, and phlegmatic. And finally, these temperaments were linked to the four humors—black bile, blood, yellow bile, and phlegm. An imbalance in the humors was the source of all disease. While this theory existed in ancient Egypt before the time of Hippocrates and Galen, these Greek physicians helped to legitimize it and were responsible for its longevity past their own deaths.

Galen (A.D. 129–210), a disciple of Hippocrates, was born in what is now western Turkey and had a long education, including at Alexandria in Egypt, where he was able to pick up and carry forward the torch of Egyptian medicine, eventually ascending to being the physician to the Roman emperor.[13] He was a strong proponent of the body's circulation being an "open" system. What does that mean? Galen held that nutrients were absorbed from the food in the intestines and converted into blood in the liver. He hypothesized that all the vessels of the body emerged from the liver. The blood then moved via the veins to all the organs, where it would be absorbed. The blood that went to the right side of the heart, instead of going to the lungs, being oxygenated and coming back, just diffused from the right side of the heart directly to the left side through small pores in the septum that separated the two sides, he posited. Essentially, he theorized that the movement of blood was one-way rather than circular. Air was directly ingested into the left side of the heart, where it mixed with blood that had diffused through said invisible pores. Galen, like others at his time, believed that the chief function of the heart was not to pump blood but to provide innate heat, and that the primary function of breathing was to cool the body.

The theories that Galen held would become the staple of medical science in the civilized world throughout Europe, spreading all the way to the Arab and Byzantine empires. Though Galen was perhaps the most influential physician-scientist of all time, far from moving science forward, Galen only reinforced preexisting incorrect notions. Galen did not distinguish himself by performing experiments that were validly executed. In fact, he never dissected a human body in his entire life. And the timing of his rise in influence could not have been worse. In the years after his death, religious forces completely took over the sciences, bringing an ignominious end to any further empirical investigation for centuries in Europe. Galen's theory of the humors was so easily coopted by theology that it would be a few thousand years until enlightenment would return to Western civilization and the Dark Ages would dissipate.

It was during these Dark Ages that the mantle of intellectual pursuit was taken up by the Arab civilization. Ibn al-Nafis (1210–1288), born around Damascus in Syria, was a polymath, like so many other intellectuals of his time, but his main specialty was the eye.[14] His investigative nature, however, led him to overcome the overwhelming influence of Galen and his own mentor, Ibn-Sina (980–1037), also called Avicenna in the West.[15] Galen had theorized that blood in the right side of the heart does not go to the lungs and come back flush with oxygen. The heart did not pump blood; rather, blood moved passively from the right to left side through small, invisible pores in the septum that separated the two sides. But of course, given that he had never dissected a human body or opened a human heart, this was all conjecture.

Even today, when we can get microscopic views of the beating heart without a scalpel in sight, there is so much an actual dissection of the heart can reveal that even the highest-resolution imaging cannot. While they are rarely performed in modern medicine, autopsies can transform disease from an existential threat to a real entity you can touch and feel. Whether that is poking the hardened muscle of the heart that suffered a heart attack or actually seeing the tiny clot obstructing a stent that had been previously placed in a patient's coronary artery, there is almost no substitute to seeing humanity's nemeses in the flesh.

Unlike those before him, Ibn al-Nafis did open a human heart, and he realized that there was in fact no connection between the right and left side of the organ. Blood that went to the lungs from the right side received vital spirit from the air we breathed in and returned to the left side of the heart to be circulated to the body.[16] While he never fully divorced himself from Galen's general ideas, he was quite clear about what he thought about prevalent ideas of the circulation: "Therefore the contention of some persons to say that this place is porous, is erroneous; it is based on the preconceived idea that the blood from the right ventricle had to pass through this porosity—and they are wrong!"[17]

Ibn al-Nafis's accounts, though, while accepted in the Islamic world, failed to convince many Europeans, including Leonardo Da Vinci, who also was housed in the Galenic view of the world. Galen's influence consumed medical science, and it persisted until an English physician, William Harvey, appeared on the scene in the seventeenth century and who debunked centuries of dogma. His story, and the reaction to his findings, have important lessons about the scientific process, the brutality of the status quo, and what it takes to overcome the toxic mix of scientific and religious ideas. *Fake news* has become a buzzword recently, but it has been around as long as there have been mouths that speak and ears that hear.

William Harvey, born in 1578, in Kent, England, went to Gonville & Caius College in Cambridge, but to receive the best medical education in the world, he had to pack his bags and travel to Padua, Italy, which one might say was the Harvard of medical schools back then. At the same time that Harvey was there, Galileo was the chair of the mathematics department. After finishing his studies, Harvey returned to England, where he eventually ascended to being the personal physician to King James in 1618.

By all accounts, Harvey was not a renegade. He did not set out to upend centuries of doctrine. In fact, he rejected many of the mathematical discoveries that were being made at that time and was fully invested in the theology of the vital spirit. What he was, though, was a scientist in perhaps the truest form. In his magnum opus, *Exercitatio Anatomica de Motu Cordis et Sanguinis in Animalibus* (*Anatomical Exercises on the Motion of the Heart and Blood in Animals*), published in 1628, he wrote, "I profess to learn and teach the anatomy not from books but from dissections, not from the tenets of philosophers but from the fabric of nature." He was interested not merely in receiving the truth but in testing it with a hypothesis in mind. And unlike the cosmos, where the truth could lie completely out of reach, you didn't have to go far to examine and investigate the human body.

Before Harvey's time, the very flow of life was thought to be linear, from point A to B, never to return. Nutrition obtained from food in the intestines was converted to blood and moved to the tissues, where it was consumed and was never to be seen again. Yet this was also the time of Copernicus, who had postulated that far from being stationary, the earth was constantly revolving in circular motion around the sun. There was something so elegant and efficient about circular movement that it must have struck a chord with Harvey.

To test his hypothesis that blood traveled circularly through the body, and that arteries taking bright blood away from the heart were in fact connected to the veins bringing dark blood back to the heart, he devised an experiment so simple yet elegant that not only could an eight-year-old design it, they would be able to understand what it meant.[18]

The heart pumps oxygenated blood into the arteries. The arteries have thick walls to withstand the pressure of the heart's pulsations and to transmit those pulsations all the way down their course. Veins, on the other hand, carry blood at low pressures, since they are not connected directly to the pumping chamber of the heart and, as Harvey observed, have valves to prevent blood from flowing back toward the tissues. Arteries and veins are connected by microscopic vessels called *capillaries,* which look like interlocked fingers surrounding tissues in their webs. It is through these thinwalled capillaries that blood can deliver oxygen and take up carbon dioxide, which is waste produced after the oxygen is used to create the building blocks of energy in the human body.

Harvey tied a band tightly around a man's elbow—so tight that it occluded both the artery taking blood to the hand and the vein bringing blood back. This caused blood to start accumulating in the throbbing artery in the arm above the band, since it couldn't cross the tight band, and the pulse in the wrist to disappear in that same artery downstream.

Harvey then repeated this experiment, but this time with the elbow band only tight enough to compress the vein but not the artery. In this case, the man still had a pulse in the wrist since arterial blood was still making its way to the hand past the elbow. Yet because blood in the veins from the hand could not return back to the heart, it started collecting there, causing the hand to become swollen and distended.

Having proved that the arteries and veins were connected, with arteries moving blood toward the fingers and away from the heart, and the veins vice versa, he then devised another incredibly simple experiment to establish that the heart was central to this connection.[19] In a still-living fish, Harvey tied off the veins draining into the fish heart. The fish heart almost immediately emptied out since it was continuously pumping blood forward, and it started accumulating blood behind the ligature on its way back. In a snake, he pinched the aorta, the great artery emerging out of the heart. Immediately, the heart became swollen and distended, a change that resolved as soon as he let go. Even though the hearts of humans and fish are not identical, how they work is similar enough to support the veracity of this experiment.

Therefore, with a band here and a pinch there, Harvey proved quite simply that all the blood in the body was traveling, constantly and relentlessly, in one big loop, over and over and over again, incessantly, in both humans and animals, driven by the heart, the captain of this crazy train.

After centuries of dabbling in dubious distortions, how would humanity even react to the truth? Galen's words and theories by Harvey's time had acquired a divine power that was above question from even the brightest of minds. What would it take for people to realize that not only was everything a deviation from the truth but manifestly false in every imaginable manner? The story of William Harvey is important because if you are an optimist, it demonstrates the natural history of the truth coming to light and being accepted for what it is. In an address in 1906, Sir William Osler said, "By no single event in the history of science is the growth of truth, through the stages of acquisition, the briefer period of latent possession, and the glorious period of conscious possession, better shown than in the discovery of the circulation of the blood."[20] But if you are a pessimist, you realize just how strong a grip falsehoods can have, especially when so many are so invested in them.

Harvey, who was incredibly powerful at the time of the publication of his work, knew that he was not immune to retribution. In *De Motu Cordis,* he wrote, "What remains to be said on the quantity and source of this transferred blood, is so strange and undreamed of that not only do I fear danger to myself from the malice of a few, but I dread lest I have all men as enemies, so much does habit or doctrine once absorbed become second nature, and so much does reverence for antiquity influence all men."

Harvey did find some supporters, but they were greatly outnumbered by his opponents, who spanned the entire European continent.[21] René Descartes approved of Harvey's theory in *Discourse on the Method* (1637), but he believed that blood did not flow due to the pumping of the heart but by the natural heat implanted by God in the heart, causing the blood to expand and move forward.[22] The one thing that was common to all those opposing Harvey was that they didn't actually perform experiments to disprove his claims. In fact, one of the only adversaries of Harvey who used physical experiments to challenge his claims actually converted to Harvey's theory of circulation, convinced by his own experimentation.[23] Eventually, though, given his proximity to the royal family and prominent position in the Royal College of Physicians, William Harvey's theory found acceptance during his lifetime. Harvey was also a careful man—he published his book in Frankfurt and not in England so as to not arouse the ire of his direct peers. He also accepted most of the theological assertions of his time and used his political connections to protect himself. He fared much better than Galileo, who was placed under house arrest and accused of heresy by the pope.

Harvey's greatest legacy, however, was perhaps not so much his discovery as how he got to it in the first place. His true gift was introducing the art of scientific experimentation and observation into medical education and research. Many of the young doctors he influenced went on to repeat his experiments and then become seeped in a tradition of generating new data through hypothesis-driven testing. While that tradition continues unabated to this day, much of what Harvey stood for appears to be under siege once again. In the Western world and particularly in the United States, anti-intellectualism and a disdain for science have begun to rear their long-dormant heads. Disruptive science is not only attacked by those for whom scholarship is but a convenient companion but by other scientists with competing financial or intellectual biases. Climate science comes instantly to mind, as many with vested interests or entrenched biases seek to redirect the march of science. Only these days, instead of pitchforks, heated battles are waged over Twitter and through legislation passed by government. While the body count is thankfully sparse, the damage to the spread of knowledge is constant and worrisome.

As we progressed toward a more accurate understanding of the physiological function of the heart and how it relates to us, a parallel and equally important journey was taking place: the role the heart plays in artistic, literary, social, and religious discourse. The heart has always played an outsize role beyond its biologic function. When most people talk about the heart, to this day, it represents something far more than a thoughtless pump, mindlessly churning blood through the body; it represents the very core of human life in its myriad layers in all cultures and at every point of human history.

The metaphorical heart, rarely swayed by the winds of time, was shaken forever by William Harvey's *De Motu Cordis*. Harvey not only changed how physicians and biologists think about the heart but how poets, philosophers, and novelists contemplate it and its role in our lives and the qualities that it represents. From an organ that provided warmth to the body, the heart now became a muscular pump, circulating blood throughout the body. This represented not just a new function but a new character.

In his book *The Language of the Heart, 1600–1750,* Robert Erickson posited that while the Galenic heart had a "strongly receptive or 'feminine' function," given that it attracted and then warmed the blood, William Harvey's heart, given its throbbing dilations and constrictions, performed a "more ejaculatory and 'masculine' function."[24] Through his scientific findings and editorial overlays, Harvey developed an "implied allegory of an erotic and divine harmony between the husband heart and the bodily wife."

From being an organ that was the key to understanding not only human nature but divine nature, the heart was increasingly seen as a laborer, a cog in a conveyer belt. Advances in knowledge about the nervous system led to the recognition that the brain was more than just a filler between the ears. It was Charles Darwin who, in 1871, took the crown from the heart and placed it firmly on the brain, calling it "the most important of all the organs." To many, the heart was no more than a mule, slogging away in the mud, carrying the load without asking questions. In *Illness as Metaphor* (Farrar, Straus and Giroux, 1978), Susan Sontag wrote, "Cardiac disease implies a weakness, trouble, failure that is mechanical."

As we continue to move forward, the long and eventually fruitful development of the theory of circulation, which overcame centuries of missteps and untruths, has important lessons for us today, leaving many unanswered questions: What do we believe in today that will be the equivalent of Galen's invisible pores in years to come? How do we even go about that search? To do that, let's look at what we know about the heart today, the culmination of a portrait centuries in the making, put together by scientists and artists alike, yet still as mysterious and ambiguous as Mona Lisa's smile.

The heart sits behind the rib cage slightly to the left of the breastbone with its tip pointing down and to the left. The human body has many valuable organs, yet few are as well protected as the heart. As big as your closed fist, the heart is unlike any other organ because it is always beating, always moving, and, to make sure that it is provided the best possible environment to be able to do that, it is surrounded by a thin, double-walled fibrous sac called the *pericardium*. The pericardial sac contains about 30 milliliters of a transparent fluid called *pericardial fluid*. The pericardium does many things—it lubricates the heart, allowing it to continue pumping while expending the least amount of excess energy. The pericardium also shields the heart from infections that might occur in the tissues around the heart. Unlike the heart, which floats like a fetus in its sac, the pericardium is attached to the tissues and bones around it, effectively anchoring the heart in place, which would otherwise just be flopping around in the chest. And finally, because of its inelastic nature, the pericardium restricts the heart from ballooning out of control.

The heart itself is made up of four chambers, two smaller, thin-walled atria on top, and larger, thick-walled ventricles below. The left and right atria are separated by a thin septum, while the ventricles are separated by a much thicker septum.

The largest two veins in the body—called the *vena cava,* one coming down from the head, the other coming up from the body—converge at the right atrium, bringing venous blood from the body to the heart. Blood flows from the right atrium, across the tricuspid valve, into the right ventricle. The heart valves are meant to prevent blood from going in reverse gear and keep blood moving in the right direction. The right ventricle, much smaller than the left ventricle, is connected directly to a large artery called the *pulmonary artery* that leads this venous blood to the lungs. As soon as the pulmonary artery emerges out of the right ventricle, pointed up toward the head, it splits into the right and left pulmonary arteries like a *T.* These pulmonary arteries then keep splitting like cracks in a frozen lake until they become tiny capillaries wrapping around *alveoli*, the tiny sacs where air drawn in from the lungs comes face-to-face with the blood without actually touching the other. These capillaries, now with blood brightened with oxygen, merge into other smaller veins, eventually ending up as four large pulmonary veins, bringing juiced-up blood back to the heart, draining into the left atrium. This blood then moves down the mitral valve into the left ventricle, the largest and most powerful part of the heart, responsible for pumping blood to the entire body, unlike the right ventricle, which only pumps blood to the lungs. With every contraction, blood leaves the left ventricle through the aortic valve and into the aorta, which then branches off into vessels leading to each and every part of the body.

The small and wispy atria and the large and powerful ventricles engage in a rhythmic dance that starts from the first heartbeat to the last. When the atria relax and dilate, causing blood to rush in from the body on the right and the lungs on the left, the ventricles are contracting, pushing blood out of the heart. They are separated by the valves, which ensure that the pressure generated in the ventricles during their contraction, called *systole,* does not travel back toward the atria, which would interrupt them filling with blood. Therefore, the atria exist to ensure that the heart is filling with blood at all times. After the ventricles are done contracting, they relax, actively sucking blood in from the atria across the tricuspid valve on the right and the mitral valve on the left. To maximize filling of the ventricles, the atria contract while the ventricles are relaxing in diastole, providing an additional kick of blood flow into the ventricles. This ensures that the ventricles are nice and full when they beat next. And because the atria are full when the ventricles contract and the ventricles are full when the atria contract, the overall size of the heart only varies by about 5 percent during the entire cardiac beating cycle. The dance between the atria and the ventricles also means that blood in the body is always moving forward, either out the aortic valve and into the aorta, or up and down the vena cava and into the right atrium.

What is important to realize is that even though the heart is always full of blood, it does not derive any nourishment from the blood that courses through it. The heart gets its own oxygen from the blood in the coronary arteries, which originate just past the aortic valve from the wide mouth of the aorta. The right coronary artery emerges from the right side, supplying the right ventricle and the inferior portion of the left ventricle, while the left coronary artery splits into two large vessels, the left anterior descending and left circumflex arteries. Of these, the left anterior descending artery supplies the entire front face of the left ventricle, all the way from the top to its pointy end, called the *apex*, and then wraps around it. The left anterior descending is affectionately called the *widow-maker*—not only is it the most common of the three coronary arteries to be affected by blockages causing heart attacks, but an occlusion in the left anterior descending is also the most dangerous since it supplies the greatest territory of heart muscle.

Disease can affect each and every part of the heart described here, from the pericardium to the electrical conduction system within the heart, and for the most part, we have figured out ways to treat, manage, and in some cases, cure, most of those pathologies. This progress represents one of the single most impressive achievements of our race.

The truth, though, is that much of what I described here, the foundation on which we have built modern cardiovascular medicine, might be completely false. What science has taught us to date so far is that nothing is absolute, yet the past fifty years have yielded more tangible progress in culling the progress of cardiovascular disease than any other time in our history. Furthermore, what the history of the heart also teaches us is the fragility and reversibility of scientific progress. Ancient civilizations went from being this close to putting the theory of human circulation together, perhaps being one tourniquet around the elbow from revealing the true nature of the cardiovascular system, to descending into almost fifteen hundred years of darkness. How can such progress be so brittle? Perhaps, as in the case of vaccines, its effectiveness at preventing diseases such as measles, polio, smallpox, and whooping cough obscures to people what we have worked so hard to overcome. Sometimes, progress can be prevented due to disinformation. Until recently, the sugar and tobacco industries were actively suppressing research suggesting that their products caused harm. Our history makes clear that we must always remain vigilant and protect what we now finally know after millennia of setbacks.

Science, too, runs the risk of becoming what it was made to overcome. William Harvey and others used the scientific method to change how we interrogate reality, not to believe what has been passed down but to empirically figure it out for ourselves; many scientists and physicians, however, cling to ideas like they are religious texts that cannot be questioned even though this was exactly what the scientific method was supposed to overcome.

For now, though, we can bask in the light illuminating every crevice of the heart. And to get things started, let's squint into some of the tiniest blood vessels in the human body. The heart is always full of blood that is used by the rest of the body, yet the blood that the heart itself needs for oxygenated nourishment fills the coronary arteries that cover it like paper covers rock. In the most important real estate in the human body, a millimeter of plaque can be the difference between life and death.

3

〜〜

THE ELEPHANT IN THE ROOM
(Sitting on the Chest)

But the heart has its own memory and I have forgotten nothing.

—Albert Camus, *The Fall*

R ajeev was on his way back home to Nepal. It was a really long flight from his home in North Carolina. He just "slept, slept, and slept" for the entire flight from Atlanta to Istanbul, he told me, where he had a long, nine-hour layover.

After shopping at the duty-free shop, he got himself a coffee and walked around the airport, looking for a good spot to settle down, plug in his laptop, and catch up on life. It was when he had finally found a quiet nook that the familiar feeling returned at the bottom of his throat.

Over the past few months, frequently when he was exercising, Rajeev would feel like his throat was on fire. "I had been having this uncomfortable sensation before, but it would usually go away," he told me. Often when he had this feeling, he would try to cough, and usually it would make things better. "I started to cough that phlegm out, which seemed to make things better in the past. But this time, it didn't seem to work."

Rajeev moved over to the restroom and kept coughing, but instead of things getting better, they started to get worse. "I felt like I was drowning . . . even as I kept breathing in huge quantities of air, I just felt like I couldn't get any air out."

Rajeev had no idea what was going on. He was in his forties and hadn't seen a doctor in almost a decade. "I had never even had a flu or fever." But this time, he just knew he was in dire straits. "I felt the only way I could stay alive was if I kept breathing very quickly and deeply."

He was hesitant to seek help, though. "I thought someone might think I was having an Ebola attack or something."

He was also still hoping all this would go away, just like it always had, and he could go home and be with his parents, yet he reached a point where he felt like he had no choice and could barely stand. Drenched in sweat and now almost in a panic, he went up to security officers, who immediately called for help. "The emergency team came quickly and put me on a stretcher. They put on an oxygen mask, but it didn't seem to help."

The team was so worried that they told Rajeev he would have to be taken to a local hospital. Rajeev, however, didn't have a Turkish visa. They immediately called an immigration official, who processed the fastest visa he had ever issued, and very soon Rajeev was in the hospital.

Rajeev never had chest pain or any of the symptoms he thought were associated with heart disease. He had smoked in the past but had quit many years ago. "My dad is in his eighties and has been smoking since he was twelve years old. His doctor just told him he has the body of a twenty-year-old," he relayed to me. Rajeev was also a bit of an athlete himself, regularly playing racquetball and lifting weights. Even the electrocardiogram that had been performed at the airport did not reveal anything wrong with his heart.

And yet what Rajeev has since learned is that what he experienced in international no-man's-land was a brush so close with death he might as well have been enveloped in the reaper's cold breath. For two days, the medical team had no answers. On the third morning, he was abruptly told he was being moved to the cardiac intensive care unit.

"They told me I'd had a heart attack."

"Did you believe them?" I asked.

"Absolutely not."

When people talk about heart disease, what most mean to talk about are heart attacks—a disease process of such mythological menace, it is as much a part of the pop culture vernacular as it is the medical lexicon. Every fourth American dies of heart disease, and one of the most dreaded manifestations of heart disease—heart attacks—affect almost a million Americans every year.[1] Heart attacks are so common, almost everyone knows someone personally who had one. And at a time when infectious diseases are decreasing, heart attacks are becoming increasingly common around the world. At the same time, though, what qualifies as a heart attack is changing. Many times, the only way a heart attack comes to be known is through a blood test. As we learn more about the heart, it is changing much of what we knew about heart attacks, why they occur, how best to treat them, and how to make sure they never happen in the first place.

And yet, even as we have made tremendous progress in helping people live through heart attacks, there is still so much we don't know about what causes heart attacks and what is the best way to treat them. Many think of heart attacks as being a modern disease, a consequence of the ills of our sedentary, overconsumptive lifestyles, yet that couldn't be further from the truth. Men and women have been clutching their chests, hoping for the lights to not go out, for as long as they have been around.

Atherosclerosis, the insidious process of plaque deposition occurring in our blood vessels, resulting in narrowing and at times catastrophic blockages throughout the body, is the root cause of heart attacks, strokes, limb-threatening leg disease and chronic kidney disease. Heart disease can take many different forms, but atherosclerosis is the process behind some of its most common manifestations, such as heart attacks. While a heart attack or a stroke strikes like a bolt out of the dark, like a starved lion hungry to finish off its prey, atherosclerosis takes its time. Atherosclerosis can take decades to develop, finally crippling its victim from head to toe in its suffocating, ever-constricting grip. Atherosclerosis kills more people than any other process around the world. Even though we have been battling atherosclerosis for a while, we might finally be starting to figure out its mysterious origins.

On September 23, 1955, on a beautiful autumn day, a sixty-four-year-old man was playing golf on the Cherry Hills Country Club golf course in Denver, Colorado.[2,3] He had been spending the last few weeks fishing in the Rocky Mountains, but the stresses of his day job hadn't let him alone; while playing, he was frequently called back to the clubhouse to take phone calls. Between games, he had a hamburger with Bermuda onions and soon enough, on the eighth hole, started to feel indigestion. He stopped playing, and later at about two in the morning, chest pains woke him up from his sleep. His doctor attributed it to acid reflux, gave him a slug of morphine that put him into a slumber so deep he didn't wake up until the next morning. He kept having pain in the morning and was taken to the hospital, where an electrocardiogram was eventually performed, and he was diagnosed with a massive heart attack. News of this heart attack spread quickly. It was a haymaker in the face of a historically strong U.S. stock market, which lost $14 billion in value over two days.

Decades before Dwight D. Eisenhower, the thirty-fourth president of the United States, had the most expensive heart attack in history, atherosclerosis had started building in his blood vessels, methodically laying down brick by brick the lethal foundation that eventually led to him being on the verge of death.

Long before a heart attack actually happens, the footprints of atherosclerosis start to appear in blood vessels.[4] Blood in the body usually moves with laminar flow, with each cell parallel to the other, like birds flying in a flock, seamlessly and efficiently. Within the body, however, there are parts of blood vessels that are more prone to shear stress, where flow of blood is not as smooth. This stress places increased pressure on the endothelium, the innermost membrane of blood vessels. The foot soldiers of the body's immune system—white blood cells—accumulate underneath the endothelium like shadowy figures behind frosted glass. Over time, these lesions start to become visible as fatty streaks, the primordial precursors of things to come. Fatty streaks are found in most adolescents in developed countries and continue to slowly progress until they become more prominent and start to take up more space in the blood vessels.[5]

The resultant irregularities in the blood vessels disturb blood flow further and result in the endothelium being damaged or defaced, causing additional cells to accumulate under the membrane. These plaques, as they are called, have a fatty center but are covered by a firm cap, which keeps all the contents of the plaque contained. Frequently, calcium, the mineral making up the bones and teeth, can get deposited on these plaques, further cementing them in place. While plaques can form in any blood vessel in the body, they seem to be predisposed to form in the coronary arteries supplying blood to the heart because of non-laminar flow causing increased shear. These plaques, by narrowing the blood vessels they form in, can restrict blood supply to various organs but are rarely fatal by themselves. That can change as soon as something catastrophic happens. If anything causes the firm fibrous cap of plaques to get disrupted, their fatty center can spew out, resulting in an explosion of activity.

As soon as the body detects the fatty core of a plaque gushing out into the blood, the coagulation cascade, the body's innate mechanism to form blood clots, springs into full gear. The coagulation cascade is meant to protect the body from injury by preventing uncontrolled bleeding. However, when a plaque ruptures, the coagulation system is fooled into activating unnecessarily, with potentially devastating consequences.

When an atherosclerotic plaque cracks open in the coronary artery, it results in a heart attack, and as many as three out of four heart attacks occur because of plaque rupture.[6] When the same occurs in a blood vessel in the brain, it results in a stroke, leading to loss of function of the part of the brain the vessel is supplying. In fact, many people who die suddenly and out of the blue do so because of plaque rupture.

Most if not all adults have plaques in some of the most critical vessels in our body. Why do some plaques rupture and others don't, and why do some people's plaques rupture more often than others? Plaque rupture rarely occurs in parts of the blood vessel with the greatest degree of plaque buildup. This makes a plaque rupture very hard to predict since the biggest plaques causing the most obstruction aren't necessarily the most dangerous. And why do plaques rupture when they do? What was it about that tranquil autumn afternoon that caused Eisenhower's ticking time bomb to go boom?

There are features of some plaques that make them more vulnerable to burst than others.[7] A plaque with a relatively thin fibrous cap covering it, or one with a large number of dead cells in its center, is susceptible to disintegrating. There are other environmental factors inside the body, such as how the blood flows in and around plaques, that can also cause them to pop.

The greatest mystery that has always been at the heart of atherosclerosis is not how it ends, with people hunkering down and being unable to breathe, being unable to see or speak or move their arms or legs, or just dropping to the ground in a heap. An even greater mystery about atherosclerosis is how it starts—how healthy endothelium goes from being well to unwell.

Over the last decade, our understanding of what forms the basis of the main cause of human death around the world has changed. The role played by our immune system—the elaborate defense mechanism always vigilantly protecting our insides against the big bad outside—in *causing* atherosclerosis is now finally starting to be fully understood. To know why inflammation—the immune system's body-wide response to external threats—might be in ways the biggest threat to human life, we have to go way back again to the very first human beings.

—⎍—

Six million years ago, our apelike ancestors roamed the forests of eastern Africa, and every day in their lives brought them to the precipice of extinction. They were on their feet and on the move almost all day. They were vegetarian for the most part, feeding on fruits, leaves, nuts, and roots.[8,9] While all these foods were mostly comprised of carbohydrates, these foods they ate all had a low glycemic index, meaning they were slow to digest and only modestly raised the sugar content in the bloodstream. As the climate changed and woodlands morphed into arid grasslands, our early human ancestors moved to the coasts. Here their diet changed; they increasingly consumed protein and fat from the animals they started hunting. Therefore, their diet went from being dominated by carbs to one that was high in protein, with a fair share of fats. This change in diet is thought to have helped our brains grow bigger, a process called *encephalization*.[10] And the rest, as they say, is history; almost three hundred thousand years ago, *Homo sapiens* started wandering the earth.[11]

Human life was considerably different back then, something with consequences for us to this day. The good times were great, but bad ones could be terrible. A hefty haul of food came once in a while, but it was never clear when the next one would arrive. Without agriculture, there was no sustained supply of nutrition. It is posited that this vacillation between feast and famine led to the selection of so-called thrifty genes, which promoted the storage of nutrients rather than a system that just let them drip away in our urine.[12] Because we consumed such little sugar, genes that decreased the potency of insulin—the hormone that reduces the concentration of sugar in the blood—were positively selected. This would be especially important for the brain—which, unlike the rest of the body, depends exclusively on sugar for energy. While it only accounts for 2 percent of the body by mass, the brain uses half of our sugar intake. To keep our bodies, especially our brains, nourished, it is more than likely that we evolved to blunt insulin, which is trying to rid the blood of sugar. This might be another reason that insulin resistance, the central mechanism of diabetes, might have been selected by evolutionary mechanisms.[13,14]

This thrifty genotype, however, has come back to haunt us, as the ready availability of food dominated by simple sugars with a high glycemic index on top of our vastly less active lifestyles may have led to the global pandemics of obesity and diabetes.[15] Obesity and diabetes are not only extremely common in rich countries, they are also becoming more common in low-income countries. When I was in medical school in Pakistan, I conducted a study of schoolchildren in Karachi, the country's largest metropolis, and found that even though a quarter of children were malnourished, another quarter were simultaneously overweight or obese.[16] Both diabetes and obesity are some of the great risk factors for developing atherosclerosis.

Atherosclerosis has been sold as the price of modernity, as the collateral consequence of a changing world, which saw us completely upend how we ate, worked, traveled, and lived in the past. We are learning now that it has been clinging to us for at least several thousand years.

On September 19, 1991, a German couple hiking at ten thousand feet in the Austrian Alps came upon a frozen body, lying facedown, with half of it encased in ice. The couple, however, continued with their hike and alerted the authorities after they reached a mountain rest hut. The next day, an Austrian gendarme was deployed for the recovery effort, but he could only half-chisel the body out of the ice before the weather soured and he had to retreat. It took another two days of multiple mountaineers chipping and hacking away with picks, chisels, ski poles, axes, sticks, rocks, and a jackhammer before the body could be released from the ice. It was then that they realized that this was not some recent climber but a mummified body. Ötzi, the Iceman, as he was posthumously named, we know now is the oldest mummified body ever found. He died almost 5,300 years ago and had been remarkably well preserved by the block of ice that was his transparent grave for thousands of years.[17,18]

Ötzi, who was likely middle-aged, died of what is perhaps the most human of afflictions—murder. Scientists found an arrowhead lodged in his left shoulder. Yet they also found something they much less expected to find—evidence of atherosclerosis in both the large arteries in the neck as evidenced by calcium deposits in the vessel. This was a startling discovery given that it represented the oldest human being ever to have been found to be affected by it. Yet even before Ötzi was dislodged from the ice, atherosclerosis had been found in the blood vessels of Egyptian mummies.

Autopsies of mummies in Europe in the early twentieth century yielded surprising results. In his paper in 1911, Marc Ruffer, a contemporary of the famed French biologist Louis Pasteur and one of the first people to perform autopsies on Egyptian mummies, commented that it was "interesting that it [atherosclerosis] was common and that 3,000 years ago it represented the same anatomic characteristics as it does now."[19] A century after Ruffer's paper, a study was published by a multinational group of scientists, who put mummies of ancient Egyptians, Peruvians, and hunter-gatherers from the Aleutian Islands off the Alaskan coast into CT scanners.[20] The researchers found probable or definite evidence of atherosclerosis in a third of the 137 mummies that they studied. While most died young, with an average age of thirty-seven years, those with atherosclerosis were older, around forty-two years of age. Only 4 percent had atherosclerosis in the coronary arteries. Yet the study left a heavy question hanging overhead—why was atherosclerosis even present in those who had a good diet, were pretty active, and did not have any of the other modern-day risk factors we associate with atherosclerosis?

Turns out that to answer that question, you have to go even further back. Since the dawn of time, what has killed human beings has not been heart disease or cancer; it has been infection. Bacteria, viruses, parasites, fungi—you name it—have haunted us at every stage of our development. The greatest killer of man is not man itself but the annoying and insidiously lethal mosquito. Infections barely left room for other things to pick human beings off. So, to survive, humans didn't have to worry about heart disease or cancer, which were not even major killers in the early twentieth century, but infection.[21]

How does the body protect itself against infection? It develops an aggressive, paranoid, hypervigilant and trigger-happy immune system led by killjoy white blood cells. And while for centuries, those mercenary cells got plenty of practice from infectious organisms finding their way into the human body, recent years, due to better lifestyle hygiene, have led to a drastic reduction in infections and subsequent deaths from those pathogens. Yet millennia of being trained in a hyperinfectious environment has overprepared the immune system to a threat that just doesn't exist anymore. Instead, the immune system has all this unused arsenal just hanging around, which it then starts to overuse on the most benign of threats. What this means for us today is that inflammation, the wall that the immune system puts up in the face of infectious threats, the body's version of the troops charging on the beach of Normandy, might in fact be our greatest nemesis.

When people think of inflammation, they usually think of an inflamed joint—red, swollen, and angry—perhaps after an infection. They usually think about how their body feels after they get the flu—feverish and flushed. I bet they don't think about heart disease or atherosclerosis or plaque rupture. I am here to tell you that inflammation is the central mechanism of atherosclerosis and that how we have evolved has led to inflammation afflicting more people than any other disease in our times.

While atherosclerosis has been found in ancient humans, it wasn't really why we died in our twenties and thirties. What killed us were infections. And what could we do to fight infections? At that point, we didn't really know about the importance of hygiene, we rarely had clean water, there were no antibiotics we could use, and we were always exposed to the hordes assembled in the worlds around us, just waiting to pounce. The only defense we had was inside us—it was our immune system. The relentless and remorseless onslaught of infections throughout our life spans kept our immune systems jacked. Evidence of this theory has now been gathered by a pioneering study in a remote nook of Bolivia. While our previous understanding of primitive civilizations was based on educated guesses at best, the Tsimane Health and Life History Project provides as vivid a window back in time as we have ever had.[22]

The Tsimane people of Bolivia are some of the most isolated people on earth. They still practice a forager-horticulturalist lifestyle, just a bit more advanced than hunter-gatherers. They depend on growing plantains, rice, and corn and hunting and fishing for food. A study funded by the National Institutes of Health and the National Institute of Aging brought together a vast team of physicians, anthropologists, biochemists, and assorted researchers to study the Tsimane from their first breath to the last. The Tsimane, on average, live to be in their forties or early fifties. To survive, the Tsimane have to hunt until they die, mostly of infections. Most of the Tsimane also carry parasitic worms in their intestines, and as a result, blood tests show that they spend a lot more of their lives in an inflamed state than those living in more modern societies. The Tsimane living in more remote areas show even higher levels of inflammation. Extrapolate what we know about the Tsimane to even more primitive human beings, which makes up the majority of our existence, and it becomes clear how a life span held hostage by contagion would select for only those with the inner fortitude to survive this onslaught.

What else shakes the immune system up from its slumber is the sort of thing that found itself lodged in Ötzi's left shoulder. Whenever there is an injury—any disruption of the sacrosanct barriers that keep our bodies and their contents intact—immune cells are rapidly deployed to the warfront. Throughout our history, violent injuries and deaths, both intentional and unintentional, have plagued us. Along with infections, traumatic injuries were the dominant driver of human mortality through much of our existence, representing another reason our immune systems needed to be hyperactive. Times have changed, though, and even as people still experience injuries, whether in car accidents or gunshots, the numbers are lower than at any point in the past. Yet the defenses that we created for those wounds remain as stout as ever before.

Injuries and infections, therefore, appear to give those with heightened inflammatory defenses a leg up on their competition, yet our circumstances have changed. Global violence is at an all-time low, even if that may not seem to be the case. Infections, with vaccines and public hygiene, are nowhere close to being as common as they were. In a sense, therefore, for modern human beings, the immune system is like a cabinet full of guns for an apocalypse that never came. While the main reason why evolution may have caused the epidemic of heart disease is by allowing us to live long enough to develop it, it is quite likely that atherosclerosis is collateral damage from an immune system misfiring after centuries of being erected for threats that lack the edge of yesteryears. The protector has finally become the predator.

From the origin of atherosclerosis, before it even becomes visible in the blood vessels, to the terminal end of its natural history, when a vulnerable plaque blows up, inflammation turns the key, changes the gear, and throttles the gas.[23] Widespread evidence supports the centrality of inflammation in atherosclerosis. Any condition that chronically raises the level of inflammation in the body can raise the risk of heart disease. This is true, as we found in an analysis I published with colleagues, even of diseases such as the skin condition psoriasis.[24] Patients with psoriasis are much more likely to have heart attacks and strokes, and this occurs because these patients' immune system is always going gangbusters, not only causing the angry skin lesions these patients have but leading to atherosclerotic plaque deposition in the blood vessels and eventually causing their rupture as well.

Inflammation, in addition to being the seed of atherosclerotic plaque, is often involved in bursting its bubble, leading to plaque rupture. Immune cells called *macrophages,* when active during a state of acute inflammation, can eat away at the fibrous caps that keep plaques intact, leading to them bursting open. Any state of heightened inflammation, such as after influenza infection, raises the risk of having a heart attack. This has led to anti-inflammatory drugs such as colchicine, traditionally used to treat gout, and methotrexate, used for patients with severe rheumatoid arthritis, psoriasis, and even some blood cancers like leukemia and lymphoma, being tested to reduce the risk of heart attacks, although results from most clinical trials have been disappointing with one notable exception.[25,26] While several drugs that dampen the immune system have failed to reduce the incidence of heart attacks without success, there has been some notable progress recently. Canakinumab, an artificially made human antibody that is a part of the inflammatory cascade, was tested in a trial of ten thousand patients against a placebo.[27] Neither the researchers nor the patients knew who was receiving the drug versus the placebo. While there was no difference in death rates, patients receiving the drug had fewer heart attacks. While the difference was small, it was statistically significant and provided the clearest proof available that heart disease was driven in large part by inflammation, and the future of heart disease treatment perhaps could mirror treatments for autoimmune diseases, such as multiple sclerosis or lupus, in which the immune system attacks the body.

Inflammation, though, cannot be the only reason people develop atherosclerosis. In fact, heart disease didn't become a major killer of human beings until the start of the twentieth century even though atherosclerosis has clearly been around for a while. While atherosclerosis has certainly been found in ancient people, it rarely led to anything serious. In fact, even though the Tsimane people have sky-high levels of inflammation, life-threatening atherosclerosis is largely nonexistent among them, and they die mostly of things the inflammatory system hopes to stave off, like infection. Answers to what is behind the pandemic of atherosclerosis in modern humans were also found through another large study. This particular study was not performed in a remote village but in Framingham, Massachusetts, twenty miles west of Boston. Research performed in this town formed the basis of much of what we know about the risk factors that have pushed modern human beings into the life-limiting embrace of atherosclerosis.

—⋀—

More than twelve years into his presidency, on April 12, 1945, Franklin D. Roosevelt (FDR) was sitting in a chair in his retreat in Warm Springs, Georgia, posing for a portrait.[28] Also present was his mistress, Lucy Mercer, unbeknownst to his wife, Eleanor, from whom the affair had been kept a secret. The United States and its allies were on the verge of an overwhelming intercontinental victory over Germany and Japan, and he had only recently successfully won a fourth term in office. Earlier that day, his guests "commented on how well he looked." According to his personal physician, Ross McIntire, FDR enjoyed perfect health. "He suddenly complained of a terrific occipital headache," wrote FDR's cardiologist, Howard Bruenn, years later. "He became unconscious a minute or two later."[29] Bruenn tried everything, including injecting adrenaline straight into FDR's heart, replicating a scene from the movie *Pulp Fiction,* in which John Travolta's character injects a syringe of adrenaline right into Uma Thurman's character's heart after she overdoses on heroin. While Uma's character recovered, FDR would never wake up, and he was declared dead within two hours.

The news came as a shock and a surprise to the American people at a most crucial time of history. Heart disease had become the leading killer of Americans, and there was little if anything that could be done to treat it. At a time when heart disease killed every other person in the United States, there was a growing sense that there was nothing that could be done about it but to sit back and put one's affairs in order. The sudden death of a sitting president only reinforced the sense of nihilistic defeat many felt at that time when it seemed like defeating the forces of Hitler was easier than the battle being waged within our blood vessels.

When FDR died, we barely knew anything about the disease that killed more Americans than their enemies could ever hope to. Not only did we not know why heart disease occurred, we barely understood how to even diagnose it, let alone treat it. There were very few who specialized in treating heart disease. FDR was far from the first sitting U.S. president to die of atherosclerotic heart disease. In 1923, when Warren Harding, the twenty-ninth president of the United States, died in a San Francisco hotel room from chronic heart failure, the only medical person he trusted was a homeopath who had been treating him with laxatives in the days leading up to his demise.[30] Even FDR's personal physician, McIntire, was an ear, nose, and throat specialist, with barely any knowledge of the disease that actually afflicted the president.

FDR was succeeded by Harry Truman, who, after successfully defeating Germany and Japan, took on the even greater and ominous challenge posed by heart disease. In June 1948, he announced the foundation of a division at the National Institutes of Health focused on cardiovascular disease, known today as the National Heart, Lung, and Blood Institute.

A question for this institute was this: How should the research funds it was allocated be used? Should they be used to figure out how to better treat those who suffered strokes and heart attacks? Certainly, that would have been a prudent endeavor—the routinely prescribed treatment for these disorders was simply bed rest. Yet the institute approached their mission from the opposite end. Instead of figuring out what to do after someone has a heart attack, the institute's leaders decided that they wanted to invest far more upstream to better understand how we could prevent people from having heart disease in the first place. And this was how the Framingham Heart Study came to be.[31,32]

To explore why people developed heart disease, the United States Public Health Service decided that they wanted to conduct a long-term study in a population that would be representative of the United States overall. Framingham, a blue-collar, mostly white town, was picked due to its proximity to Harvard Medical School, which was home to Paul Dudley White, the most famous American cardiologist of his time. The study, the likes of which had never been performed, enrolled its first patient on October 11, 1948, and monitored its first group of 5,209 people aged 28–62 years between 1948 and 1952. The first research findings from the Framingham

Heart Study were published in 1957, and the study has been ongoing ever since.[33] The most recent round of the study enrolled the grandchildren of those who had participated in the original iteration of the study.

Perhaps Framingham's greatest contribution has been the introduction of the term *risk factor* into how doctors and patients think about disease.[34] Instead of waiting for disease to develop, Framingham moved doctors to start coming up with ways to prevent disease from ever getting established in the first place by modifying the risk factors that led to its onset.

One such risk factor Framingham revealed was hypertension. When the heart beats, it sends a pulse through the arteries. The blood pressure, usually measured with a cuff on the arm, provides a sense of how the pressure in the blood vessels in general is. The systolic blood pressure, which is the higher number, represents the pressure in the vessel the pulse generates. The lower number, the diastolic blood pressure, represents the pressure in the blood vessel when no pulse is passing through it. While it sounds simple enough, and is probably measured billions of times every day, to date, few know how to take a blood pressure correctly. Shockingly, when medical students were recently tested on the steps required for accurate blood pressure measurement, only 1 of 159 incorporated all eleven elements.[35] These steps include assessing blood pressure after five minutes of rest with the patient sitting with their legs uncrossed and using the appropriate cuff size. Measuring blood pressure, however, is something that is increasingly being done at home by patients and their caregivers, as finally many people have realized how it might be one of the most important pieces of information we can obtain from our bodies even when it isn't assessed in the most accurate fashion. We know today, after stumbling in the dark for almost a century, that lowering blood pressure can save more lives than any other clinical intervention known to mankind.[36]

William Howard Taft, the twenty-seventh president of the United States, was likely the first serving president to have his blood pressure measured.

In a letter forwarding results from an examination by a Boston physician in 1910–11, Taft wrote, "He said my blood pressure was 210—whew!"[37] A normal systolic blood pressure is between 90 and 120. Taft's blood pressure would be considered a medical emergency these days, but back then, it resulted in a sigh of relief. Taft was far from the only American president struggling with high blood pressure. Woodrow Wilson, who was next to take office after Taft, had a series of devastating strokes because of high blood pressure that left him completely debilitated. His wife, Edith Wilson, hid him from public view, even from his own cabinet, assuring them he had a nervous breakdown while effectively taking over the day-to-day work of the president.[38] FDR's ailments, too, were almost certainly due to severe hypertension. However, FDR was diagnosed with hypertension, and heart failure due to hypertension, only a year before his death, at which point his blood pressure was noted to be 186/108.[39]

Despite being found to have what we now know to be a critical piece in the development of atherosclerosis, even the most privileged Americans of their time, the presidents, received no treatment for high blood pressure. If anything, most prominent physicians of that time thought that lowering blood pressure would in fact be harmful. In 1912, Sir William Osler, the famous Johns Hopkins professor, told physicians in Glasgow that in patients with atherosclerosis, "the extra pressure is a necessity—as purely a mechanical affair as in any great irrigation system with old encrusted mains and weedy channels."[40] He actually assured a patient that "it was a very good thing for him that his engines had kept up a pressure of about 180mm." In 1937, Paul Dudley White wrote, "Hypertension may be an important compensatory mechanism which should not be tampered with, even were it certain that we could control it."[41] In fact, the elevation of blood pressure was (and is still) referred to as *essential* hypertension, given that a greater force was thought to be essential to help blood reach all the important organs in the body. John Hay, a British physician went a step further, writing, "The greatest danger to a man with high blood pressure lies in its discovery, because then some fool is certain to try and reduce it."[42]

The significance of high blood pressure and its relationship with an increased likelihood of heart disease, stroke, and death was realized by another party, with a much more direct financial stake in understanding the relationship—life insurance companies. At a time when the leading medical minds were dismissing the need to measure blood pressure, in 1914, the medical director of the Northwestern Mutual Life Company wrote, "The sphygmomanometer is indispensable in life insurance examinations, and the time is not far distant when all progressive life insurance companies will require its use in all examinations of applicants for life insurance."[43] In a report published in 1925 by the Actuarial Society of America, the direct relationship between both rising weight and age with increasing blood pressure and the association between hypertension and death were described.[44] These findings, however, failed to pique the interest or curiosity of the leading scientific minds of that time, yet the insurance companies kept persevering. In fact, decades later, when the Framingham study was threatened with its funding being cut, life insurance companies helped bail it out, seeing how important the actuarial benefits of the study were.

In 1957, ten years after it was started, the first paper from the Framingham study was published. The study showed that hypertension was strongly associated with an increased risk of developing heart attacks.[45] Heart attacks were so dangerous back then that a third of Framingham residents died immediately of the heart attack, and only about half eventually survived them. Framingham, however, popularized the concept of a risk factor, as separate from disease, and further research published in 1965 indicated a strong link between high blood pressure and strokes as well.[46]

The Framingham study investigators thought their job was done after they began publishing their landmark findings but quickly realized they had run into a wall—that wall was their fellow physicians. The overwhelmingly strong data they had generated failed to change the practice of either the most preeminent doctors of their time or those running mom-and-pop-style clinics in the country. And all this time, people continued to die of untreated high blood pressure by the millions—after the Second World War, every other person died in part due to hypertension.[47] Even in the 1970s, when some medical textbooks started to recognize the importance of blood pressure, they focused on the lower number, the diastolic blood pressure, even as the Framingham investigators continued to show that it was the systolic blood pressure that mattered a lot more. Yet it wasn't until the 1980s and 1990s, after large clinical trials proved them right, that the medical community fully embraced the findings from Framingham that had been published sequentially over many decades and had long before been supported by life insurance companies.

Today, however, the debate about blood pressure has swung fully in the opposite direction. The current dispute raging in academic journals (and on Twitter) these days is not about how high it is acceptable for people's blood pressure to be but what the lower limit of recommended blood pressure is. We have come full circle from a time when almost no one cared about blood pressure, to an era where almost no adult is spared the diagnosis of hypertension because of how low currently acceptable blood pressure has been deemed. I first learned about this controversy, like so many others, when I opened my laptop one early morning and a push notification appeared on my desktop: one of the largest studies funded by National Institutes of Health, the Systolic Blood Pressure Intervention Trial, called the SPRINT trial, had been stopped early, *The New York Times* announced.[48] Most studies are stopped prematurely when a safety committee sees a signal of harm or futility, preventing additional subjects from being hurt. In this case, though, the reason was quite the opposite. The trial, which looked at the effect of very aggressively lowering blood pressure, even below 120/80, showed that the benefit of such aggressive lowering was overwhelmingly positive. These results were considered so strong by the National Institutes of Health that they didn't even wait to present the results at a research conference or in a journal article. They released the information in a press release, which was then followed by a notification-worthy piece on the front page of the *Times*. When the blood pressure guidelines were updated in the wake of these results, overnight, more than thirty-one million Americans found themselves newly diagnosed with hypertension.[49]

It took decades for hypertension to be recognized as a legitimate risk factor for heart disease, but science eventually triumphed over dogma. The history of heart disease, like so many others, makes it clear that sometimes the biggest impediments in the progress of science are the gatekeepers and opinion leaders of their respective fields. Yet an expert is by definition wedded to the status quo, and as their expertise grows, so does their relationship with the existing body of knowledge upon which their authority is recognized. In medical science, detours from the truth bear a heavy human cost, and a century of unchecked hypertension likely led to the deaths of millions upon millions of people from heart attacks and strokes. And all this knowledge of the ills of high blood pressure leads us to the most important question of all: What can we do to fix it?

Mary was the picture of health. Thin and petite, she had gone eight decades without seeing the inside of a hospital, and yet over the last few months, she had been to the emergency room multiple times after getting scary high blood pressure readings. It just didn't make sense to her—she and her family even compared the measurements of the home blood pressure machine with the one brought in by emergency medical services to make sure it was working right. Soon enough, she found herself sitting across from me in clinic, nervously fidgeting in her chair, hoping someone could figure out how to treat her blood pressure.

High blood pressure can cause heart disease in so many ways that it is today the leading cause of death and disability worldwide.[50] But how does it cause so much debility? The forceful flow of blood in the vessels can cause increased shear stress on the sensitive inner lining of all blood vessels, the endothelium. This stress results in micro-injury, which triggers the body to activate its response to injury—inflammation. And inflammation leads to atherosclerosis, which leads to heart attacks and stroke. Extreme bouts of high blood pressure can cause blood vessels to burst open, and this can affect the most important vessels in the body like the aorta or those supplying the brain. Moments before Roosevelt had a hemorrhagic stroke, his systolic blood pressure was noted to be greater than 300. The extreme blood pressure caused a vessel in his brain to tear open, filling his skull with blood, leading to his sudden death.[51]

By placing a stranglehold on blood vessels, high blood pressure results in the heart pumping into a circulatory system that has fully clamped down, causing it to work much harder. Initially, the heart does what any other muscle in the body would do when it is asked to work harder—it grows thicker. A big heart, though, while a compliment in everyday parlance, is frequently a precursor to heart failure. A thick and muscular heart, as it continues to keep working harder and harder, can frequently burn out, at times ballooning out and becoming dilated and wimpy.

To beat blood pressure, though, we must first understand how hypertension even happens. The puppet masters that control how relaxed or taut the blood vessels are, are the two bean-shaped organs that sit on either side of the belly just behind the navel and close to the spine—the kidneys.

In a word, the life's mission of our kidneys is to achieve one thing—*balance*. Far from being an agent of change, kidneys are hard at work to achieve sameness. The two things that kidneys attend to the most are the two reasons they hold the keys to how stressed each and every blood vessel in the body is: kidneys care about how much blood volume there is in the body and about the composition of that volume.

When we think of the human body, we tend to, I guess naturally, anthropomorphize it. We think of us as a person, but the kidneys see us as a mixture of salts in sequentially connected tubes. The human body is, lest we forget, a vessel that is 70 percent water. Kidneys are always scanning the blood passing through them to make sure they have the right balance of electrolytes. And of all the electrolytes—like potassium, calcium, and chloride—kidneys care most about sodium.

Kidneys also care a lot about how much volume there is in the human body, and they are one reason we don't just swell out of proportion. Say you haven't had water in a while and become dehydrated. This could lead to there not being enough fluid in your blood vessels, which could lead to your blood pressure dropping, causing you to feel dizzy and light-headed because there is not enough pressure in the blood vessels to maintain adequate flow to all parts of the body. Ultimately, low blood pressure to organs such as the brain could lead you to lose consciousness and possibly even die. What prevents this from happening every single time you haven't had some water to drink is the kidneys.

Kidneys keep tabs on salts and nutrients passing through its narrow tubules like ICE agents at JFK Airport. There is one salt that kidneys really look out for, and that special salt is sodium. Kidneys use sodium to get a sense of how well hydrated the body is—too much salt usually means that there is not enough water around to dilute it. This causes the kidneys to hold on to water until the concentration of sodium drops into the normal range and it is just right again. Too little sodium means that the body might be overflowing in water, and it might be time to open the floodgates and let the extra water out until the sodium level is more concentrated.

Now imagine if you indulge in a delectable, ferociously salty serving of fried chicken and a side of collard greens sautéed in fat. All the sodium in your meal goes straight into the blood and fools the kidneys into thinking that the body is dehydrated, causing it to hold on to extra fluid, and raising the blood pressure. In fact, many people's feet will get visibly puffy right after they have a salty meal. Salt restriction, therefore, to many is the keystone of blood pressure management. In fact, in FDR's time, severe limitation of salt was one of the only ways blood pressure could be lowered.

Having already established that the world around us is nothing but an ensemble of threats to our existence, perhaps none of this craven horde is quite as insidious as salt. Born of the union between the positively charged sodium and the negatively charged chloride ion, what makes it so dangerous is just how irresistible it can be. In many cultures, salt is as integral to being as language. The draw of salt is far from benign as the addictive nature of salt and pathologic salt craving is only now being recognized.[52,53] In fact, our relationship with salt might not be as ancient as we imagine. For most of history, human beings consumed only about 0.25 grams of salt a day, and that is the level that our bodies have been trained to best tolerate. The average person around the world today consumes 4 grams of sodium, almost double the World Health Organization's recommended daily salt intake of 2 grams. Why does this matter? Salt intake, by contributing to high blood pressure when consumed above this recommended level, is estimated to account for 1.7 million deaths around the world.[54] Many more suffer from heart failure, heart attacks, strokes, aortic aneurysms, and disease of the arteries in the legs. So if we were to think of salt as a drug, it could be the most dangerous one around. For context, all illicit drugs account for about 190,000 deaths worldwide.[55] And salt doesn't only kill over a long period of time; a salt overdose can have immediately fatal consequences.[56]

After undergoing brain surgery, a nineteen-year-old woman in France started to have seizures. Rather than seeking medical treatment, her loved ones were convinced that she was bewitched. Her religiously inclined family took her to a local cleric, who recommended an exorcism.[57] The exorcism started at 11:00 in the morning in the presence of her parents and brother. The many "treatments" she received included severe flogging with a reed. By the time the exorcism ended around 5:00 in the evening, the girl could barely breathe and lost consciousness. She was taken to a nearby hospital, where she died. What had killed her was not the flogging but the salt water she was forced to drink during the ritual. The sudden rapid ingestion of salt caused her lungs and brain to fill with fluid. Her brain got so swollen that it started to try to come out of her skull. The cleric was later convicted in a French court for torture. A twenty-year-old woman in Israel developed depression after giving birth.[58] She, too, was forced into a ritualistic ceremony attended by family and loved ones to ingest salt water, eventually leading to her death.

So, if salt ensnares like a drug and kills like a drug, why is it not regulated like one?

In 2016, the United States Food and Drug Administration (FDA) issued nonbinding recommendations to the food industry to lower salt content.[59] Turns out that 75 percent of the salt in our diets doesn't come from the shaker; it comes in processed, packaged, and restaurant-made foods.[60] In fact, in addition to the more obvious offenders—canned soups, pizza, and deli meats—the other three greatest contributors of salt in our diet are less obvious—bread, deli meats, and chicken.[61] The FDA's guidelines, though, are soft at best. This might reflect some data on the other end of the spectrum, which suggests that very low amounts of sodium in the diet might be harmful.[62] The existence of this contrary data, showing that salt restriction might in fact be bad, has been used to perhaps justifiably temper the wrath of regulators.[63]

The big questions that many concerned about their patients and people concerned about their health struggle with is quite simple: How does one survive without salt? Salt, it is said, is the only rock that human beings consume, and it seems almost an essential ingredient to one of our primal, everyday pleasures. In the Talmud, the central text of Rabbinic Judaism and the primary source of Jewish religious law and theology, it is said, "The world can live without wine but it cannot live without water; the world can live without peppers, but it cannot live without salt."[64] Answers to this question cannot be found in historical texts or research papers, so I turned to the one person I knew, for whom this answer was a matter of life and death—my wife, Rabail.

Rabail was in her early twenties in 2004 when she learned that her father was having a heart attack.

"He was in the middle of a conference, and right after lunch, he started to feel nauseous. He felt like something was pulling his chest," she told me. The person he was in the conference with didn't help because she thought that he was showing symptoms of food poisoning.

"She felt he needed fresh air, so she put him in a car and drove him around amid busy traffic with the windows down for forty-five minutes. Instead of getting better, he only got worse. She eventually took him to a hospital."

When he reached the hospital, the medical technician who first looked at his electrocardiogram was nonplussed and told him he could go home. His pain continued, and when they had the supervising physician review the same electrocardiogram (EKG), they got a very different reaction. "When the senior doctor saw the EKG, he went completely pale. He told my father that he could have died in the car and was having a major heart attack." He went on to have a procedure to have his blocked artery opened later that day.

My wife and I have been married for many years, and this was really the first time we talked about this in such detail. "We were all so scared. He was so young," she told me. "I thought he would lose himself—he was so energetic, so full of life—he was at the peak of his career, and it felt like it would all go away."

My father-in-law was not the sort of person one would think would be at risk for a heart attack. He was lean, didn't smoke, didn't have diabetes—it seems that his only vice was that he liked salty food. His doctors told him to use as little salt in his food as possible. "When he was growing up, he had two saltshakers at home, always sitting on the table," she recalled. "With every bite, he would add salt on top."

Rabail, who has now written a cookbook and is an unbelievably talented chef to my unparalleled delight, didn't make much food back then. "Ammi [Mother] would do all the cooking, and she just started to boil everything," she recalled. "We would be sitting around the table, then a plate of discolored boiled veggies would arrive, and Abbu [Father] would become upset and sometimes leave the table."

Her father was just sick of feeling like a patient. Less than a month after a serious heart attack, he had started to rebel, and Rabail knew she had to do something and took charge of the kitchen. "The question wasn't how he could eat better—it was how all of us could eat healthy."

"As you slowly reduce salt—it's like caffeine—you just stop needing it more. Your flavor buds reset. When people are told to reduce salt, often they reduce everything."

Rabail started to improvise. "Instead of making oil and salt as my primary cooking base, I began making pastes out of fresh vegetables, yogurt, herbs, and spices and cooked my meat and legumes in them. I also embraced lemons and used their juice as a flavor enhancer. I was suddenly making all these great dishes, all with a minimal amount of salt, some even salt-free but full of flavor." To offset the reduction in salt and oil, she began to amp up the spices, herbs, and greens she was adding. She was careful to avoid premade, salt-heavy seasonings, most of which contained too much sodium. She also regularly used sour tamarind pulp to give the food a nice tangy kick. "Salt masks everything, and when you start using lesser amounts, you really begin tasting the natural savoriness of meat, beans, grains, nuts, and vegetables."

Rabail's nightmare seems a long time ago now; it's been more than ten years since her dad had a heart attack, and he has been in great health since. Reducing salt in the diet, however, while a good first step in our efforts to fight the clutches of hypertension clawing down on our blood vessels and causing heart disease, might not be enough. In fact, the evidence that salt restriction leads to better health outcomes is not that strong, not even for conditions such as heart failure, which have traditionally been thought to be very salt-sensitive. This was more than clear to the scientists and researchers in the middle of the twentieth century, who were watching every other person die of heart disease, in large part due to high blood pressure, with salt restriction being the only available treatment. A fascinating discovery, however, would lead scientists to eventually develop medications that could stop this pathway in its tracks, and it came from the darkest recesses of the dense Brazilian rain forest.

The kidneys are the unsung heroes of the human body. If there were ever a Buzzfeed article called "The Best Organs in the Body—You Won't

Believe Which One Is Number One!" probably the kidneys won't be in the top five. They are not as obviously cerebral as the brain, nor as obviously busy as the heart, nor as indispensable as the lungs, yet they are always at work behind the scenes, making sure all the other flashy viscera can keep basking in the spotlight.

In addition to the relative concentrations of all the different electrolytes in the body, the kidneys really care that there is enough volume of blood in the body. As soon as the kidneys detect that there is not enough blood flowing into them, they set in motion a cascade of actions that raise the blood pressure. This effect was first discovered by Harry Goldblatt, a pathologist in Case Western Reserve University in Cleveland, Ohio.[65] In 1934, Goldblatt built a silver clamp and used it to partly restrict blood flow to one of the kidneys in the dogs he was experimenting on. This caused the dogs' blood pressure to rise. This discovery was a quantum leap in blood pressure research since it now gave researchers a model they could use to test therapies on. What they would uncover over the next few decades was that when the kidneys note a reduction in blood flow coming in through their tollbooths, they secrete a hormone called *renin*. Renin leads to the production of angiotensin. Angiotensin causes constriction of blood vessels, thus raising the blood pressure to normal.

It would make sense, then, that blocking the renin-angiotensin pathway might be one of the most effective means to lower blood pressure. In fact, this pathway is frequently hyperactive in some people, leading to both high blood pressure and retention of water, even when neither is needed. Not only does this lead to one being hypertensive, but the inappropriate retention of body fluid—which can lead to excess accumulation of fluid in the body—is a central mechanism driving heart failure. These discoveries in the 1950s and 1960s were missing the final step, though—the creation of an actual medication that could disrupt this nexus and prevent millions from dying of high blood pressure. That final step would be unearthed serendipitously in the Amazon jungle.

In the banana plantations of southwest Brazil, workers face a fearsome, hair-raising workplace hazard—*Bothrops jararaca*—also lovingly referred to as the Brazilian pit viper. A swift bite of the viper causes its victim to instantly drop to the ground. In fact, the indigenous people of Brazil would collect its venom and paint the tips of their arrows with it. Why was the viper venom so potent? Brazilian researchers found in the 1960s that it caused a catastrophic drop in the victim's blood pressure. Eventually, Sérgio Ferreira (1934–2016), then a research student, traveled in the 1960s to the London lab of famed British pharmacologist Sir John Vane with a vial full of Brazilian pit viper venom in his pocket.[66] Vane was able to convince his colleagues both in the UK and across the pond to continue to try to unravel the secrets of the virulent venom. In fact, one of Vane's friends at Cornell University injected a synthetic version of the venom directly into his patients and found that it was effective at lowering blood pressure, though not too effective to kill them, thankfully. A decade more of research, mostly directed at trying to develop a compound that could be ingested in a pill rather than require injection, resulted in the development of the first in a groundbreaking family of medications—angiotensin-converting-enzyme (ACE) inhibitors.[67] Captopril, the granddaddy of many more medications, all ending in *pril*—enalapril, lisinopril, and quinapril—to name a few, was discovered in 1975, and to this day, this family of medications forms the centerpiece of treatment for not only blood pressure but heart failure.

Other medications have also been developed to lower blood pressure. Diuretics are a category of drugs that lower blood pressure by causing kidneys to lose extra salt, with fluid following the salt in the urine. When the kidneys lose salt, water follows, causing one to urinate the extra fluid and therefore lowering blood pressure. If anything, these days we have too many medications to choose from when it comes to lowering blood pressure. In some cases, though, people can have blood pressure that just doesn't respond to medications, no matter what kind. People with so-called malignant hypertension are particularly difficult to treat. In fact, one in ten people with hypertension have high blood pressure despite being on three blood pressure–lowering medications or more. My patient Mary, the eighty-year-old elderly woman sitting across from me in clinic, was one such patient. She was on multiple medications, including an ACE inhibitor and a diuretic, but continued to have spikes of high blood pressure that sent her rushing to the emergency room.

Was there anything else I could offer her?

Yes and no.

An important interlocutor of blood pressure in the circulatory system is another widespread parallel system in the body—the nervous system. The peripheral nervous system, which includes all the nerves outside of the brain and spinal cord, has two moods. To experience one of its moods, go and have a nice big feast (or imagine having one), and consider what you feel. You feel nice and relaxed, you could sink into that couch, you could even experience what is commonly referred to as a "food coma." Why does one feel this way? Because the body wants to optimize itself for digestion of the food by redirecting the blood to the gut. This mood is mediated by the parasympathetic nervous system. The coma-like feeling one might feel after a big meal occurs because the parasympathetic system causes the blood pressure to drop, and in rare cases, it can even lead to people fainting after a massive meal. The yin to the yang of the parasympathetic system is the sympathetic system, which can go into immediate berserk mode if, say, you get startled in the dark or if you see your computer screen go blue while you are in the middle of an unsaved manuscript. Not only does the sympathetic nervous system send your heart racing, it raises the blood pressure in your body.

How does the sympathetic nervous system raise blood pressure? Well, there are sympathetic nerves that line renal arteries, which take blood to the kidneys. When the sympathetic nervous system is activated, it causes the renal artery to constrict, reducing blood flow to the kidneys.[68] This fools the kidneys, which then react as they would if one is dehydrated or losing blood—they activate the renin-angiotensin pathway, therefore increasing blood pressure.

Back when the only treatment available for treating hypertension was a low-sodium diet, doctors were desperate to try anything. One agent, for example, that was commonly used briefly was potassium thiocyanate, now widely considered a poisonous compound. Why? Because users would frequently lose their minds before dying.[69] Much more widely accepted was the use of surgery to treat blood pressure—surgeons would actually cut the nerves of the sympathetic nervous system.[70] This surgery, while useful in reducing blood pressure in some patients, also had significant side effects. The sympathetic nerves are responsible for causing us to sweat, so patients would not sweat in the legs and other areas where the innervation was dissected. Paradoxically, they would sweat excessively in parts that were still left, like the face or head. Some men would be unable to have an erection or ejaculate. The most common side effect was actually low blood pressure when people were on their feet.

Almost a century after surgical ligation of the sympathetic nerves was first developed, researchers found a much safer way to target the sympathetic nerves in the kidneys. Instead of approaching the nerves from the outside with a scalpel, they developed a catheter that could use ultrasound or radio waves to basically neuter the nerves innervating the renal arteries. The catheter could be introduced into the body with a small nick in the leg. And best of all, there were barely any other nerves affected; therefore, the complications were minimal. When this procedure was tried on patients in Europe, their blood pressure dropped precipitously.[71]

So why aren't we performing this procedure willy-nilly? Well, the European trials had one weakness. There was no sham control in the trial. What does that mean? When a clinical study evaluates the effectiveness of a new procedure, it needs to compare patients receiving the new treatment against another group who are very similar other than that they are not getting the procedure. That comparison group is called a *control arm*. To make sure that patients in both groups are similar and are not any healthier or sicker than each other, which would affect the results, the patients are randomized—as in they are randomly put in either the control or the intervention arm.

The final step that ensures the validity of the results from a trial is important—it's called *blinding*. If patients or their doctors knew, for example, that they had received the denervation procedure, versus, say, just medications, they might treat them differently, both consciously and subconsciously. While previous trials were randomized and they had a control arm, they were not blinded. How could one, in fact, hide the fact that a procedure had been performed?

Well, that's where a sham procedure can help. In the pivotal trial of renal denervation performed in the United States, called Symplicity HTN-3, patients in the control arm only had pictures of their renal arteries taken but did not get their nerves zapped.[72] They had no way of telling the difference. In 2014, I was in attendance at a cardiology conference in Washington, D.C., where the results from the Symplicity HTN-3 trials were to be announced. On the main stage, with thousands in attendance, epic entrance music accompanied Deepak Bhatt, one of the most prolific cardiac researchers in the world, as he walked onto the podium to announce the results of the study. When the results were announced, there was an audible gasp in the erstwhile riveted-silent crowd. Between the renal denervation and sham control arm, there was no difference, not even a smidge. While smaller sham-controlled studies recently presented have been more positive, the treatment is not recommended until further evidence is generated.

Where does that leave me with my patient, now on three medications, and still with high blood pressure?

I rechecked her blood pressure myself as she lay down on the bed, and my eyes widened—it was 205/120.

She had brought a diary of all her blood pressure readings. What struck me was how even though she had some blood pressures that were super high, like right at that moment, she also had readings that were much lower. Something was off.

I had her sit up and rechecked it. It was 185/100. I then had her stand up and stood close to her. I rechecked it a third time. It was 120/80.

I asked her if she felt dizzy and she said no.

I told her next time her blood pressure was too high, she should try standing up. She had autonomic dysfunction, which meant that her body's nervous system had gone haywire. The more upright she was, the lower her blood pressure would be. I told her there was a chance she might have to sleep in a chair, to make sure her blood pressure wasn't too high at night when she was sleeping. More medications or procedures weren't the answer. But more than anything else, I told her to not worry, to think about what great health she was in, and to focus on herself and how she felt and not the numbers. In an ecosystem overwhelmed with information and technology, sometimes that's easier said than done, for both patients and their doctors.

When Rajeev was told by the doctors in Istanbul that he'd had a heart attack, he didn't really believe them at first. "I got violently angry," he said. "I said, 'What are you talking about?'"

They found so much disease in his coronary arteries that they told him he would need open-heart surgery. "Going from never having seen a doctor to needing bypass surgery was quite a shock . . . For me, it was all in reverse. Only then did I get a primary care physician."

I had been listening quietly but felt compelled to ask him if he thought that if he had sought regular, preventive care, perhaps this could have been avoided.

He was silent, and he told me he wasn't sure if it would have changed anything.

Rajeev, who had never seen a doctor in his life before, was going to see more than his fair share now. He flew back to the United States from Turkey and had open-heart surgery. When he woke up the day after in the intensive care unit, he had tubes in both lungs draining out blood. "The first night after surgery was the most painful time of my life."

Things got better, though, and he was back at work before he knew it. A year passed, and he told me of a morning when he was rushing to work. "I was late, so I walked very fast. I was almost running upstairs with my backpack, and for the first time since my surgery, I got the burning feeling in my throat."

It was the same feeling he'd had in the airport, and it was learned soon after that of the four vessels that the surgeons had repaired, two were already blocked again.

"I thought of my body as my greatest asset," Rajeev told me, now sounding a bit rueful. "My body is my enemy now."

Too often, we wait for tragedy to occur before we act. Too often, people think of getting flood insurance after half the basement is submerged. I have lost count of the number of people who stop smoking only after they are in the emergency room, strapped down to a gurney, having a life-altering heart attack. Even though heart disease often appears to strike out of the blue, it has often been smoldering for decades in the shadows. It can be difficult to activate and engage people for risk factors like high blood pressure that don't cause any immediate discomfort like, say, a fractured leg would.

Restricting salt, losing weight, and mild exercise can help lower blood pressure for some, but for many more, it will not be enough. The good thing is that today we have better options to control blood pressure than ever before, and with almost all blood pressure medications having been around for a while they are now generic, so the treatment of hypertension won't bring anyone to financial ruin anytime soon. On the other hand, many people don't like taking medications. With results from the landmark SPRINT trial showing that when it comes to blood pressure, the lower we can get it safely, the better, this means that every patient and their doctor need to be having long conversations about what this means for them, not in moments of crisis but hopefully long before that plaque ruptures in the heart or the brain.

Blood pressure, though, is just one of many risk factors that can mark us for heart disease. Perhaps the greatest threat to our ability to not only live long but to live well is what we put in our mouths. It has been said before, but when it comes to the health of the heart, it is incredibly true—we are what we eat.

In addition to hypertension, the parallel discovery of cholesterol as a core component of atherosclerosis was a journey also marked by triumphs, both by clinicians at the bedside and by scientists in the laboratory. And just like high blood pressure, the story of cholesterol is characterized by as many dead ends as speedways. Few medications have been as controversial as cholesterol-lowering statin medications. No day goes by without these medications, the most commonly prescribed drugs in the United States, being simultaneously declared our saviors from all sicknesses or the determinant of all our deficiencies. And like every compelling story, that of cholesterol has its fair share of backstabbers, fearmongers, snake oil salesmen, and—of course—superheroes.

4

—⋀—

YOU ARE WHAT YOU EAT

It is strange how often a heart must be broken,
Before the years can make it wise.

—Sara Teasdale, *The Collected Poems*

One night, Brandon, a young man in his early twenties with not a care in the world, started feeling like he couldn't catch a breath. He went to the emergency room in his hometown's small rural hospital in North Carolina. The doctor in the emergency room performed an electrocardiogram, and as soon as the heart rhythm strip started to print, he took out his phone and called the one person he knew could bail him out.

I was busy working in the cardiac intensive care unit (CICU) at my hospital when the ringtone I had now come to dread started to sound. It was the default ringtone of the phone carried by the doctor covering the CICU, a phone whose number was on the speed dials of almost every emergency room physician within a few hundred miles. The ER doctor told me that Brandon likely had pericarditis—inflammation of the pericardial sac surrounding the heart—a condition that mostly occurs after a viral infection and is treated mostly with over-the-counter anti-inflammatory medicines like ibuprofen. The fax machine, a sight still common in hospitals, started to slowly sputter out Brandon's EKG. I took a look at it, and sure enough, it did look like it could have been pericarditis. There was nothing on the EKG suggesting that he was having a heart attack or anything else life-threatening. I told the emergency room doctor to have Brandon sent over to our hospital via ambulance. He told me he would reach us in about a half hour.

As the emergency department doors opened, the ambulance's blinding lights flashed as Brandon was rolled in on his gurney. I was waiting for him and just wanted to lay eyes on him, make sure everything was okay, and then have the doctor managing the patients in the wards take over. When I actually saw him, he didn't pass the most critical prognostic test in modern medicine—the eyeball test.

Brandon looked like he was in distress. He was cold but was drenched in sweat. I had the skeleton crew hook him up to the electrocardiogram, and when the heart rhythm showed up, it might as well have been drawn by the angel of death. On his EKG, which looked nothing like the one he'd had in the other hospital, he had a pattern commonly referred to as *tombstones*. Tombstones indicate that there is a part of the heart where the supply of blood has been completely cut off. It usually means that the person is having a massive heart attack, almost certainly due to an atherosclerotic plaque rupturing in one of the coronary arteries and completely blocking blood flow.

This was not a moment to dally or dither—as soon as I saw those tombstones, I knew that he was having what is called an *ST elevation myocardial infarction* or STEMI—the classic heart attack manifested by an elevation in the *ST* segment of a patient's EKG due to complete obstruction of blood flow in one of the coronary arteries. Without thinking, I asked one of the nurses to activate the cardiac catheterization lab. She called the hospital operator, who immediately sent an urgent page to the entire team, who were at their various homes with their pagers handy. As all those pagers went off at the same time and all the team members proceeded to reach for their car keys and head straight for the hospital, only one of them actually called me on the way. It was the cardiologist who would be performing the procedure. The entire team assembled, and within minutes, Brandon was being rolled to the cardiac catheterization lab. The very first glimpse we received of his coronary arteries on the x-ray machine confirmed our suspicion—there was a fresh blood clot lodged in the mouth of the left anterior descending artery supplying the entire front wall down to the tip of his heart. The interventional cardiologist passed a wire through the clot and then slid a miniature stent down to where the plaque had ruptured and used a small balloon to deploy the weblike metal structure in Brandon's lifeline.

Blood flow returned to his heart and the tombstones disappeared, but much of the damage had already been done. The part of the heart supplied by the erstwhile blocked vessel was barely moving, and much of the muscle there had died. The heart is so sensitive to oxygen deprivation that it can start dying permanently within minutes. His blood pressure bottomed out, and it was clear he was developing very severe heart failure. The interventional cardiology team then deployed a large balloon that sat just outside his heart in the large artery coming out of it—the aorta. The balloon—extending all the way from his navel to the middle of his chest—started to beat inside his aorta. When his heart squeezed, pushing blood out into the aorta, the balloon deflated, sucking blood forward and reducing the pressure the heart was beating against. When the heart was filling with blood and was relaxed, the balloon inflated, pushing blood back toward the heart, so that it would fill the coronary arteries that emerged right at the spot where the aorta came out of the heart. This helped improve the blood supply in the coronary arteries. As soon as the intra-aortic balloon pump started to beat, his blood pressure improved, and he was transported from the cardiac catheterization lab to the CICU.

All this time, as his life hung in the balance, I wondered, *Why did a twenty-one-year-old man with no prior medical problems even have a heart attack, let alone one this massive?* The answer, I would find out soon, was cholesterol.

—⩗—

Everyone, *everywhere* knows about cholesterol today. Growing up in Pakistan, everyone around me knew that cholesterol was bad. Very, very bad. Back when my siblings and I were kids and chicken *karahi* was served for dinner and there was a layer of amber floating on top, we knew that it was bad, because there was cholesterol in all that oil. The more advanced among us went even a step further. Not only did they know of the bad cholesterol, they knew of a good cholesterol, too.

After I started my training as a cardiologist, almost everyone I knew personally wanted to talk to me about cholesterol. For a fact, I know the cholesterol levels of my entire family and several other close relatives. Cholesterol confessionals can occur at any time and any place and sometimes can take unexpected turns.

My wife and I were out for dinner in Raleigh with friends, who, like us, also had a baby daughter. We picked a Lebanese fusion restaurant, which didn't disappoint. Just thinking about the fluffy bread they served with olive oil takes me to my happy place. Just as the entrées arrived, my friend told me that he had a problem. He told me that he had gotten his cholesterol checked and it was high. I wasn't too worried about him; he was thin and lean and exercised regularly. He pulled up the results on his cell phone and passed them on to me. I took the phone, practicing my inner reassuring voice, telling him he should enjoy the dinner.

When I saw the results, though, I was left astounded. His bad cholesterol was almost twice the normal limit. I asked him whether he'd followed up with his primary care physician after he'd gotten the results, but he told me he never went back. I wanted to tell him not to worry, but I just couldn't. I told him that this was serious, that he might have to take medications, potentially for life. Almost certainly, he had a genetic disease that predisposed him to having a very high cholesterol level called familial hypercholesterolemia, the same disease Brandon had that caused him to have a heart attack.

The kebabs he had ordered remained unattended. I tried to urge him that things would be okay, and while he told me he was okay, he wasn't. Eventually, I had to finish his food for him. While there are some who couldn't care less about their risk factors, there are some on the far other end of the spectrum. My father-in-law is one of them. Ever since his heart attack, he is über-watchful and in many ways the ideal patient. He watches what he eats, exercises regularly, and takes his medications. His question for me is if his bad cholesterol is *too* low.

The really interesting thing about cholesterol is that while many facets of medicine and health exist almost entirely outside of popular discourse, cholesterol is very much public property, like mammograms and pap smears. When it comes to cholesterol and the medications that treat it—statins—the people make their voices heard and are very much part of the conversations that surround them.

With so many voices, it has become increasingly difficult to filter the signal from the noise. News reports are populated by divergent information about the supposed benefits and risks of statins and the best way to change one's diet to reduce the risk of heart disease. One day, fat is bad, and the next day, it is good. One day, statins cause people to develop dementia, and the next day, they are being tested to reduce the incidence of dementia. How can one find the truth in a tweet storm? Whose voice can be trusted, especially when it comes to food or pharmaceuticals, where a lot of big checks and stuffed pockets are involved? More than almost any other part of medicine, cholesterol and statins have a monumental #fakenews problem, and it is one we simply can't blame the Russian troll army for.

To understand the present and to forecast the future, we have to start by pursing through our past. The story of cholesterol is in fact the story of science. This journey is punctuated by exhilarating rushes into the future all too often interrupted by whiplash-inducing collisions as well as some disheartening reversals.

—⋀—

High cholesterol, by accelerating atherosclerosis, is responsible for millions upon millions of deaths, but for researchers, cholesterol has been a gift that keeps on giving. More than ten thousand research papers a year are published that mention cholesterol. A grand total of thirteen Nobel Prizes have been awarded to biologists and chemists for their study of cholesterol through the years, and there might be at least one more on the way. All this is to say both how important this one molecule is to the state of human health and how even this amount of investigation has left people at times with more confused looks than wide-eyed nods.

François Poulletier de la Salle, a prominent French researcher, became the first person to isolate cholesterol in 1758.[1] Interestingly, Poulletier was not interested in heart disease. Instead, he was busy crushing golden gallstones, dissolving them in warm alcohol. Gallstones are mostly made of cholesterol crystals, and he initially thought that it was a type of wax. The term *cholesterol* was coined by another French researcher in 1815, by combining *chole*, which means *bile*, the fatty liquid that fills our gallbladder, and *stereos*, which means *solid*. More than thirty years later in 1847, a German pathologist's eye was drawn to a "yellowish-white greasy mass" in the wall of an eighty-four-year-old's aorta during a routine autopsy.[2] That mass was atherosclerotic plaque, but the pathologist, Julius Vogel, was not the first person to note its presence. When anatomist Jakob Wepfer died in 1695, in an interesting twist of fate, his own son-in-law, also an anatomist named Johann Conrad Brunner, performed his autopsy.[3] Brunner found severe atherosclerosis in his father-in-law's aorta, describing its appearance as "rotten like fruit."[4] However, it was Vogel who discovered that these plaques got their color from being full of cholesterol.

The science of atherosclerosis and cholesterol kept moving forward. Rudolf Virchow, the German polymath and physician-researcher extraordinaire, asserted in 1858, "In some particularly violent cases the softening manifests itself even in the arteries not as the consequence of a really fatty process, but as a direct product of inflammation."[5] That means that more than 150 years ago, inflammation, atherosclerosis, and cholesterol were all linked together. Yet there was a fatal flaw in Virchow's inference—he posited that the deposition of cholesterol in the blood vessels in atherosclerotic plaques was a wholly *passive* process, a natural consequence of aging, rather than a disease process that was *actively* brought about by dietary cholesterol consumption. Virchow, who came so close, never made the connection between cholesterol and heart disease. It would take another hundred years before the causative link between heart disease and cholesterol would be made. In fact, pure cholesterol was often consumed in the early twentieth century as a cure for all sorts of ailments, including tuberculosis, jaundice, and anemia, among others.[6]

Unbeknownst to much of the rest of the world, a Russian scientist in the early twentieth century had leaped right into the future and made many discoveries that it would take the rest of the world another half century to accomplish. Nikolay Anichkov was a pathologist who, starting in 1913, achieved a series of breakthroughs by feeding rabbits a whole lot of cholesterol.[7] Anichkov traced the progression of cholesterol and its intercourse with atherosclerosis from its origins. Anichkov discovered that even before the earliest visible lesions of atherosclerosis developed, white blood cells were invading blood vessels, where they transformed into fatty foam cells that gave rise to fatty streaks. He found that cholesterol entered the vessel walls from the blood, and the more cholesterol there was in the blood, the more atherosclerotic plaques developed. The cholesterol Anichkov fed these rabbits was dissolved in sunflower oil—while these rabbits all developed profound atherosclerosis, rabbits fed only sunflower oil without any added cholesterol did not. Crucially, he also found that early atherosclerotic lesions could regress if dietary cholesterol was reduced. Sadly, despite thirteen scientists winning Nobel Prizes for cholesterol-related research, the most trailblazing one, Nikolay Anichkov, never did.

Even though Anichkov published his work in both German and, eventually, English, he had difficulty shaking the established "senescence hypothesis"—that atherosclerosis was an inevitable consequences of growing older, rather than an acquired condition that could be worsened with excessive consumption of cholesterol and other risk factors. Not only were people cowering in the face of heart disease, waiting for its unanticipated strike, researchers had accepted the inevitable march of atherosclerosis as one they could witness but not avert. As much as they had surrendered to the disease, they also surrendered to dogma.

Overcoming this status quo would require someone with unparalleled scientific acumen and fierce ambition backed by the will needed to ram head-on into the established way of thinking. That man was Ancel Keys, who lived to be a hundred years old and is a central figure in the heated debate that rages to this day about what we eat and how that affects us. To many, he is a hero, who used empirical science to save millions of lives, and to his detractors, he was a conflicted fraud. Who was he really?

Ancel Keys almost single-handedly changed prevailing views of the ills of cholesterol. Born in 1904, Ancel was identified as a genius of sorts from a very young age.[8] At eighteen, he was found to have the highest IQ of one thousand or so of his peers in California. He left school and worked in a mine, in a lumber camp, and as a crewman on an ocean liner that was headed off to China before he returned and received a master's degree and two doctorates, one in biology from the University of California–Berkley, and the other in physiology from King's College, Cambridge.

Keys got his start by winning a contract to design the famous K rations for paratroopers, which, through a combination of biscuits, chocolate, and dry sausage, crammed 3,200 calories into a pocket-sized package that could fit in a paratrooper's pocket.

After the Second World War, the world of nutritional research was squarely focused on how to overcome nutritional deficiency to ensure that military-aged men were ready to spring into action at all times. Keys was the lead investigator of one of the most dramatic studies in nutrition science—the Minnesota Starvation Experiment—designed to study the effects of famine and starvation and the best methods to rehabilitate the famished.[9] The study was offered as an alternative to military service for conscientious objectors—they could either go fight in the war or allow themselves to be actively starved for months. In 1944, thirty-six white men who had been vigorously screened to be both physically and mentally healthy were enrolled. Over the course of the study, which lasted for a year, most of the men were starved to prunes until they began to resemble survivors from concentration camps. The study also offered a gruesome insight into the psychological effects of starvation—almost all the men experienced extreme emotional distress and depression, with one chopping off three of his fingers with an ax.

Yet as events unfolded after the war's end, given the epidemic of heart disease, it became clear that underconsumption was not going to be as big a threat as overconsumption. In fact, Keys, who had since moved to Minneapolis, noticed this most starkly in some of the businessmen he knew in the area, many of whom were dying prematurely of heart disease. One of the important observations that Keys made was that the risk of heart disease was much lesser in the subjects in the starvation study.[10] This signal bolstered observations from other scientists who had noted that the incidence of heart disease was very low in non-Western societies, such as Indonesia, Libya, and China. It wasn't clear if there was anything in the environment that caused more Westerners to have heart disease or whether it was something in their diets. In his own travels, Keys had noted that heart disease was less common in countries where the average level of cholesterol was lower. In 1958, therefore, to try to see if there was a link between diet and heart disease, Keys launched one of the most ambitious studies of his time—the Seven Countries Study.[11]

Keys's landmark study included more than twelve thousand men in their forties and fifties from the United States, Finland, the former Yugoslavia (Serbia and Croatia), the Netherlands, Italy, and Japan. Strikingly, he showed that there was an almost direct relationship between the level of cholesterol in the blood and heart disease, regardless of where one lived. These findings helped bolster the conclusion from studies from

Framingham that cholesterol was bad, very bad. The Japanese, for example, had the lowest risk of heart disease, which the study suggested was associated with low cholesterol levels. These results, followed for half a century since the study started, have shown a strong and consistent relationship between cholesterol and heart disease.

Subsequent studies showed that when Japanese people migrated to the United States and their diets became more Americanized, they experienced rates of heart disease similar to their new countrymen and -women.[12] The important question was whether these observations were *correlative* or causative. Did cholesterol cause heart disease in the way that smoking causes heart disease?

To prove that cholesterol causes heart disease, you would need to design a trial in which you could give one group of people more cholesterol and the other ones less and then show if one group did better than the other. Sounds easy, but it isn't—getting people to take a medication is easier than having them alter their entire diets. Nutritional studies, therefore, are notoriously hard to do unless you have a captive audience.

Well, the veterans' hospital in Los Angeles had a bright idea.[13] They ran a dorm for healthy but destitute veterans who lived in the facility and exclusively ate in one of two dining halls. The researchers made no changes in one hall but in the other hall used vegetable oil instead of animal fat, although the overall fat content was kept the same. The study included eight hundred men over eight years, who were examined by doctors with no idea if they were getting the modified or regular diet. At the end, when researchers looked at heart attacks, there was no difference, but if you combined that with strokes and arterial disease leading to amputation, both of which are due to atherosclerosis, the risk was 31 percent lower in the veterans getting the modified diet. However, because people at that time did not link strokes with cholesterol, which we know to be the case today, the results were not considered impressive.

Another group of researchers in Finland, overseeing two large psychiatric hospitals, performed a similar experiment at the same time, which replaced the animal fat in milk with soybean fat.[14] The experiment lasted twelve years, and the diet modification was switched midway from one hospital to the other, and in sum, patients receiving the modified diet had lower cholesterol and fewer heart attacks.

Both the veterans' study and the Finnish study were published in 1968 and 1972, respectively. You would think that this would be enough to close the case, but you would be wrong. As late as 1979, George Mann, a biochemist and physician at Vanderbilt University, in an interview in *People* magazine, called out the "heart mafia," deeming the link between dietary cholesterol intake and heart disease as "an unwholesome conspiracy."[15] In *The New England Journal of Medicine,* when describing the scientific consensus backing the link, he wrote, "Galileo would have flinched." The article was titled, "Diet-Heart: The End of an Era."[16] What would it possibly take to push the vast majority of people and doctors, both of whom still remained on the fence, to believe that dietary cholesterol was truly deadly?

A mountain of evidence started to build up, particularly in the United States, where in the 1960s, the American Heart Association advocated for a cholesterol-restricted diet given the overwhelming evidence that cholesterol was linked to a higher risk of heart disease and stroke, including from the Framingham Heart Study.[17] However, opposition to cholesterol's causative role in atherosclerosis persisted widely. In 1979, Sir John McMichael, one of the most prominent British cardiologists of his time, in an article in *The British Medical Journal,* called the recommendation to reduce dietary cholesterol "propaganda," going on to write that atherosclerosis is a "wear-and tear disease" and warning that "reducing blood cholesterol by diet or drugs may have injurious effects."[18]

It became obvious that a blockbuster study would be needed to not only get detractors to put down their pitchforks but to convince the lukewarm masses. Showing an effect, any effect, just with changes in diet has always been and continues to be very difficult to demonstrate in clinical studies.

While all of us know of that one uncle who came off all their blood pressure medications after they reduced salt intake, or that aunt who now only has stevia-sprinkled brownies and doesn't have to take diabetes medications anymore, many large clinical studies that enroll thousands of patients and measure changes over years have traditionally not found dietary changes to be effective or durable. Finally, the concept of blinding, the concealment from both the study participants and the researchers so as to avoid biasing either, is almost impossible in a diet-based trial.

The National Institutes of Health realized that unless a trial was successfully performed, no amount of correlative data would be useful. The only problem was that all the drugs that existed at that time were suboptimal. Clofibrate was a drug that had been around since the 1930s and no one really knew how it worked, but it seemed to lower cholesterol. However, its effect was very modest, and it caused such complications as gallstone formation, stomachaches, and muscle damage. Another was niacin, a B vitamin, which caused a lot of discomfort among patients, most commonly flushing-reddening-itching-tingling of the face. The researchers, therefore, settled on a medication called cholestyramine. Cholestyramine is not absorbed into the body at all but works by absorbing the cholesterol-rich bile produced naturally by the gallbladder from the intestines. This causes the liver to make more bile, which needs cholesterol for its synthesis and can therefore lower cholesterol levels.

Another reason researchers picked cholestyramine was because it had the safest risk profile given that it is not absorbed into the body at all. The caveat was that the medication came in a grainy powder form that had to be dissolved in water; the patients had to drink two packets three times a day. Given that the seven-year-long study was recruiting almost 4,000 men with heart disease and elevated cholesterol levels, none of them knowing whether they were taking the medication or placebo, the researchers were perhaps foolhardy.[19] In fact, they had to screen half a million men to get to their sample of 3,800 after several years of enrollment.

A failure of this trial would be exactly what cholesterol disbelievers were looking for. But the trial made it, squeaking over an imaginary statistical bar, but only *just*.[20] Patients using cholestyramine, over about an average of 7.5 years, experienced a reduction in cholesterol levels by only about 13 percent but experienced a 19 percent reduction in death from heart disease or a heart attack compared to those taking the placebo. The effect would have been even stronger had more patients actually taken the medication, given that many couldn't tolerate the recommended dose, given how awful it was to take.

This trial, called CPPT—Coronary Primary Prevention Trial—was the keystone of a century of research into cholesterol coming together, leading to a much wider adoption of the "cholesterol is bad, so we should lower it" hypothesis. And one could say that even with all this progress, the finish line was nowhere to be seen. Sure, cholesterol is bad, now most agreed, but there was almost no good option to treat it. The medications available all had significant side effects, and it would be hard to get people outside of a research study to take them. The meds weren't that effective either—in the CPPT trial, while heart-related events were lower, mortality was similar between both groups receiving the drug or placebo. If lowering cholesterol wouldn't help you live longer, why bother taking terrible medications for life trying to do so? The weak results meant that the largest cholesterol drug trial to date, costing the NIH $150 million, couldn't silence critics like George Mann, who now claimed—without proof, of course—that the researchers had "manipulated the data."[21]

Even the best possible trial could not make up for the fact that the treatments available were just terrible. Dietary restriction, on the other hand, while showing promise in some rigorous studies, was notoriously ineffective in the real world. The CPPT had helped push the lipid hypothesis forward, but its implications for patients were limited given how difficult taking the medication was.

It became clear that an advance as distinct as, say, the iPhone was needed. Such an advance would be produced by a Japanese biochemist who was studying fungi in petri dishes, trying to find the next blockbuster antibiotic. Even in his wildest dreams, he never could have imagined what he would stumble upon.

Born in 1933, Akira Endo, in his own words, grew up in a "rural farming family in northern Japan," and found himself fascinated with molds and mushrooms as a child.[22] He dreamed of one day becoming the next Alexander Fleming. Fleming (1881–1955), a studious microbiologist, was perhaps not the tidiest. He was investigating a common bacterium in petri dishes. One day when he showed up to his lab, a bacterial colony had been destroyed by fungus, which had contaminated one of the samples. When he cultured that fungus, he found that the mold juice that it produced had killed bacteria. He called that juice *penicillin*.

Akira Endo joined a Japanese pharmaceutical company, hoping that one of the molds he was studying would one day help him discover the successor to penicillin. When he came to New York for studies in the 1960s, there were aspects of American life there he found very alien. "I was very surprised by the large number of elderly and overweight people, and by the rather rich dietary habits," he wrote. "In the residential area of the Bronx where I lived, there were many elderly couples living by themselves and I often saw ambulances going to take an elderly person who had suffered a heart attack to the hospital."[23]

Endo thought that the same fungi that produced penicillin might also produce substances that could reduce the production of cholesterol, which was part of bacteria's cell membrane. Back in Japan, his team tested more than 3,800 types of fungi before they hit pay dirt.

Cholesterol reaches the blood through two ways—one, obviously, is through one's diet. The other is through the liver, which actually makes cholesterol. Why does the liver need to make cholesterol? Well, that's because cholesterol is a fundamental ingredient for all living things, humans especially. Cholesterol, a critical part of the membrane of each cell, is a key ingredient in many hormones and substances such as bile, which assist with the absorption of food and are an essential component of the human brain. The liver's production of cholesterol was likely necessary when fat was an infrequent component of our diets, but now that we have more than our fair share of cholesterol in our everyday foods, this production is probably not that necessary. The liver, though, hasn't adapted to the changes in our diet and continues to produce cholesterol even when there is enough of it in our foods. Even if you have a ton of cholesterol in that greasy hamburger and upsized fries, most people's livers keep churning out cholesterol. This is one reason many people's cholesterol levels remain elevated even when they have religiously cut down on cholesterol-containing stuff on their plates.

Endo tested this substance in animals, every one of whom, except rats, showed significant lowering of cholesterol. The reason it didn't work in rats was because the enzyme that this drug blocked would rebound after a while in rats only, nullifying the beneficial effects. Endo teamed up with a Tokyo-based physician and began testing it in humans and early results were very promising. And then suddenly, everything came to a screeching halt. Some dogs treated with doses hundreds of times higher than necessary had developed what was thought to be intestinal cancer but was later found to be a noncancerous change occurring in the cells because of the enormous doses being used.[24] Even as work at Endo's company stalled out of an abundance of caution, another pharmaceutical company, Merck, developed a similar compound and, after finding no signal of risk in their studies, continued with the development of their product. That product was called lovastatin, the first statin drug to ever reach the market in 1987. Akira Endo had not discovered the next blockbuster antibiotic—without knowing it, he had discovered perhaps the most important medicine since penicillin.

When it hit the market, lovastatin itself did not have the strongest data, but that soon changed. The first major study of any statin was the Scandinavian Simvastatin Survival Study, called 4S and published in

1994, which, incidentally, included 4,444 middle-aged people with heart disease, half of whom got a statin and the other half of whom received a placebo.[25] After five and a half years, patients taking the statin had a 30 percent reduction in the chance of dying, compared to those taking the placebo. Presumably, given that the survival curves continued to diverge between the statin and the placebo group, this difference would only have gotten bigger if the trial had gone on longer.

The 4S trial was no fluke, and it was exactly the sort of study that shook not only medicine but human life at large. That was because high cholesterol affects so many people, most of whom try but fail to normalize it with dietary changes. Even within a regulated research setting in which participants volunteer to enroll and are subsequently egged on by research coordinators and staff, the potential benefits of dietary interventions are unfortunately not very substantial.[26,27] What this means is that statins are today the most commonly prescribed medication in the United States and perhaps around the world. Some in the cardiology community have even advocated for them to be put in the water supply. While the vast majority, including myself, would never ascribe to that viewpoint, at this point it is hard to deny that they are some of the most important means to improve and prolong life we have ever developed as a species.

Thirty years on from being first available to patients, statins are also perhaps the most extensively studied medications in history. Just recently, a group called the Cholesterol Treatment Trialists (CTT) published a paper in the British medical journal *Lancet* in which they pooled data from more than two dozen randomized controlled trials with hundreds of thousands of patients each followed over several years.[28] They only picked clinical trials that were of high quality, with a minimum of one thousand patients who were followed for at least two years. The group centered at Oxford University includes research collaborators from all over the world.

This paper confirmed what each and every individual trial had shown but did so in a much more expansive and thorough manner. The researchers showed that benefits of statins are quite substantial and consistent.

Statins reduce the risk of heart attacks, strokes, the need for cardiac procedures, and perhaps, most importantly, deaths from heart disease in almost every patient group—men and women, diabetics and nondiabetics, young and old, smokers and nonsmokers, people with low and high cholesterol, low and high blood pressure, and those with and without prior heart disease. The greatest benefit is provided to those at the highest risk—those with cardiac risk factors such as hypertension and diabetes, those with very high cholesterol, those who are older, and most of all, those who have already had bad things happen to their hearts. There is a reduction in risk of future problems in people across the risk-profile spectrum. On average, in high-risk patients, statins achieve an absolute reduction in the rate of adverse events by 10 percent, on top of everything else one can do to reduce the risk of adverse cardiac events. This may not seem like a lot at first, but one in ten people not having a heart attack or stroke is a really big deal. Statins are so effective that no medication since their development thirty years ago has so far been shown to be better than they are, and it is incredibly difficult for any medication to show benefit when it is prescribed to someone already taking a statin.

When I emailed Akira Endo, who is eighty-four years old and retired, I never expected to hear back, but I did. According to him, it is clear what the greatest achievement in heart health is: "I think that cholesterol metabolism and prevention and treatment are the biggest advances." On whether he was taking a statin, he wrote, "Both my wife and I have taken statins for more than ten years. I cannot tell you which one."

Endo and his wife are just two among hundreds of millions taking statins. How common are statins these days? In a study I performed with my research team published in *The Journal of the American Medical Association: Cardiology,* we found that almost forty million Americans older than forty, which is more than one in four, use a statin and that this proportion is going to be one in three soon.[29] While this may seem like a lot, in patients who had experienced a heart attack or had confirmed significant disease in their coronary arteries, a third were not using any statin. Almost half of stroke patients weren't using statins either. These patients are most likely to benefit from a statin, and yet a very large number of them are still not using what can be certifiably said to be a lifesaving medication. The reasons many patients don't take statins have as much to do with physicians not prescribing them as patients being wary of taking them.

We also found that almost $17 billion are spent annually on statins in the United States, but this price is coming down even as the number of statin users increases. Why? Well, that's because in the last decade, the patents for each and every major statin have expired, meaning that they are now all available in inexpensive generic form. So even though they were big moneymakers for many drugmakers for decades, their average price has plummeted in recent years. Pfizer's atorvastatin (Lipitor), for example, is the bestselling drug of all time but came off patent in 2011. As of 2014, in another analysis, we found that only 5 percent of patients using atorvastatin were using brand-name atorvastatin, while the rest had all transitioned to the much cheaper generic version.[30]

And yet, of all the shiny, colorful confections in doctors' candy stores, nothing riles up and infuriates a large and incredibly loud segment of the masses like statins. To many, statins are an elaborate, multinational plot funded by Big Pharma and fronted by bespectacled, white coat–wearing physician-scientists. Conspiracies, amplified by the internet and social media, are a hallmark of modern human society. There is, for example, a growing number of people who believe that the earth is flat. They have societies and "research" conferences; they are really into it. But when it comes to conspiracies involving health and medicine, while it is easy to forget the forest for the trees and get mired in the nerdy details, the fact that lives are at stake is always present to me.

Is there any truth to the claims that harms from statins exceed their benefits? And what is it about statins that has made them a target of so much vitriol? Answers to these questions do not necessarily have anything to do with the heart. In fact, they require us to better understand the human mind, how it is connected to what we feel, and how the collective of human minds we call society and culture comes to be.

When I was working at the Beth Israel Deaconess Medical Center in Boston in 2014 as a hospital physician, I didn't really have an office; I used the computers stationed on the patient ward, and I liked one more than the others because it had two monitors. One day as I walked in to work at around 7:00 a.m., in front of that computer was an overstuffed, unmarked yellow envelope addressed to me. Curious, I opened it and quickly realized what it was.

A few days earlier, I had written an op-ed for *The Wall Street Journal* decrying the fact that so many parents in the United States were not allowing their children to receive measles vaccinations, which in turn had led to a spike in cases of this hypercontagious disease.[31] The envelope was a cornucopia of vaccine conspiracies with a typed note specifically addressed to me. Instinctively, I looked around but saw no one who wasn't supposed to be there. Someone had to have known where I sat and worked and dropped it there. It was one of the creepiest things to ever happen to me.

Statins and vaccines have many similarities—both are ubiquitous, especially in high-income countries, and are preventative therapies. While statins are certainly not as effective at preventing diseases as most common vaccines are, there are many vaccines that don't provide blanket immunity either, such as the flu vaccine. The parallels are really clear when it comes to the sort of reactions they elicit.

Statins do have some side effects associated with them. While in rare cases, about five to ten patients out of one thousand treated with a high-intensity dose of a statin for five years will develop diabetes, most of these patients are already at risk for diabetes and get pushed over into a diabetic range a bit sooner than they otherwise would be.[32] Of these patients who develop diabetes, the sum benefit of statins, and their prevention of future heart events, exceeds that of discontinuing the statin. Patients with statins also are at risk of developing inflammation of their muscles. Patients who develop this condition, called *myositis,* will have an elevation of an enzyme in their blood, which signifies damage to the muscles. This damage can resolve as soon as the statin is stopped. No medication is perfect, and by this account, one could argue that acetaminophen and ibuprofen have side effects that are far more dangerous than statins. In sum, even accounting for these rare effects, statins are one of the safest drugs available for almost any indication.

What occurs much, much more commonly is patients experiencing generalized aches and pains in their body. In clinical practice, this is the most common reason people stop taking statins. I have had many patients who have dropped statins because of these symptoms, and I am sure many readers may know of someone who has experienced similar issues. When a patient has such symptoms, I will usually try to reduce the dose of the statin or switch to another statin until I find one that works. However, there is something very curious at play when one looks into the data.

When you analyze studies that look at people being given statins under normal circumstances in clinic, muscle pain and weakness occur in between 10 and 25 percent of patients, which is a lot.[33,34] Now, when you look at the totality of studies in which patients did not know whether they were getting a statin or placebo, there is actually no increase in aches or weakness.[35]

Umm, what?

That's right—there is not a single major trial that shows that statins significantly increase the risk of muscle pains and weakness that occur without any test-confirmed evidence of muscle damage compared to placebo. In fact, in one very interesting trial, when patients were taking a statin but they didn't know whether it was a statin or placebo, there was no increase in achiness or weakness.[36] As soon as patients found out that they were taking a statin, suddenly they were much more likely to report weakness and pain than those taking a placebo.

Over time, we have learned a lot about placebos. *Placebo,* which is Latin for "I shall please," used to refer to professional mourners hired to stand in for absent family members at funerals. The history of the placebo effect runs deep in medicine because, until recently, *all* of medical care was essentially placebo. In fact, in a way, the placebo is the most widely tested therapy in medicine, given that it is administered in most well-designed clinical trials. We now know what makes a better placebo. Heavy, pricey, invasive, and brightly colored placebos are more effective than placebos that are light, noninvasive, and inexpensive.[37,38] Surprisingly, we know a lot about people who take placebos, too. For one, patients in clinical trials who more regularly take their placebos than those who don't actually live longer![39] Why? Well, people who more regularly take their placebos—unknowingly, of course—are also more likely to engage in other healthy behaviors more religiously. We also know that a placebo works—wait for it—even when patients are told they are getting a placebo.[40] Why? Well, the phantom pill is only a small part of the placebo effect. There is perhaps no placebo more powerful, more effective, and more dynamic than the physician or nurse. Any doctor or nurse can treat, but the great ones can *heal.*

While some of the symptoms that patients taking statins experience may indeed be from the drug, a sizable population is almost certainly experiencing the nocebo effect.[41] While everyone knows about the placebo effect—when patients experience unexpected benefits from just the idea of taking a medication—fewer know about the nocebo effect. The nocebo effect is the evil cousin of the placebo effect—it encompasses any negative symptoms that patients may experience even if they are taking a placebo medication. The nocebo effect can be produced by any and every type of medication. Take beta-blockers, for example, which are lifesaving for people with atherosclerotic heart disease and heart failure. Each and every medical or nursing student is taught repeatedly that these lifesaving drugs can cause depression and increase fatigue. Turns out that if you look at the data from clinical trials, beta-blockers don't cause any more fatigue than the placebo and, in fact, improve depression and depressive symptoms.[42] Yet most patients who are started on a beta-blocker are warned of these two symptoms, increasing the chances that they will go on to experience them.

Statins are the most commonly prescribed medications in countries like the United States, and tales of their side effects often precede them. In fact, I know many patients who won't even start a statin because of all the negative information they have heard about them on television or from the internet. In fact, there is data to suggest that news stories that have incorrectly portrayed statins in a negative light are associated with increased heart attacks and deaths presumably due to fewer people taking them in light of those stories resulting in a reduction in the protection they offer in countries as diverse as the United Kingdom, Denmark, France, Australia, and Turkey.[43]

I don't have to refer to research to know the price that patients might pay if they don't receive the best possible preventive treatment. I remember once taking care of a woman with rip-roaring coronary artery disease. She had very limited flow in every vessel supplying her heart. She would need heart bypass surgery. It was very unusual for a woman in her fifties to have such widespread disease in her heart. The only thing that suggested why she had a heart attack was that her cholesterol was very high. I looked through her list of medications and did not find a statin. To my surprise, statins were listed in her allergy list.

When I asked her about what allergic reaction she had, she told me that she developed muscle aches after starting on one. She stopped using the statin, and her doctor didn't try another one to see if that would be tolerated instead. I was trying to figure out if we could try something else, but before we could do that, she ended up having a cardiac arrest and, despite our best efforts, died.

While death is inevitable, it was clear that it came too soon for her. She and her family could never have anticipated it. Every time a patient takes an unfortunate turn or experiences an untoward medical event, most physicians perform a personal inquest. And for that patient, it seemed like the only thing I kept coming back to was that missing statin. Could it have saved her? I wasn't sure. A statin could have prevented her from having perhaps such severely high cholesterol and resultant atherosclerosis. There is research that suggests that among patients who have had heart disease, patients who are unable to tolerate statins have a 50 percent higher risk of having a recurrent heart attack.[44]

The nocebo effect, like the placebo effect, serves a very specific protective function. It represents our bodies preparing for sensations before they hit us—the nocebo effect is us responding to an expectation of discomfort before we experience it. Therefore, when patients receive a sugar pill and they are warned that they might expect to feel exhausted, more than a fifth may feel it even though they are ingesting nothing more than a suggestion. Similarly, the reason patients receiving statins in trials don't demonstrate greater aches and pains isn't because they don't feel those symptoms; it is because a similar number feel symptoms receiving the placebo. The nocebo effect is represented by specific patterns of stimulation in our brains and is magnified by our expectations—the nocebo effect is more pronounced after a more expensive drug, given that recipients may have had more optimistic expectations of benefit, compared to a cheaper sham drug.

These findings raise some important questions. Are patients who experience bodily weakness and aches after taking statins mostly feeling these symptoms because they have been warned by their doctors that they might do so? And if so, should doctors not forewarn their patients about muscle aches and weakness so as to avoid the nocebo effect?

I, for one, do believe that some patients probably experience true statin-induced muscle weakness or pains. Research suggests that patients who experience symptoms in their thighs, for example, are most likely to be experiencing true drug-related symptoms rather than those caused by the wear and tear of regular existence or the nocebo effect.[45] I have changed my practice and now make it incredibly clear when starting a patient on statins that it is exceedingly rare for patients to not tolerate these medications and indicate what symptoms are more suggestive than others. If a patient has been on a statin in the past and experienced intolerance, I try to persuade them as kindly as possible to give statins another shot, maybe at a lower dose or maybe with another type of statin because anything is better than the converse.

The war on statins goes far beyond just aches and pains. A loud and rancorous segment of the population would rather believe that statins are worse than cyanide, that they cause side effects such as dementia and permanent muscle damage. Even more importantly, statin deniers are making arguments against the entire foundation of the lipid hypothesis—claiming that cholesterol is good and lowering it is bad. At a time when the competition for attention is measured through clicks, tactics employed by quacks can be far more effective than those employed by nuanced academics. What is really at the heart of statin-induced hysteria, and what does it say about the future of how medicine and society will interface?

One day, when I was in medical school, I was sitting on a bench at the hospital gym lifting weights when I heard a high-pitched clicking sound in my back. A surge of excruciating pain seared through my entire body, and I almost immediately collapsed. Luckily, there were people around me who made sure that the weights I was lifting didn't fall on me. I felt extreme pain throughout my back, and my friends put me into a wheelchair and rolled me to the emergency room. An MRI revealed that I had prolapsed a vertebral disc in my lower back, and it was pinching my spine. A neurosurgeon gave me the choice to try to rehabilitate my back with exercise or go under the knife. A colleague told me that once your spinal column is opened by a surgeon, it is never the same again. I decided that I would exercise my way out of this hell.

For years, I was in pain at every given moment from when I slept at night to when I woke up in the morning. All the things I loved—playing basketball and lifting weights—I had to stop. I involuntarily lost almost thirty pounds. Pain became my unwavering companion, and I was prepared to have it as a constant presence in my life for as long as I would live.

I began an aggressive exercise regimen that many times made me hurt even more. Several times during the day, alone in my room, I just kept stretching and flexing and extending my back. I became a frequent flier in the physical therapy room; I practically lived there. Through all this, I never took a pill, not even an ibuprofen or acetaminophen. The pain was a message my body was trying to give me, and I didn't want to blunt it. More importantly, though, as a doctor, I realized that when it comes to medications, there is no such thing as a free lunch. Dealing with medication complications all the time had trained me to be wary.

I, of course, am far from the only one averse to taking medications, yet we live in unusual times. Many note that the pill-popping culture has reached its zenith in modern society.[46] Overmedicalization has led to an overdependence on medications. People want pills to lose weight, to not lose an erection, to not lose hair, to not lose their tempers, to not be in pain, to never, ever be in pain. Consequences of this culture are all around us—the opioid epidemic almost certainly was triggered by overprescription and overuse of opioid pain medications.

Pharmaceutical companies are anything but innocent bystanders, and if anything, they have seen an unprecedented windfall from a culture they have helped create. This is especially true of the United States, one of the only countries in the world where pharmaceutical companies can advertise directly to patients, many of whom are vulnerable due to their sickness. The overuse of drugs is leading to another crisis. An analysis of Congressional Budget Office data I published along with Kevin Schulman, a business school professor and physician, in *The New England Journal of Medicine* showed that drug costs are the fastest-rising sources of Medicare expenditures and that they might bankrupt the U.S. health system.[47] When it comes to statins, I have published research showing how the U.S. health system spends billions of dollars on brand-name statins, even after that same drug is available in a cheaper, generic form.[48] I am of the opinion that no matter what pharmaceutical companies say, it is hard to deny that their ultimate loyalty is to their shareholders.

Skepticism about drugs and drugmakers, to me at least, is healthy, and this skepticism is particularly pointed when it comes to cholesterol-lowering drugs. Before 1987, the year the first statin was approved, the last drug to be approved by the Food and Drug Administration to lower cholesterol was called triparanol, all the way back in 1960.[49] Scientists had previously discovered that the hormone estrogen lowered the risk of heart disease in women and also resulted in lower cholesterol. When given to men, however, estrogen had a strong feminizing effect. A pharmaceutical company based in Ohio, Richardson-Merrell, developed a "nonestrogen estrogen," a nonalcoholic beer of sorts. By blocking a late step in the liver's cholesterol production pathway, it prevented cholesterol from being formed. Triparanol was patented in 1959 and was released into the market the very next year.

As soon as patients started to take triparanol, many reported extremely disturbing side effects ranging from nausea, vomiting, blindness from cataracts, a change in the texture of skin to a fishlike scale, and a paradoxical *increase* in atherosclerosis. How could this happen?

Turns out that Richardson-Merrell had known that triparanol caused all these awful side effects but had forced their safety officer to falsify the reports that had been submitted to the FDA. Even though she refused and quit her job rather than do something unethical, Richardson-Merrell went ahead and gained approval for their poisonous drug based on forged data. Triparanol, while blocking the production of cholesterol, increased production of another compound that deposited in the eyes and skin and accelerated development of atherosclerotic plaques. Richardson-Merrell pled guilty and paid a fine, although it is speculated that they made a lot more money selling their drug to the half a million Americans who had taken it in the two years that it was on the market.

The triparanol catastrophe has been relegated to dusty history books. No one teaches it in medical school or even to cardiologists in training, but it helps explain why many suspect pharmaceutical companies of nefarious behavior.

In this regard, though, statins represent a triumph of sorts. Three decades of data from all over the world, from both clinical trials and from routine clinical use, from different manufacturers, among all races and ethnicities and age groups, confirm that statins are safe and their benefit extends across all sorts of divides. Episodes like triparanol have led to the institution of more stringent safety assessment procedures, and the FDA has served as a robust gatekeeper, protecting Americans from bad drugs reaching their pillboxes.

These days, if anything, one could argue that it is in pharmaceutical companies' interest for people to *not* take statins. Because statins are common and generic, they have become very cheap with little margin for profit. Remember the bad drugs we had even before statins were available, drugs like niacin, cholestyramine, and fibrate drugs? Turns out they are still available and are actually used in some patients who can't, or won't, take statins. In an ironic twist, an analysis I performed with my team of national U.S. data showed that companies actually make more money on these ineffectual drugs because, one, all the statins are now generic; two, statins are so commonly sold, they don't need to be exorbitantly priced to reap a profit; and three, because so many companies make generic statins, competition to lower prices is rife.[50] Companies would rather have patients take these other drugs, or newer statin alternatives, on which they can make some serious moolah.

Another broad front that conspiracy theorists have erected is an attempt to discredit the science at the heart of cholesterol-lowering and its role in causing heart disease. A weak link in the science of cholesterol is something many people have heard about. Frequently, people hear about good cholesterol and bad cholesterol. You would think that increasing good cholesterol would be great—but it hasn't panned out in clinical trials. The story of good and bad cholesterol illuminates what to many is the messy side of science. To understand heart disease, it is essential to first understand the science *behind* the science of heart disease.

5

—⼁⼂—

THE METHOD IN THE MADNESS

Your vision will become clear
only when you can look into your own heart.
Who looks outside, dreams; who looks inside, awakens.

—Carl Jung

When we eat food, all of it is digested from the intestines into a special vein that leads straight to the liver. The liver is not just a recipient of nutrients; it makes its own, too. Cholesterol, in fact, is largely produced in the liver. The liver packs cholesterol into microscopic shuttles made out of protein and transports it to the rest of the body. The most important of these shuttles is called low-density lipoprotein (LDL), carrying most of the cholesterol in the blood. While LDL, for the most part, is just benignly transporting cholesterol through the body, it can also sometimes undergo a dastardly mutation. Inflammation can cause LDL to become oxidized. Once oxidized, LDL deposits cholesterol in the walls of the blood vessels, resulting in the buildup of atherosclerotic plaques. LDL, unsurprisingly therefore, is colloquially referred to on dinner tables, in wellness magazines, and websites as *bad* cholesterol. In fact, most times when cholesterol goals are being discussed by doctors or patients, they are usually talking just about the LDL levels.

Yet the truth is that not all cholesterol is bad, for just like LDL, which takes cholesterol from the liver and sends it around the body, at times being deposited in atherosclerotic plaques, there is another type of cholesterol-carrying shuttle that evacuates cholesterol from the body back to the liver.

Back in its early days, when the connection between cholesterol and its various lipoprotein shuttles was still being carved out in the blank sands, some conflicting results started to emerge. While it was clear that as the levels of the total cholesterol and most of the cholesterol-carrying lipoproteins rose, atherosclerosis became more apparent, there was one such lipoprotein that seemed to have the opposite effect. The story of good cholesterol, namely high-density lipoprotein (HDL), was dramatically first narrated in a conference at the National Institutes of Health by Donald Fredrickson, a researcher. He began by saying, "This is the story of an island, a family, and a strange malady."[1] This sounds more like the start of an intergenerational magical-realism novel than a scientific case presentation.

This strange malady in a family on an island was noted in the back of the throat of a five-year-old boy who was a member of this clan and was getting his tonsils excised. Before his enlarged tonsils could be removed and thrown disdainfully in a bucket, the physician made a striking observation. His tonsils were bright orange and bulbous. After they were cut out, additional testing revealed that they were bursting with cholesterol-filled white blood cells. The case took a mysterious turn when the boy's sister was found to have the same enormous orange tonsils. Researchers had no idea what the disease was or how it was caused, so they named Tangier disease after the small island of Tangier in Chesapeake Bay that the siblings originated from. This disease is so rare that it is likely that there are more people researching it than there are actual patients who have it. Yet this island, the family that inhabited it, and the malady that afflicted them opened the back door of cholesterol's life cycle, revealing how it eventually leaves the body.

Even though their bodies were full to the bursting point with cholesterol, researchers noted that the siblings barely had any HDL. This finding confirmed other research showing that as atherosclerosis went down, HDL levels, unlike LDL or any other cholesterol-carrying molecules, went up instead of down. Finally, it was discovered that people with high levels of HDL had much lower rates of heart disease. In fact, some of the strongest data about the relationship between elevated HDL and lower rates of heart disease came from the still-ongoing Framingham Heart Study.[2] Not all "cholesterol," thus, was to be feared.

Turned out that to counter LDL, there was a whole army of molecules in the body whose sole purpose was to effectively excrete cholesterol from the body. As opposed to LDL, which takes cholesterol from the liver to the rest of the body, HDL served the opposite purpose—bringing cholesterol *back* from the rest of body to the liver, where it would be expelled from the body after being converted into bile in the gallbladder and excreted into the intestines. The smallest and densest of lipoproteins, HDL, is the most benevolent.

This finding has since spawned an entire industry aimed at improving people's HDL. HDL has become the "how much do you bench" of middle and older age. People compare each other's HDL like teenage boys comparing the size of their biceps, as if nudging that good cholesterol up would be the key to everlasting life. A patient told me about how he would have his HDL checked every few months. His HDL number was like the credit score of his heart: a good number would make his day; a bad one would throw him into a tailspin of despair.

There was encouraging data to back this notion up. Exercise increased HDL and also resulted in a reduction in risk of future heart problems. Stopping smoking, too, led to HDL increasing and the risk of heart disease plummeting.[3] Many food items, including moderate amounts of red wine, increase HDL.[4] Just recently, a study was published, sponsored by the Almond Board of California, touting predictably that almonds increased HDL.[5] But before you swipe your credit card and buy that bumper bag of organic, non-GMO, cage-free almonds from your local megastore, I suggest some pause, because unlike the road to lower LDL, which has been relatively linear, the path to improving HDL might well be considered, at least today, to be a road to nowhere.

HDL was supposed to be the Good Samaritan who stopped by the bumpy blood vessels and sucked out cholesterol from atherosclerotic plaques, taking it back to the liver so that it could be dumped out of the body. And in people who exercised, people who lost weight, and people who stopped smoking, their HDL increased, and they had fewer heart attacks and strokes. It seemed like it would be the perfect target for researchers and pharmaceutical companies to develop medications for.

A drug that predated even statins and was known to effectively increase HDL was niacin, which happens to be a vitamin. While it was clear that niacin was not superior to statins by itself, the manufacturers figured that it might be useful to see if adding niacin on top of statins might help patients further reduce their risk of atherosclerotic heart disease. The results of their first trial, called AIM-HIGH, were published in 2011, and in about 3,400 patients with low HDL, niacin failed to show any benefit even though it resulted in the HDL level rising.[6] Instead of being defeated, the manufacturers figured that the reason the trial failed was because they had perhaps not aimed high enough, and there were too few patients in this trial. So they performed another trial, HPS2-THRIVE, which had a whopping 25,673 patients.[7] The results, published in 2014, showed that not only did raising HDL with niacin in these patients have no benefit, there were serious side effects like infections and bleeding from the drug.

Drugmakers figured that maybe there was a better way to increase HDL. Rats, it had been noted, almost never got atherosclerosis no matter how much cholesterol they were fed. They also had super-duper levels of HDL. Turned out that rats lacked an enzyme called CETP. This enzyme is a primary mover and shaker in the process that leads to cholesterol being excreted from the body. What if this enzyme could be turned off in humans? That would effectively prevent the human body from moving HDL to the "recycle bin." There was already some evidence that people with low levels of this enzyme had a slightly lower risk of heart disease.

With a frenzied zeal, some of the largest drugmakers in the world designed clinical trials to see if drugs that inhibit CETP would increase HDL and reduce the risk of heart disease. The trials were resoundingly successful in demonstrating that CETP inhibitors in three studies, with a combined forty-one thousand people, were great at increasing HDL.[8] When it came to whether they improved actual patient outcomes, none of the three trials showed any benefit in reducing heart disease and one of the trials resulted in a higher risk of death. A fourth trial, conducted recently, called REVEAL, which enrolled thirty thousand patients, showed that while the addition of a CETP inhibitor on top of a statin might have some very modest benefit after it was taken for about four years, it was almost certainly due to the very small improvement in overall cholesterol levels rather than the whopping increase in HDL.[9]

But how could this be? Is good cholesterol really good? If so, then why won't making it better reduce the risk of heart disease? And if not, what does that say about the decades of science that had supported that notion? I have many patients who come into clinic having worked hard to exercise more and eat better with the hope that their HDL will have improved. What should I, as their doctor, tell them? Is good cholesterol meaningless?

Once during a routine health exam, the nurse asked if I would like to have my cholesterol profile checked. I hesitated to have the blood test drawn, but she told me they would give me a free box lunch, so I agreed. When I got my results, I was startled. My LDL level was great, but my HDL was shockingly low. I ran on the treadmill several times a week and I ate carefully. And yet, my low HDL almost conferred a higher risk of future heart disease than almost anyone else similar to me who did not have a low HDL. What could I do for my low HDL cholesterol? And if I didn't know the answer, which I didn't, what could I tell a patient who came to me seeking help for a similar issue? The story of HDL cholesterol offers a window into the greater science of heart disease, which provides the sharpest view into the steep challenges facing the entire scientific enterprise.

Our relationship with the truth has always been complicated. Human beings have always claimed they want the truth, and nothing more or less, and yet a study of history finds us running actively from the truth for most of it.

The greatest barrier to truth, of course, was faith. Faith that the pharaohs were gods, faith that the color of one's skin made one better than the other, faith that one gender was more superior to the other. Faith required us to both believe what the eyes could not see and to unsee what they could.

For almost a millennium, the leading physicians of the world believed in humors; they believed there were invisible holes in the heart connecting the right to the left side; they believed there was air in the arteries, not blood; that the brain cooled the body while the heart kept it warm; and that high blood pressure was *essential,* among other beliefs. The heart was the seat of emotion, and not just as a metaphor.

And then, science happened. Science replaced faith as the lens through which many of us observed the physical world. And science gave us ample evidence of its outputs for us to retain our trust in it. The human life span, which first doubled from twenty to forty over hundreds of thousands of years, did so again from forty to almost eighty in just 150 years. The scale of this life extension is so dramatic, so unprecedented, that scientists haven't been able to replicate it in a laboratory with bacteria or cells. People experienced these benefits regardless of gender, nationality, sexual orientation, race, or ethnicity. Even in countries where people don't live as long as in higher-income countries, they have made progress in leaps and bounds. Therefore, science in many ways transcended any and all of those lines that otherwise crisscross and divide human society.

Science's ascent, while unhindered economically, has received some major setbacks in its role as the undisputed world-champion truth-wielder. HDL cholesterol comes to mind when it comes to the science of the heart, but it isn't the only one. What type of diet is best to reduce the risk of heart disease seems to change fortnightly. In the field of basic science, in which scientists study the most intricate cellular mechanisms of health and disease, a huge controversy has occurred because many influential experiments cannot be replicated. The social sciences are equally wrought by an inability to replicate seminal studies. What is going on here? Who can we trust anymore if not science and scientists?

An important reason driving this turnaround might be a widening trend of scientific findings either being refuted or their effect diminishing in experiments over time. This effect has also been referred to as "regression to the mean," pointing to initial outlier results slowly being overturned by outcomes much closer to the average over time.

When it came to HDL, it turned out that, while indicative of risk, it might be more of a marker of risk but not really a target. Pushing HDL up, it turns out, likely doesn't change risk for heart disease, at least with the medications that have been rigorously tested to date. And the reason things like exercise, weight loss, and stopping smoking reduce the risk of atherosclerosis is probably not related to HDL levels but to the myriad other changes they cause in the human body or the fact that the people likely going through the rigors of lifestyle change are also partaking in other healthy behaviors not being captured. Newer research performed even more cleverly than ever before—using a methodology called Mendelian randomization—questions the very association between HDL and risk of heart disease.[10,11]

To understand the grand rise and fall of HDL and how it fits into our larger understanding of the sickness and wellness of the heart, we must first interrogate the science that forms the basis of everything we know. One of the most important distinctions in science is the one at the core of some of the most hair-raising reversals in modern science—the difference between observational and interventional science and the distinction between causation and correlation.

—∿—

Growing up in Pakistan, one of the most exciting things I could get my hands on was *Reader's Digest*. I could never afford a new copy, so I frequented the bazaars where old, weathered magazines spotted with chai stains were frequently sold in bulk. I bought them for the jokes but lapped up entire issues. It seemed like every other week, a new story seemed to upend one that was published just recently. In one issue, alcohol was bad; in the other, it was good. In one, caffeine was bad, and then it was good in another. These days, such reversals don't take place on a monthly basis; they seem to occur every day.

We are living in times where there has been a dramatic erosion in how people view and trust societies' core institutions. Cell phone videos have provided grainy-vivid images of police brutality, often directed toward minorities. Social media opens windows into the deranged thoughts of some of the most influential people in the world. The public's trust in the government has hit record lows.[12] Similar trends are noted in how people view the media.[13]

Scientists, particularly medical scientists, on the other hand, enjoy some of the highest approval ratings among Americans. According to a recent Pew Research Center poll, 84 percent of surveyed Americans had a great or fair deal of confidence in medical scientists, beating out every other group in the poll.[14] Yet there are growing threats to that confidence. I see those threats everywhere around me, and, often, I find them in my email in-box or in a hastily put-together envelope I find in my mailbox.

And while there are many to blame for this slo-mo shipwreck, part of it goes back to the very heart of it—the scientific method. And nowhere is this more apparent than in the science of the heart.

How a scientific study is designed can define what type of findings can be generated from it and what they might mean. But research is complicated, and how most research is written makes it even harder to understand. Back when I first tried to read a medical paper, the complexity almost made me gag. It is almost redundant to say that the devil is in the details in research studies. For many studies, the devil doesn't even make it to the paper and might in fact find life in the supplementary materials that often go unread.

Probably the most important thing to know about any research study is whether it was a trial or an observational study. An observational study might, for example, survey a bunch of coffee drinkers at Starbucks and look at their grades in college. This study might conclude that people who drink more caffeine do better in college. But this observation could be incorrect since there are other differences that might be present between those drinking coffee at Starbucks and those not, such as perhaps greater resources.

To study whether coffee actually improves college performance, you would have to perform a double-blind, randomized, controlled trial, in which a randomly selected group of students starting college are selected. One half of the group would be randomly selected to drink caffeinated coffee, while the other group would be randomly selected to drink decaf. Neither the students nor researchers would know whether someone was in the caffeine versus decaf group. And then these groups would be followed over time and their scores in exams, or whatever other metric was deemed a suitable indicator of academic success, would be recorded.

The problem, though, is that conducting such trials is expensive and time consuming. Performing observational studies is much easier, and therefore, the vast number of studies that you read about in both the mainstream media and academic publications are in fact based on observation. Many love such research because they can generate catchy headlines like PEOPLE WHO HAVE SEX FOUR OR MORE TIMES A WEEK MAKE MORE MONEY.[15]

There is a much darker side to this type of coverage, though. At the turn of the century, small observational studies noted that patients taking statins also had higher rates of dementia. These studies led to headlines such as IT'S NOT DEMENTIA. IT'S YOUR HEART MEDICATIONS in *Scientific American,* the oldest continuously published monthly magazine in the United States.[16] This led to many people stopping their statins, something that has been linked to an actual increase in the risk of heart disease.[17] On the other hand, promising but observational data also noted that statins *reduce* the risk of dementia.[18] What can one conclude about the relationship between statins and dementia based on these completely divergent findings?

The problem with observational data is that it can rarely if ever prove that A *causes* B. It can tell us quite convincingly that A is more common when B occurs, or vice versa, but it can almost never prove that A *makes* B occur. A famous example is that people who have lighters in their pockets are more likely to get cancer. While that is almost certainly true, it isn't because lighters cause cancer. It is because people with lighters are much more likely to smoke, which *causes* cancer. Things like these have led to the origin of one of the often-used phrases in modern parlance, used to put the kibosh on many a rowdy online debate—*correlation does not imply causation.*

In the "lighters cause cancer" correlation, smoking is what's called a *confounder,* in that it is affecting the results even though we aren't measuring it. Another example might be found in the link between suicide and gender.[19] The number of men and women who die from suicide is fairly similar, which could lead one to conclude that suicidality is equally common among both genders. However, if you go a step further, it becomes apparent that women are much more likely to attempt suicide. The confounding factor here is how the two genders differ in how they attempt to take their lives. Men, unfortunately, end up using means that are much more effective, primarily guns, to kill themselves, while women are more likely to overdose on pills. So even though more women are attempting suicide, because of their different methods of going about it, men sadly end up being more successful.

Confounding factors are the Achilles' heel of observational research. It is likely that patients taking statins have more atherosclerosis to begin with, which is associated with higher rates of dementia, making it appear as if statins cause dementia when it is just an association. Furthermore, what if patients who take statins are more likely to be people who want to take care of their bodies, and exercise and eat well, and it is these lifestyle factors that might reduce the onset of dementia. There is just no way to tell in an observational study.

Egregiously confounded correlations, however, are all around us, and if you collect enough data, finding a relationship between any two unrelated phenomena is easier than ever before. There is, for example, an almost linear relationship between per capita cheese consumption and the number of people dying by getting tangled in their bedsheets, or the marriage rate in Kentucky and the number of people who drowned after falling out of a fishing boat.[20]

The human mind works in a way that is always making connections, especially with things that happen one after another and are therefore linked temporally. I remember when I was in medical school in my native Pakistan, many people swore that homeopaths were better at treating viral infections than doctors were. Turned out, though, that when people got sick, they would go to physicians first who would prescribe anti-inflammatory medications, but when patients got frustrated at not getting better, they would go to homeopaths. However, by this time, their infection had already begun to cycle through and would have gotten better anyway, but the mind connected getting better with the things the homeopath prescribed.

The father of correlation is a man whose name is associated with the statistical test still commonly performed to see if two things are more likely to occur together or not. Karl Pearson (1857–1936) was a British polymath who was a foundational figure in modern statistics and helped quantify the degree to which two separate statistical occurrences might be linked.[21] An example of a correlation he gave is that while smallpox rates might be higher in Africans than Europeans, leading one to the conclusion that smallpox is highly correlated with the color of one's skin, the likely confounding factor was the different rate of vaccinations in those two populations.

We need to see these relationships because they might be essential for our survival. After all, as the adage makes clear, smoke is highly correlated with fire even though smoke doesn't actually cause fire. The truth is that even though it is easy to disregard correlations and say they are meaningless, reality is far more complicated. The fact is that whenever A causes B, A will almost certainly always be highly correlated with B, too. We have talked about lighters and lung cancer, but something else that is highly correlated with lung cancer is smoking itself. And yet, it was the tobacco industry that cried *correlation, not causation* when the link between tobacco smoking and lung cancer first emerged. If anything, lack of correlation can almost certainly be proof for a lack of causation.

Another stumbling block to the interpretation of observational studies is what's called *reverse causality*. Consider the fact that in many studies, patients with lower weight have a higher risk of dying.[22] These paradoxical studies, several in patients with heart disease, confused many, given that overall, among otherwise healthy subjects, higher weight is bad. But here's the deal—many illnesses cause patients to lose weight. So now if you look at these patients, you may incorrectly assume that lower weight is worse, when in fact that might not be the case, since that lower weight may be indicative of some serious illness, such as cancer. Similarly, there is data that many cholesterol skeptics quote that low LDL cholesterol actually is bad in older persons.[23] Could that be true, or is that merely an effect of people with higher LDLs not making it to older age or the LDL level in older age not reflecting the cumulative effect of LDL over one's lifetime? This would be important to know since many use these data in patients older than seventy-five and extrapolate that to everyone, claiming that there is no link between elevated bad cholesterol and heart disease.

So how do we figure out answers to one of the most basic things in heart disease? Does bad cholesterol, or LDL, *cause* atherosclerosis, or is it merely correlated with it? And what about good cholesterol? Is it merely elevated in healthy people, or does it actually play a hand in the natural history of atherosclerosis? Answers to these important questions are finally coming to us because the real story may not be the sausage. It may truly be how it gets made.

—⋀—

In 1756, Great Britain and France began a war waged across several continents today called the Seven Years' War. The war ended in 1763, with Britain's emergence as the greatest power of that time and for many years to follow. This victory came at a great price. The British navy recruited almost 185,000 sailors during that time, and almost 133,000 of those went either missing or were killed by a mysterious disease. The disease started with weakness and soreness in the arms and legs and progressed to pain and dryness of the mouth, easy bleeding, and death. The ailment had been described since the days of the ancient Egyptians and Hippocrates, but no one really knew what caused it. Many posited that the common features of life on the ocean—physical hardship and the naval diet—caused the body's digestive system to fail. Some even took to drinking sulfuric acid in hopes that the caustic poison would wake up the intestines, though it only succeeded in injuring their guts.

Among the myriad of untested therapies, citrus fruits like lemon and orange were frequently used. The evidence for their effectiveness, though, was merely anecdotal. James Lind, a Scottish physician aboard the HMS *Salisbury*, a fifty-gun warship, was done with young sailors dying aboard his ship, yet he wasn't sure what to do. Scurvy killed far more of his men than the enemy could ever hope to. He knew of at least six treatments available but wasn't sure if any of them really worked, so he devised an experiment.[24] He selected twelve sailors with very similar symptoms—all of them "had putrid gums, the spots and lassitude, with weakness of the knees." He put them all in one place in the holds and gave them all a similar but terrible diet like water gruel sweetened with sugar for breakfast and fresh mutton broth for dinner. He then, supposedly at random, gave them the treatments he knew of. He gave two cider, two sulfuric acid, two vinegar, two seawater, two a mixture of nutmeg and garlic, and finally, gave two lemons and oranges. The results were remarkable—of the entire group, the patients who received lemons and oranges were fit for duty within a week and began nursing the others to health. This was, for most intents and purposes, the first "controlled" clinical trial performed in human history. He described these results in his book *A Treatise of the Scurvy*, published in 1753, but it took another fifty years for citrus to become the accepted treatment for scurvy.

Clinical trials don't necessarily answer *why* A causes B—two hundred years passed since Lind's trial before the Hungarian Nobel Prize winner Albert Szent-Györgyi discovered vitamin C (ascorbic acid), the deficiency of which causes scurvy.[25] Yet clinical trials remain the best bet we have at establishing that A *does totally cause* B. James Lind's experiment was important because he ensured that all the subjects in the trial were controlled, meaning both patients getting the intervention and those getting other therapies were similar. Bad things happen when experiments are not controlled. Suppose the patients getting citrus were sicker than those getting seawater, who had a milder deficiency. In that case, the patients receiving the citrus may have fared worse simply because they were sicker to begin with.

Clinical trials have evolved greatly since Lind's experiments. An important issue with clinical trials was that somehow, the hand of the treatment had to be hidden. Why? The expectation of harm or good from a treatment can cause real physiological changes in people receiving therapies. Hope is not just something that makes you feel better; it can actually make you better. The medicinal term used to describe this hope is *placebo*. Even well-regarded therapies such as acupuncture have now been shown to be almost entirely placebogenic.[26]

The placebo effect is still highly prevalent in medicine. Even when you take a medication such as ibuprofen, known, for example, to reduce pain, just that knowledge and expectation of betterment can enhance the effect of the active ingredient of the medication. In fact, when modern medicine was emerging, the prescription of placebos was taught widely, even in places like Harvard Medical School, and was seen to be a necessary but altruistic deception.

Following wider recognition of the placebo effect, it also became clearer that there was a need to separate the actual effect of the treatment from the expectation of benefit that comes with any intervention being re-searched. In the eighteenth century, a common means of improving aches and pains and other ailments was to strap metal rods to the affected part of the body, with the belief that the electromagnetic properties of the metal rods would make everything better. John Haygarth, a British doctor, set out in 1799 to really test whether these expensive rods were able to draw out disease, as they were purported to do. In addition to strapping the metal rods to five patients, he switched them out for wooden panels and found that there was no difference between the two "treatments." He wrote about these findings and perhaps gave away his conclusion in the title of his now prescient book, *Of the Imagination, as a Cause and as a Cure of Disorders of the Body,* published in 1800.[27]

The introduction of the placebo-controlled, randomized clinical trial was a monumental step in the history of medical science, which cannot be emphasized enough. Up to this point, medicine was a supernatural art at best. It was finally being transformed from eminence-based dogma into an evidence-based science. Some doctors and researchers still have a difficult time admitting that they might be wrong, their experience unfounded, their clinical observations biased, their anecdotes irrelevant, and their in-stincts off-kilter. While a few doctors are like that to this day, the placebo-controlled trial was the first major step in a journey that is still ongoing in the battle between anecdote and evidence, both within and outside academia.

Today, though, the clinical trial enterprise, particularly in heart disease, is hitting new roadblocks. Newer medications are becoming increasingly expensive to develop, with a controversial analysis showing that it takes more than $2 billion to develop a good drug and the pipeline of promising therapies for heart disease is dwindling.[28] To show a benefit, trials need to be increasingly large, to the point that the only organizations with the in-centive and resources to do these studies are pharmaceutical or medical device companies. To foresee the future of heart science and its highlights, from exciting therapies that use mechanisms from stem cells to the bacteria in your gut to fight atherosclerosis and heart disease, we first have to hit the lowlights of science. And no lowlight is lower, dimmer, and darker than the crimes committed under the guise of science in the small Bavarian town of Dachau.

It is hard to look back at what happened in the Dachau concentration camp as science. It is perhaps simpler to just look at it for what it was—a vile campaign of dehumanizing violence perpetrated by the Nazi regime.[29] The "experiments" that they performed could easily be considered cold-blooded torture and murder. In fact, they were so grim, no amount of words can express how heinous they were. Twins were sewn together in an attempt to see if they could be conjoined. Head injury was simulated by hitting children with mechanized hammers. Naked bodies were frozen to death to assess the effect of cold immersion on the human body.[30] Inmates were purposefully exposed to mustard gas, malaria, and poison. Most who underwent these experiments, many of whom were children, died; the survivors were frequently executed.

While the "medical experimentation" of the Nazis is perhaps the darkest episode of experiments conducted in the name of science, and most scientists distanced themselves from these cruel and inhuman acts as much as possible, they were far from isolated. In fact, the Nazi experiments were very natural extensions of the type of science frequently being performed in the United States and Europe at that time.[31] As much as we would like to separate Nazi experimentation from mainstream scientific work, a broader look reveals that it was an extreme version of much that was being done in the guise of research.[32]

Before the Second World War, scientific progress was on a tear, and things like consent and humane treatment of subjects were largely seen as hurdles to scientific progress. Prostitutes in Germany were unknowingly infected with syphilis while cancer cells were being injected into patients in New York City.[33] Many researchers argued that the ends justified the means, but Henry Beecher, an anesthesiologist at Harvard Medical School and one of medicine's most famous whistle-blowers, argued, "A study is ethical or not at its inception. It does not become ethical merely because it turned up valuable data." He went on to ask, "Whoever gave the investigator the godlike right of choosing martyrs?"[34]

With the advent of the controlled trial, another frequent ethical slip was the deprivation of treatment to patients in the control arm of trials. Before a trial is started, scientists today are asked to determine if there is scientific equipoise. What does that mean? Well, imagine there is a new treatment for dementia, and you want to perform a randomized trial for this new treatment. What type of treatment will patients in the control arm get? Is it ethical to withhold the treatment being studied from the patients getting the placebo? With dementia, given that there are almost no evidence-based treatments for it, it may be fair to provide no additional treatment to the patients in the control arm. Now consider an experiment that was performed to test the effectiveness of penicillin in military servicemen with strep throat. It was already known at that point that penicillin was an effective treatment for strep throat, yet a group of servicemen received the placebo in the trial and went on to develop complications such as rheumatic fever and kidney disease from untreated strep throat.[35]

The truth is that before the Great War, academics and physicians the world over were in awe of the Nazi regime's scientists, particularly as they set out to involuntarily sterilize anyone they deemed unfit for reproduction. American scientists and journals were falling over themselves to praise this movement, with one editorial in *The New England Journal of Medicine* in 1934 proclaiming, "Germany is perhaps the most progressive nation in restricting fecundity among the unfit. . . . The individual must give way before the greater good."[36] Involuntary sterilization, which was heavily directed toward immigrants and minorities, was legalized in almost half the American states, and even after the end of the Second World War, twenty thousand individuals underwent this procedure without their consent by 1963.

The scientific community has been hesitant to police itself, and nowhere is this more evident than in perhaps the longest unethical research study of all time.[37] In 1932, the United States Public Health Service wanted to study the natural history of untreated syphilis. It enrolled several hundred black sharecroppers in rural Alabama under the pretense of giving them free medical treatment. These men were followed for almost forty years even though syphilis could have been easily treated. These men were never told they had the disease and ended up passing it to their spouses. Some even had children born with congenital syphilis, and others ended up dying of complications of syphilis.

What finally led to the termination of the study had nothing to do with the medical establishment. In fact, even after some physicians complained that this study was unethical, the Centers for Disease Control and Prevention and the American Medical Association insisted that the study was necessary for scientific advancement. It wasn't until one of the key whistle-blowers leaked details of the experiment to the press that decisive action was taken. The study broke in *The Washington Examiner* on July 25, 1972, and the next day was on the front page of *The New York Times*.[38]

The fact is that in medical circles, the study was far from secret, and reports from it had been published almost fifteen times in medical literature. In fact, in 1965, a young doctor just out of medical school, Irwin Schatz, after reading one of these results in a medical journal, wrote a letter to the researchers in charge of the study, expressing his outrage. "I am utterly astounded by the fact that physicians allow patients with a potentially fatal disease to remain untreated when effective therapy is available," he wrote to them.[39] But the letter fell on deaf ears, and the authors of the study never responded to him. It wasn't until the press got ahold of this experiment that it blew up, leading to the study's termination and widespread reforms in the regulations governing medical research and informed consent.

The medical scientific community, since they enjoyed godlike status in ancient Egypt, can be reluctant to introspect. Even today, when it comes to some of the greatest challenges facing medical care, such as soaring prices, overuse of medical procedures at the end of life, transparency in clinical care and research, conflict of interest, and free dissemination of research and education, the academic establishment continues to be reactive and regressive rather than proactive and progressive.

The distrust that studies like Tuskegee engendered continues to this day and in many ways might even be becoming more widespread. Many, particularly minorities, continue to be very distrustful of physicians prescribing statins.[40] When it comes to heart disease, many in the public imagine a worldwide global conspiracy. They imagine a deep-state version of the medical-industrial complex, which meets regularly in a circular meeting room at the top of a skyscraper, where they plot the demise of mankind, the deaths of all their enemies, and a road to intergalactic domination paved in gold bullion.

The truth is less dramatic.

Yes, there is fraud in medicine. Yes, there are studies that are unethical. But what dominates the vast majority of modern science and represents the real existential threat to its persistence is not insincerity—it is incompetence.

Since its earliest descriptions in ancient Egypt, heart failure has been associated with a weakening in the function of the heart. The strength of the heart's pumping function is usually described by the ejection fraction, the amount of blood the muscular left-sided ventricle of the heart pushes out. When the ejection fraction is 55 percent or more, it is considered normal. While many patients with heart failure have a reduction in their ejection fraction, almost half of patients with heart failure actually have normal ejection fraction. In these people, the heart muscle is very stiff, leading to very high pressures in the heart, resulting in the classic symptoms of heart failure even though the contractile function is normal. Both types of heart failure are equally efficient killers of men and women—patients older than sixty-five years of age admitted to the hospital with either of these live for only an average of two more years in the United States. There is one big difference: there is not a single proven treatment for patients with heart failure with preserved ejection fraction, unlike heart failure with reduced ejection fraction, which has a wide array of both medications and devices proven to reduce mortality. The search for a treatment, any treatment, hasn't been for lack of trying, though, and this one time, we came pretty darn close.

The National Institutes of Health decided that it needed to jump to the rescue of patients worldwide by funding a very large multinational trial, TOPCAT, which sought to test a promising and inexpensive medication, spironolactone, in patients with heart failure with preserved ejection fraction. The randomized, double-blind trial included 3,445 patients, half of whom were in North America and the other half were in Russia and Georgia. The results, published in 2014 in *The New England Journal of Medicine*, were very disappointing.[41] Spironolactone, sadly, did not improve outcomes in heart failure patients with preserved ejection fraction.

While scientists were rummaging through the disappointing results, they stumbled across a very curious funding: the patients enrolled in Russia and Georgia were very different from those enrolled in North America. How? Well, the Eastern European patients appeared to have very little of the sequelae of disease like heart attacks that heart failure patients usually have. In fact, some even wondered whether these patients even had heart failure to begin with. A subsequent analysis testing the urine of patients from both North America and Eastern Europe found that many patients in Russia or Georgia had no trace of the medicine in their urine, meaning that they were either not taking the medication or were never prescribed the medication in the first place.[42] Why did this matter? Well, if you just looked at the patients in North America, the drug that was tested, spironolactone, did in fact reduce the risk of death from heart disease, cardiac arrest, and hospitalization due to heart failure by about 18 percent compared to patients receiving the placebo.

The TOPCAT tragedy, which has likely deprived the proper appraisal of perhaps the only worthwhile medication available for heart failure with preserved ejection fraction, is the harbinger of things to come. Clinical trials in the United States are becoming superexpensive. In response to this, many clinical trials are now either exclusively performed outside the United States or mostly include patients outside the United States. This, however, comes at a cost. It is easier to do research in many other places, such as in South America or Eastern Europe, because it is cheaper to do research there, though the quality of the research apparatuses is not as robust as that in the United States and other higher-income countries. This has important implications, particularly for patients with heart disease. Furthermore, many trials are performed by for-profit clinical research organizations who may be more invested in profits than science.

While TOPCAT failed to produce what is called a positive result, there is another force that is throwing science askew—too many positive results.[43]

One of the biggest goals of any research study is to find out if a result that it generated represents "truth" or random chance. So let's say I design a study to find out the relationship between drinking coffee in the morning and being run over by a dump truck, assuming that there would be no difference between the risk of being run over in the morning or in the evening. I then look at two hundred people who bought coffee from a café at 7:00 in the morning. Suppose I find that ten of these two hundred people were run over. Now for comparison, I look at two hundred people having coffee at 7:00 in the evening and find that only two of those were run over. This means that 5 percent of coffee drinkers in the morning, compared to 1 percent in the evening, were run over by a dump truck. Running a simple test shows that there is only about a 4 percent chance that this difference is by chance if in truth there is no difference between that risk at morning or night in the data analyzed. Under modern scientific convention, if something occured <5 percent of times by chance, resulting in a *P value* of less than 0.05, it would be considered a "statistically significant" finding.

The P value tells us nothing about the actual relationship between two events. It doesn't tell us why those morning coffee drinkers are getting run over or how. It doesn't tell us if the coffee had anything to do with the risk of being run over, nor does it tell us if it is the early-morning hours that might lead to more people being run over. Maybe it's just the area outside the café or simply a vengeful dump truck driver? The P value doesn't even tell us how much more likely coffee drinkers are to be run over in the morning than at night. All it tells us is about the chances in the data analyzed that this finding is totally random when in fact there is no difference in truth. Another issue is this: What if there are three people instead of two who are run over at 7:00 in the evening, with the new risk being 1.5 percent? Now suddenly, the P value is 0.087, higher than the magical threshold of 0.05, and therefore the finding is not considered statistically significant. One way to increase the likelihood of significant results is by increasing the number of data points or subjects in the study. Say I now look at four hundred people in the morning and four hundred in the evening, yet the risk of being run over remains the same (10 percent versus 1.5 percent), now suddenly the P value for this comparison is 0.008.

Why is this a big deal? Remember the landmark CPPT trial back in the 1970s, which first showed that lowering cholesterol could reduce the risk of heart disease?[44] Well, the P value for that squeaked just under 0.05. Also, they performed another statistical leap by performing a single-tailed t-test rather than the conventional double-tailed test, effectively lowering the hoop to get the P value under 0.05. In fact, the P value was so close to 0.05 that they never even wrote the actual value in the paper, merely referred to it as less than 0.05.

If the P value for CPPT were 0.05 or more, it would have set the world of heart disease back by almost a decade. We now know that the relationship between lowering LDL cholesterol and the risk of heart disease is very robust, based on dozens of trials and data that we have generated since then, but it took some wily statistical engineering to get the P value to a point where it would magically be considered significant.

The P value, however, has become such a focal point of medical research that we have witnessed a pandemic of statistical significance in the last few decades. And it is this trend that has led to more heart science being reversed than any amount of fraud or malice that we know of.

The P value is one of the reasons many scientists concluded, and many millions more believed, that statins cause dementia. The P value is one of the reasons many also concluded that statins can reduce the risk of cancer. Subsequent studies have shown that statins do neither of those things, but the only reason researchers were emboldened to come to those conclusions was because in their observational research, the P value for those relationships was less than 0.05. Yet the quality of the results is only as good as the quality of the study used to derive those findings. And scientists and universities and journals and journalists that make hoopla about shoddy findings are all to blame for the mixed messages everyday people seem to be getting from science, particularly that of heart disease.[45]

Journal editors and reviewers love P values. Journal editors love P values because they know their readers love P values. And authors, myself included, know they have to comply. And if you have research, if you don't emblazon your paper with P values, editors and reviewers will frequently ask for them to be prominently displayed. And if you have research that did not show a lot of significant differences, chances are that research will never see the light of day because you would be hard-pressed to find a journal to accept the research. Whenever I write a paper and analyze the results, I am secretly praying for significant P values, knowing that they might be the difference between a paper being published or being shuttled to the recycle bin. In effect, the P value has become the arbiter of truth in research. That, however, couldn't be further from the facts.

The P value has led us down many dead ends, primarily because it can be used at times as a shortcut to entrust meaningfulness to findings. The fact is that I would rather trust a finding with a P value of 0.06 in a randomized controlled clinical trial than a P value of <0.0001 in an observational study. If what you seek is truth, and if what you abhor is random chance, the P value is only one small piece of the puzzle, yet that is not how most view this conundrum, and changes in medicine and computing are about to make P value fever a whole lot worse.

Never have we had greater data available about every aspect of what we do than we do today. In fact, the proliferation of numbers has led to the emergence of what has been called Data Rich, Information Poor (DRIP) Syndrome. Personally, I have helped lead analyses that included at times hundreds of thousands of patients. Almost each and every relationship between two different groups of patients within these databases can be statistically significant but totally worthless in real life. Why? With large data sets these days, the P value for even the smallest differences can be very low, even if the actual difference between the two results is miniscule and meaningless.

This has come to such a head that just recently, some of the leading statisticians in the world recommended lowering the bar for significance from 0.05 to 0.005, effectively making it much harder for findings noted by chance to be considered "significant."[46] But by putting even more of a focus on the P value, this doesn't solve the fundamental problem that a P value doesn't tell you anything meaningful about why two different things might be related if at all.

Like almost everything else, medical science is a rat race. And in heart science, the rats are even more jacked up. Cardiology is the most competitive field among internal medicine specialties, and therefore we have a lot of extremely talented people vying for a limited pot of grant funding. The way to get grants is to publish research, and the research that is much more likely to get published is one that is layered with significant P values the way a professional wrestler is with body oil. And if you are a smart rat with any hope of finding a way out of this maze (into the next maze), you will do what it takes to highlight the statistical significance of your research. And because most researchers, especially early in their careers, are rewarded for quantity over quality, you can see why the medical literature would be inundated with so many erroneous findings.

P values and the culture of mass-produced research have led to the very foundation of science being shaken. Many of the highest-profile studies performed, especially those such as basic lab experiments and psychological research, cannot be replicated when other researchers have tried to do so.[47] Even when some studies are successfully replicated, the effect is less strong than initially reported.[48] Within heart disease, this is true of the use of medications to reduce kidney complications from cardiac catheterization, and studies that showed superiority of tiny balloons to relieve tight spots in coronary arteries when compared to medications in patients with stable angina.

Perhaps there was no other time in the past when humanity was more inundated in sham science than in the era of #fakenews. If you read the news, you would think that the most dangerous things you could do to your heart are watching sports, sleeping too much (or too little), and perhaps most distressingly, having very low levels of LDL cholesterol.[49,50,51] It is not just research; as soon as people have any kind of symptom, before they ask almost anyone else, they google it.

We live in an era where the only form of gratification that is acceptable is the instantaneous kind. When my daughter was two, she couldn't talk but knew to immediately punch the Skip Ad notification as soon as it became active before her YouTube video played. We used to read books, then moved down to long-form articles back when no one called them *long form*, then smaller articles, and now we can barely make it through a 280-character tweet without scrolling forth.

This, of course, grates against the very nature of science, which is very iterative. Almost every single research paper ever written ends with, "More research is needed." Science is like a tunnel, and just when you see the light at the end of it approaching, it turns out it just leads you into another tunnel, burrowing deeper and deeper. When we think we are out of the tunnel, it is more likely to be an optical illusion. It's like sitting in a train and thinking you are moving, when it is just the trains around you going back and forth while you are still inactive at the station. Science is like a journey with no beginning or end, just one long, never-ending middle.

The incremental process at the heart of science, which produces new knowledge, is fundamentally opposed to the chief platform on which new knowledge is communicated and subsequently consumed—the internet. The internet is a beast that constantly needs to be fed, and in turn it serves up our appetite with pellets of code dressed as posts, tweets, status updates, and essays, both short and long.

Loath as they may be to admit it, most doctors and researchers also get most of their information not from scientific conferences or medical journals but from the internet, just like everyone else. And why wouldn't anyone turn to the internet, when seeing a doctor can be so expensive. In fact, there is evidence to suggest that it is not just that the *Times* covers influential and highly cited articles but that articles become influential and highly cited because they are covered by the *Times*.[52]

Here's the catch, though. Research suggests that newspapers and websites are more likely to cover lower-quality observational studies than well-designed randomized controlled trials.[53] In fact, studies that receive greater coverage are less likely to be replicated and confirmed.[54] And oftentimes, those reversals are less well documented than the initial erroneous findings.[55] Now why might that be?

Observational studies are more likely to bring to light new relationships that might make for interesting headlines, like the finding that statins reduce the risk of cancer (they don't). And when observational studies are covered, their limitations are rarely brought up.[56] Subsequently published meta-analyses—papers that pool the cumulative research that has occurred in an area—that might go on to refute those early, exciting results are just not as sexy. In fact, research suggests that at least half of research studies that you may read about in a newspaper are not confirmed subsequently.[57]

Press releases from universities and labs often exaggerate findings, and some researchers are happy to follow suit, and journalists fall prey to this tantalizing bait.[58] Some journalists might lack the technical expertise in the field they might be covering, so they then have to rely on established experts in the field. Being an expert, however, doesn't mean that a person will offer a fair opinion, given the epidemic of conflicts of interest in medicine. Medical drug and device companies pay millions of dollars to experts who they often use to sway opinions their way. "It upsets me when they [journalists] quote conflicted people," said Rita Redberg, editor of *The Journal of the American Medical Association: Internal Medicine,* and advocate against financial conflict of interest in medicine, when I sat down with her for an interview recently. "Sometimes they [journalists] get the wool pulled over their eyes."

Researchers writing erstwhile boring papers have been shown to be using increasingly hype-worthy language that might be taken out of the notorious boxing promoter Don King's playbook. As one reporter for *Vox* wrote, "As reporters, we're biased toward what's new and exciting. But in science, truth takes time."[59] No wonder that a study showing individuals unable to bear the burden of stressful episodes are at higher risk of depression was widely covered; the many studies refuting that initial link bit the dust, dying in ignominy.[60]

We live in times where reality imitates reality TV. With politics having succumbed a long time ago to the vicarious appetites of a national audience fed on juicy morsels on television screens and infant/cat/dog-does-weird-thing YouTube videos, science might be next. Both scientists and journalists are asked to produce incessantly, and while many times they get it right, at times they can leave behind a mess that no one has the time to clean up, because both the scientists creating the science and the journalists covering it are pressed to move on to the next potentially viral project.

Where does that leave the poor person who just wants to live a long and healthy life, who wants to do the right thing for themselves and their family, who doesn't want to drop dead of a heart attack like Uncle So-and-So? Where can they turn for the truth, and where is the science behind the science of heart disease headed? And while science isn't broken by any stretch, there are cracks in its very foundation that are creeping up. And unless we plug them, the dam holding back the Sea of Untruths and False Hopes might shatter into a million pieces.

Progress in biomedical science has fundamentally changed what it means to be human, and nowhere is that more evident than in our endeavors to overcome the ailments of the heart. A living repository of these advances is Eugene Braunwald, a cardiologist and professor at Brigham and Women's Hospital and at Harvard Medical School, who was born in 1929 but is more active in research today than any prior time in his life. "The advances in cardiology and cardiac surgery have exceeded everyone's expectations," he told me. "They are basically a miracle." Just since the middle of the twenti-eth century, we have seen an almost threefold reduction in the death rate from heart disease. And even though there is more we can do since heart disease continues to kill more than any other disease on the planet, it is im-portant, too, to realize what we have achieved. And after being at the cutting edge of heart science for decades, Braunwald is more excited to be a researcher than ever before.

"I hear discussions around treating heart attacks and it brings me back fifty or sixty years and I recall how little we could do for these patients, and how much more effective our management is today," he said, "I see the great sweep of history . . . I am a very lucky person, because very few people have that."

With that said, something is awry at the heart of this ship. One of the fundamental things science has to get right is to make experiments more replicable. The reason much research from labs isn't replicated isn't be-cause there was a malevolent hand at play. One way to understand this problem might be to probe the travails of Walter White, the chemistry-teacher-turned-drug-baron antihero of the television series *Breaking Bad*, who was responsible for the most lucrative experiment in the fictionalized world of methamphetamine production. While there were others who knew his recipe, few if any could replicate the blue hue his product was famous for. Why?

Well, for one, no one really knew exactly what Walter White was doing. And while research papers have detailed methods sections, too many times there are steps that go missing or that might be so simple that they may never make it into the document. Second, Walter White didn't want people to find out how he made his special recipe and therefore purposefully didn't provide access to that knowledge to others. Such fears exist in research, too, where people are very protective of access to data, particularly from clinical trials, because researchers either worry someone else will analyze the same data and draw conclusions contradictory to what was previously found or that they will not have the statistical training to properly analyze the data and thus reach incorrect conclusions. In fact, the editor of *The New England Journal of Medicine* (in)famously called people who use previously gathered information "data parasites." While the editor subsequently retracted this statement and changed his position to strongly supporting data transparency, the comment stirred so much controversy that a scientific group actually launched an annual research award called the Research Parasite Awards for scientists who have repurposed data originally collected from other investigators to generate novel findings.

Biomedical research is also fundamentally different from chemistry and other elemental sciences. The most important reason why replication is an issue in medical research is because of the innate variation of biological materials. "No two populations of cells, no matter how well you characterize them in a plate using a set of markers, will be absolutely identical," said Joseph Loscalzo, a professor of cardiology at Brigham and Women's Hospital and Harvard Medical School, when I talked to him. "You have to distinguish between *replication* and *duplication*." While duplication implies that the results of an experiment are reproduced identically, replication of an experiment should mean that the broad findings and trends are shown again without perhaps being the same as the initial data. Medical experiments are bound to show a similar variation, given that they deal with the most labile of biological organisms—humans.

Take, for example, the wide variation in side effects that people experience from even common medications such as statins or beta-blockers; every time one takes a medication, it is akin to a scientific experiment, with the medicine being the reagent and the patient being the substrate. But when scientists make tall claims and do not delineate the inherent limitations of their work, this ends up harming science. "When we overstate the case and misrepresent the facts, we are less and less credible to the public and policy makers," Loscalzo added.

So as we move forward and try to figure out how to make sense of science, how to make sure scientists don't look like chumps when a ballyhooed research finding doesn't pan out, all of us, including docs, researchers, journalists, and everyday people, need to remember one thing—there is no silver bullet in medical science anymore. There is no one paper that can dictate our understanding of any aspect of what we do. If we look at any one study to draw our conclusions, no matter how small the P values might be or how biologically plausible the idea sounds, we can easily be led astray if we don't widen our lens. "The number of landmark papers are few and far between," said Howard Bauchner, editor in chief of *The Journal of the American Medical Association*, when I spoke to him. "It is the cumulative weight of evidence that changes practice."

When it comes to heart health, we face a different challenge altogether. While for many other diseases, such as Alzheimer's dementia, autism, or some forms of metastatic cancer, the search for a breakthrough is vigorously under way; in heart disease, many of the breakthroughs already exist. "The management of hypertension didn't exist when I was an intern," said Eugene Braunwald, but over his professional life, he has seen things change dramatically. "Now we have a family of drugs that are quite effective and well tolerated by hypertensives, and . . . they cost pennies a day."

Many of the greatest risk factors for heart disease are silent killers, though. Conditions such as high blood pressure, diabetes, and high cholesterol produce no symptoms at all and can exist for years if not decades before unleashing what can be a fatal strike such as a heart attack. However, even as treatments for heart attacks have gotten better, they aren't perfect. "In the past, patients may have died of acute myocardial infarction [heart attack] or stroke," said Braunwald. "Now they live through this, but that doesn't mean their hearts are normal." In fact, treatments for heart attacks lead many to be able to survive, but with heart failure. Therefore, prevention is the best possible treatment for heart disease.

Yet here lies the tallest hurdle of all—getting patients to trust their doctors. When patients come to me and they feel good but have some lab values that don't look so hot and maybe blood pressure that is not where it should be, they have to both be convinced that these things that cause no symptoms are truly bad, and in some instances, even after lifestyle changes haven't worked, that they will have to take a pill every day, which might cause side effects, at times with no end in sight. In short, they have to trust I have their best interest in mind. Increasingly, that trust is shaky. Science was supposed to quash the faith healer, the homeopath, the snake oil salesman, who has in their possession the elixir of eternal life and answers to the questions allopathic investigators are wary of broaching. In a recent study, Americans ranked twenty-fourth out of a survey of twenty-nine industrialized countries in how trusting they were of their doctors in a survey.[61] Who is to blame, and what really is at the heart of this wedge that has opened up between doctors and their patients, especially in America?

In the book *Hippocrates' Shadow: Secrets from the House of Medicine*, David Newman, an emergency room doctor in New York City, explained why patients don't trust their doctors anymore, making a case for a return to a time when doctors were fully present for their patients rather than busy ordering tests or writing prescriptions.[62] In an interview, he explained, "The shadow idea also refers to the many secrets, conscious and unconscious, that we use as coping mechanisms and, oftentimes, as cover."[63] A blurb by a well-known physician announced that the book could "help us get back to the essence of what good doctors do: be with patients in healing."

So one day, a few years after he wrote the book, Newman found himself at the side of a twentysomething-year-old woman who had come into the ER after a routine shoulder injury.[64] The nurse gave her morphine for pain, but Newman gave her even more sedating medications using the general anesthetic propofol. She lost consciousness, but when she woke up, she felt a burning sensation on her face and found Newman groping her breast. He was masturbating and proceeded to ejaculate on her face. It was later revealed that Newman had previously been cited for sexual assault by patients, who had claimed that Newman had groped their breasts while performing unrelated evaluations for headaches and colds, yet no discernable action had been taken then.[65] One of the victims said that she had previously told her daughter that she should only trust her and the doctor with her body. "What do I tell her now?" she asked after Newman entered a guilty plea, getting only two years in prison for his serial violations.[66]

The irony of a doctor proselytizing about enhancing patients' trust turning out to be a sexual predator is a bit too on the nose, and even though Newman does not by any measure represent the medical profession—there is one very important reason why this story matters. Doctors like myself are human and carry all the same faults, foibles, and flaws as all of us do. Even as most are kind, generous, humble, and empathetic, some can be distracted, selfish, and lazy, too.

Most doctors, though, the vast majority, are good people who came into this profession that requires more than a decade of training because they wanted to do good work. Those who stay in academics in teaching or research positions sign up for an income two or three times lower than what they might get paid if they went into private practice. And over time, even though they can still be quite self-confident and arrogant, they have been brought down from the heavens so that they can be among the common folk.

The singular focus that many clinicians have on the magical effects of modern allopathic medicine, however, can obscure a major aspect of what they do—the human aspect. A huge contributor to the therapeutic effect of almost everything we prescribe has nothing to do with what's in the pill or what we are doing with stents in someone's heart. It has everything to do with how physicians listen to patients, how they examine them, how they connect with them as human beings, and how they respond to their symptoms, allay their fears, reassure them that they are in the best of hands and that all their concerns will be addressed.

In building therapeutic relationships and honing their non-pharmacologic healing, doctors are falling behind others who are disparaged as quacks—homeopaths, acupuncturists, faith healers—who have little evidence-based drugs to dole out but many of whom are great at what many in my profession disparagingly refer to as the "touchy-feely stuff." The fact is that it is the "touchy-feely" things that doctors and patients share that represent the most enduring legacy of medicine, connecting medical students training today to the most ancient practitioners.

The reason we don't have more research on some of the most basic aspects of the patient-doctor relationship—what is the best way to reassure patients with stable chest pain that may not be life-threatening, what is the association between how much eye contact doctors make and how likely patients are to trust them, whether white coats enhance or distract from the therapeutic relationship—is because there is no large corporation whose shareholders' well-being depends on this work.

Winning the trust of our patients is probably most important when it comes to taking care of their hearts. Even if scientists don't produce a single further innovation in heart disease, we have all the tools to cut heart disease down to size severalfold, which is why heart disease needs less of a breakthrough therapy than cancer and is taking on all the contours of an information war. To win the battle for people's hearts, doctors need to win over their minds.

Well, this is where this humble snake oil salesman will offer you his hand so we can both figure out what is truly at the heart of the matter and what we can do to make it right.

The growing distrust of science has been weaponized, and I don't have to turn on the television to see a slow but steady reversal in the public's sureness in science. Long before they came with pitchforks against statins, they came for something far, far more effective—vaccines. I saw the irrational fear of vaccines firsthand when I treated a girl with measles in Atlanta, who went on to inadvertently infect a plane full of people, because her parents had not given her the measles vaccine. I see it in many patients who will not even try a statin because they have heard so many awful things about it. I see it in patients who won't quit smoking because they know of so many people who smoked but never had a heart attack.

In fact, the irony of medical distrust is that it is directly proportional to how effective at prevention the suspected agent is. How so? Before vaccines, you didn't have to open a history textbook to witness a case of polio—polio affected everyone, from halls full of kids unable to breathe from paralysis to people like Franklin D. Roosevelt, who had late onset of polio at the age of thirty-nine and was left paralyzed from the waist down. And then the polio vaccine happened, and outside of a couple of war-ravaged regions of Pakistan and Afghanistan, polio joined the likes of smallpox, measles, pertussis, and rubella as diseases that were totally pulverized with vaccination. However, as the living reminders of why we need vaccination vanish, opposition to vaccines grows because people don't even see the diseases they have almost wiped away and have therefore forgotten the reasons we need to keep taking them.[67] In behavioral economics, this is referred to as *availability heuristic,* meaning that we are more likely to think of something happening simply based on how easily it comes to mind. And because we see kids getting vaccines much more commonly than kids getting polio, we are much more likely to think about the adverse events associated with vaccines than the diseases they prevent. Doctors are not immune from availability heuristics; doctors who have graduated more recently have less favorable views of vaccines than those graduating earlier even as vaccines have become both safer and more effective.[68]

While statins are not as effective at preventing heart disease as vaccines are at preventing infections, certainly, along with diet and exercise, they are one of the best things we have to prevent heart disease right now. Their widespread use, coupled with a reduction in fatal heart attacks in younger people, though, has led to an epidemic of statin skepticism—especially because while the statin is fully present, the heart attack or stroke that it may prevent remains invisible.

In the age of the internet, skeptics of modern medicine have many distinct advantages. They don't need to do research, they don't need to be nuanced, they can say whatever they want and overpromise to their heart's content. Many of the people who gravitate toward such alternatives are those who are already in the best of health, who are engaged, and who just want to do what's right for themselves. In fact, a recent study of cancer patients using alternative medicine found that while they were healthier at the outset than patients not using alternative medications, they were also likely to die sooner.[69]

And in our current world, facts and information—far from convincing people otherwise—can have what has been called the *boomerang effect*.[70] Researchers have found that when presented with facts that counter their views, people hunker down even more into their preconceived positions. When parents who distrust vaccines are presented with information showing the lack of an association with autism, they become even more resistant to vaccination.[71] And while there is some disagreement about how entrenched the boomerang effect truly is, it does raise important questions about how best to convince people to accept facts.

When confronted with disagreements or distrust of their intentions, doctors frequently turn to what they think is their greatest resource—knowledge—for it is what they have worked for so many years to attain. Yet perhaps that might be less effective than they think. As is becoming increasingly clear, humans are far from rational beings—they are far more likely to make decisions from the metaphorical heart than the metaphorical brain. So for example, when it comes to encouraging people to improve their lifestyles or take preventive medications, we frequently talk about facts while ignoring the reality that rarely do people make decisions in unemotional, aseptic vortices. In fact, vaccine researchers have found that the principles of purity and liberty are often the main drivers of parents choosing to prevent their children from getting immunized and that addressing their concerns is likely to be much more effective than traditional means of communication, which focus on education and stimulating a sense of altruism.[72]

When modern medicine focuses too much on things like tests, procedures, and medications, the disease that is being treated or prevented can get buried in the details. Providing patients information and evidence is extremely important, but such communications cannot be divorced from the human consequences wrought by heart disease.

Current incentives encourage researchers that the next step after performing a research study and publishing it in a leading journal is to obtain a grant for another study and then publish that in another journal rather than ensuring that the initial research actually gets disseminated and implemented. For physicians, often we see our job as making recommendations and writing prescriptions rather than enforcing them. The limitations of our current approach are being increasingly felt as too much research goes unused and unread and too many prescriptions go unfilled. We are very good at making the sausage and not so good at making sure those who need it actually can eat it. How the sausage gets made is obviously messy, it is obviously imperfect, but it is also what has gotten us to where we have seen unprecedented reductions in heart disease.

What is missing in the science of the heart is the story of those whose lives are irreparably affected by atherosclerosis. Storytelling, the most human of arts, is the bridge that can connect scientists and physicians to those whom they seek to help and heal. We need to be able to tell the stories that we have learned from our patients to those who we hope will never experience such an event in their own lives. We need to let patients see as much of our worlds as physicians and researchers as we ask them to lay bare theirs.

6

THE PASSION OF THE HEART

Life will not break your heart. It'll crush it.

—Henry Rollins

He was watching television when it started. It wasn't pain, he told me, it was pressure.

It felt like he couldn't catch a full breath, that there was something sitting on his chest. *An elephant? Maybe a smaller animal . . . a dog? Maybe a large dog. That sounds about right. But what is a large dog doing sitting on my chest?*

He stayed around and watched television for a while. *These things usually go away.* This one didn't. He wasn't sick, never had been. His blood pressure had been elevated when he'd seen a doctor a few years earlier, and he was started on a small dose of a blood pressure medication. His cholesterol level was just above normal.

He had never been to the emergency room before, never been admitted to the hospital. The pressure in his chest grew intense, now traveling to his back. He had been an engineer but didn't really do much now that he was retired.

Eventually, almost two hours in, he broke. He drove himself to the emergency room, and he told the nurse at the front desk that he felt like a large dog was sitting on his chest.

There are only two types of people who come to the emergency room—those who have chest pain and those who don't. More than eight million people arrive at the emergency room every year with a chief complaint of chest pain. After abdominal pain, it is the most common reason people leave everything they are doing and make the dreadful, unwanted trip to the emergency room. For the vast majority of patients, it is nothing to worry about. For a few, the cause of their chest pain could kill them within moments.

By the time I saw him, he wasn't looking so hot. The way he described his pain—*pressure*—he corrected everyone, was almost like he had stepped out of a medical textbook. His heart rate and blood pressure, though, were stone-cold normal. I dutifully unfurled my stethoscope and placed it on his chest. I marched it down his breastbone to his left, then just below his nipple, then pushed up into his breast. *Lubdub, lubdub.* I was left nonplussed. I heard nothing resembling the sound the wind makes when it is whistling through bare-naked conifers, suggesting that there was no turbulent flow across his heart valves.

I then asked for the single most important piece of information that would help me proceed. I asked for his electrocardiogram. In this veritable ocean of information on a single piece of paper, there was not an astray ripple, an aberrant undulation. A blood test looking for particles called troponins, which can be elevated when there is ongoing damage to the heart, showed no abnormality. Troponins are proteins found in heart muscle that can leak into the bloodstream if the heart muscle begins to die after its oxygen supply is interrupted. While there are other blood tests that can also show damage to the heart, troponins are the most accurate test available.

I asked that he be given nitroglycerin, a medication that relaxes the coronary arteries, increasing blood flow to the heart. Pain from restricted blood flow in the heart usually responds to nitro, but it didn't touch his pain.

As his life flashed before his eyes, my decade of medical training blazed before mine. There were a few things that I needed to immediately make sure he didn't have that were not a heart attack but could have been somehow evading diagnosis: a ruptured aorta, a punctured lung, and a blood clot in his lung. To any of these, he was what a pin is to a boisterous, bludgeoning bowling ball—they could topple him over in an instant. I was most afraid he might have an aortic dissection, a tear in the aorta that could unzip the largest blood vessel in his body. The only treatment for such a dissection is urgent surgery.

Along with the emergency room team, I decided to get an urgent CAT scan, which thankfully didn't show a torn aorta. The man was getting no better, though. He had broken out in a sweat and was now throwing up into a plastic bin. It was just about then that we got a call from the radiologist. He told us that he had seen something neither he nor any of his colleagues had ever seen on a CAT scan. We would learn later that this was the first time anyone had ever seen this on a CAT scan. With eight million annual visits to the emergency room for chest pain in the United States alone, annually, you would think we would have figured it out. We hadn't. The CAT scan showed that a part of the heart was not receiving any blood, confirming what was our initial suspicion all along: the patient was having a heart attack.[1]

The heart attack is the most classic of all heart diseases. In fact, when people talk about heart disease, almost always they are talking about heart attacks. But heart attacks, called *acute myocardial infarctions* or simply *myocardial infarctions* in doctor-speak, are changing, too. What constitutes a heart attack is different from what was a heart attack perhaps ten or twenty years ago. How we diagnose heart attacks and then go on to treat them is also in flux.

We all deal with headaches and joint pains all the time, but the one pain that is perhaps the most serious of all is that which occurs in the chest. What is the nature of this pain, what can lead to it, what are the red flags that need to be looked out for, and what can be done to figure out if it is something serious that warrants perhaps calling 911? This is important because even as more and more people are coming to the hospital, often urgently, with chest pain, there is a parallel reality—fewer and fewer people with chest pain are actually having a heart attack. This is occurring even as the very definition of what constitutes a heart attack is being greatly expanded.

Is pain a sensation or an emotion?

To the ancient Greeks, it was something else. To the ancient Greeks, pain was a passion. What we call chest pain was called *passio cardiac proper*, with the words *passio* (passion) and *poena* (pain) sharing the same Indo-European root.[2] This made sense—the heart was of course the source of all emotions.

In many religious cultures, pain has always been purposeful, and every ounce of pain in the present world, believers are promised, will be counterbalanced by joy and levitation in the next. It was the only way that an unjust world would make sense, with the poor and downtrodden hopeful for another world, another existence, where the tables would be turned and those who hurt would be whole, and those who caused hurt would be the ones to feel it. The heart was more than just an organ but the very essence of what makes us human, a cosmic battleground for the war between good and evil.

Over time, though, pain of all sorts has become increasingly common in modern societies. In fact, pain was considered widely as the price for modernity and civilization in the nineteenth century. In 1892, the American neurologist Silas Weir Mitchell applied a particularly vulgar racial tinge to it. "The savage does not feel pain as we do: nor as we examine the descending scale of life, do animals seem to have the acuteness of pain-sense at which we have arrived."[3] He was far from alone—the German philosophers Schopenhauer and Nietzsche both agreed that sensitivity to pain was directly related to intelligence and degree of "civilization."[4] These pronouncements were made even before the first major painkiller, aspirin, had been discovered.

Part of the reason the desire to quash pain has occurred is because of the changing nature of our relationship with pain. Pain has always been the most visible hand of many diseases and maladies secretly brewing inside, and in truth, pain was considered neither a sensation nor a feeling. It was divine retribution; it was the heavens striking down upon humans with great vengeance and furious anger. Pain was not to be buried under the ground but experienced fully. Pain was not within the purview of physicians but of holy men. Where there was pain, there was sin, and no sin could ever go unpunished. And pain was necessary, for those who endured it could also find redemption from their vices. C. S. Lewis wrote, "All great religions were first preached and long practiced in a world without chloroform."

It was in fact first the Renaissance and then secularism that led to a sea change in how we viewed debility, with pain being at the front of the row. During the Renaissance, medical science first began as an extension of religion; the study of disease was merely a glorification of the divine and a means to master nature and to unlock the codes of the universe. In time, though, it jettisoned off completely, until the only reason medical science existed was for medical science itself. Man, according to Francis Bacon, became the architect of his fortune and assumed both control and responsibility for his existence.

Even though the aversion to pain and the yearning for a completely pain-free existence preceded anesthesia and the availability of painkillers, this desire found a perfect vehicle in those two agents. Breakthroughs in general anesthesia had been ignored multiple times before it was finally accepted after the landmark public demonstration by the dentist, William Morton, in what is now Massachusetts General Hospital, in 1846. This discovery spread like ether throughout Europe, unlike previous instances, when cultural and societal norms around the experience of pain and its ties to supernatural hands made it almost immoral to try to suppress it.[5] By the nineteenth century, in most industrialized countries, pain came to very much be viewed as a natural and physiological sensation rather than a metaphysical instrument of justice and heavenly intervention. And as this social revolution began to explode, a German pharmacist isolated a compound from opium. He named this compound morphine, after Morpheus, the Greek god of dreams. The overhaul of how pain was dealt with was summed up by the Dutch anthropologist Frederik Buytendijk (1887–1974), writing in 1957, "Modern man takes offense at many things that used to be accepted with resignation. He takes offense at growing old, at a long sick-bed, frequently even at death, but certainly at pain. Its occurrence is inacceptable."[6,7]

The unacceptability of pain, even a pinch, reached fever pitch by the end of the 1990s, when a concerted campaign was begun to overcome the epidemic of untreated pain in the United States. Public health organizations such as the Joint Commission, which accredits hospitals, and the Veterans Health Administration, in an effort to make pain "visible," advocated for pain to join the ranks of heart rate, blood pressure, breathing rate, and temperature as the "fifth vital sign."[8] Books were written chiseling pain assessment on to the Mount Rushmore of medical evaluations.[9] Therefore, when I started medical residency training in Boston, I was taught to ask every patient I saw, "Rate your pain on a scale of 1 to 10—10 being the worst pain you have ever experienced in your life." Almost automatically, I would get a 10 from many of the patients I saw, some of whom would be writhing in pain, others eating a hamburger and watching television. I wanted to refine my system, so I threw in some gruesome imagery, adding with "10 being the worst pain in your life, as if you are being stabbed with a knife," and yet it still didn't change the responses I got. I kept upping the ante until 10 became being agonizingly having your entire body crushed by a rampaging locomotive. Now I would get the occasional 8 or 9, although I still got more 12s and 15s.

This emphasis on pain management, of course, was one of the greatest factors leading to the opioid painkiller epidemic. Many of those writing clinical guidelines and at the helm of the "Make America Pain-Free Again" campaign were also getting paid by the companies that made opioid painkillers.[10] In fact, in a study where the pain scale was followed rigorously, it led to many more adverse events from painkillers in the hospital.[11] And a more recent study showed that opioids were in fact no better than over-the-counter medications like acetaminophen at relieving moderate to severe chronic pain.[12] Almost all medical associations like the American Medical Association and the American Academy of Family Physicians, therefore, now explicitly do not endorse pain as a vital sign as all of us try to dig out of the opioid epidemic, which is killing more Americans than the HIV epidemic at its peak.[13]

Americans feel more aches and pains than anyone else in the world and consume almost 30 percent of the world's medicinal opioid supply. The medicalization of pain, perhaps, was a mistake. Perhaps the best treatment for pain is not allopathic but humanistic. With religion in retreat, the secularization of medicine has provided us a greater impetus to treat a sensation we clearly still don't fully understand. Today, it is not a stretch to think that opiates, which by themselves have led to a reduction in the life span of Americans, fill the spiritual void many feel, adding another layer of prescient truth to Karl Marx's saying, "Religion is the sigh of the oppressed creature, the heart of a heartless world, and the soul of soulless conditions. It is the opium of the people."

As our relationship with pain continues to evolve, now at hyperdrive in the wake of the opioid epidemic, what remains most vexing about pain is the lack of an objective test, at least to differentiate life-threatening pain from pain that, despite its discomfort, might not be the harbinger of an acute illness.

Throughout the rise and subsequent fall of pain, the pains of the chest have retained their position as perhaps the most important pain of all. The accounts of men and women having chest pain litter the works of writers and scientists throughout the span of civilization. However, as atherosclerosis became an increasingly efficient assassin, the descriptions of chest pain, too, started to change and began to sound much more familiar to what the heart feels in modern times.

William Harvey (1578–1657), the British physician, once described a knight who, after reaching middle age, "made frequent complaint of a certain distressing pain in the chest, especially in the night season; so that dreading at one time syncope, at another suffocation in his attacks he led an unquiet and anxious life."[14] Andreas Vesalius (1514–1564) wondered whether a "sad feeling and pain in the heart" was associated with heart disease, yet the connection between chest pain and heart disease wasn't made until the late eighteenth century.[15] Even William Heberden (1710–1801), the British physician who laid out the first description of *angina,* thought that it was because of a disorder in the stomach. Even when people did start to understand that the classic type of chest pain that all of us fear does in fact occur because of heart disease, some thought it was a "neuralgia" while others thought it was from "exhaustion of the heart muscle."[16] The descriptions of chest pain in the nineteenth century varied, with some experiencing the pain every day for years without taking a deadly turn and others collapsing in an unceremonious heap.

There were several prevalent theories making the rounds, and one of them was the distension theory, which grew in popularity because of how common a completely unrelated disease had become—syphilis. Many times when autopsies were performed on people who had died after chest pain, no clear reason could be found. However, many happened to have syphilis, which, in its very advanced forms, caused the aorta, the largest artery in the body emerging from the heart, to transform from a smooth, silky vessel into a tree-bark-like surface. It was thought that chest pain occurred because of distension of the aorta and the stretching of the nerves that innervate it.

One of the people to put all the pieces together was James B. Herrick, a physician in Chicago, who became very interested in angina when one day, while making rounds as an intern in 1889 in Cook County Hospital, he came upon a patient and "saw him sitting erect in a chair, pale, the picture of anguish."[17] Around that time, the only treatment for angina was an inhaled drug called amyl nitrate, nowadays used primarily as an industrial cleaning agent or as a recreational drug to produce a rush during a rave or sex.

"After a few inhalations, a look of incredulity came over him. As breathing more freely, he relaxed from his tense attitude, tears came into his eyes, and, with the courtesy of the old-world peasant, he grasped my hand and kissed it. I was almost as incredulous as he; it was too good, too marvelous, to be true."

Amyl nitrate has a long and exciting journey of its own and was the first of a large and growing family of medications called *nitrates* that remain an essential part of a physician's arsenal to this day. It all started with the Italian chemist Ascanio Sobrero (1812–1888), who discovered a liquid called *nitroglycerin*.[18] When Sobrero tasted this liquid, it gave him a severe headache, which is now thought to be from dilation of the blood vessels in the brain. However, nitroglycerin was so explosive that he kept it a secret for many years until its knowledge passed along to one of his students— Alfred Nobel (1833–1896), the Swedish chemist who bequeathed his fortune and name to the Nobel Prizes. Nobel used nitroglycerin to invent dynamite, exporting it the world over, becoming one of the richest men of his time on the back of a most violently destructive compound. At the same time, though, physicians in England had started to use nitroglycerin and amyl nitrate for angina with encouraging results.[19] Ironically, one of the most well-known users of nitrates for relief was Nobel himself, who had developed significant angina.[20]

Amyl nitrate was dangerous because frequently it would drop users' blood pressure so steeply that it would reduce the blood reaching the coronary arteries, making things even worse by actually reproducing the lack of oxygenation—ischemia—that it was meant to prevent. But nitroglycerin had a more reliable effect and is, in fact, one of the first things that is popped into a patient's mouth as soon as they start to have chest pain.

Many patients with angina never leave their house without a few pills of nitroglycerin in their pocket, just in case their chest pain recurs. One hundred and fifty years later, its effect can still bring tears to one's eyes.

During an overnight shift at the hospital, I was paged about a patient who had started to have chest pain. The man had severe disease in all his coronary arteries and was in fact waiting for heart bypass surgery in a day or so. When I entered his room, he was gray as a ghost. I had known him to be a stoic minimizer—he wasn't one to complain but it was clear how sick he was just by looking at him. I wanted to start a nitroglycerin drip through the IV, but his blood pressure was too low. Nitroglycerin relaxes the blood vessels and can really make blood pressure plummet. The next measure was a pretty drastic step up—he would need a long balloon placed in his aorta to offload some of the pressure against which his heart was beating. Before he got consigned to that procedure, I wanted to at least give medication a shot. I asked the nurse to slowly start the nitroglycerin drip but to stop it if his blood pressure dropped. The nurse started the drip, and his blood pressure remained steady. I told her to crank it up until he was chest pain–free, and astoundingly, as she increased the dose of nitroglycerin, not only did his chest pain go away, the pink hue returned to his skin and his blood pressure actually *increased*. By relaxing the coronary arteries, nitroglycerin gave his heart the oxygen needed for it to finally be able to supply the body and restore the normal state of blood pressure throughout.

In the 1970s, almost two centuries after it was discovered, it was realized that nitric oxide is actually produced by the inner lining of human blood vessels and intestines. Nitric oxide relaxes blood vessels and is one of the key molecules that maintains the normal function of the body and circulation. It has far-reaching effects that almost no one could have anticipated. In the early 1990s, a new nitrate compound being tested in the town of Sandwich in the UK failed to show any benefit in relieving hypertension or angina. It did, however, produce a very unexpected side effect.[21] Men using the drug reported they were having robust and sustained erections. While researchers initially dismissed this concern, soon they performed a specially designed trial to study the effect of this drug on erections, especially in those with erectile dysfunction. Soon men who hadn't been able to maintain an erection and have sex in years were able to.

"I was as surprised as anyone when my research on a potential treatment for heart disease revealed a side effect that sparked a sexual health revolution," recalled Ian Osterloh, a physician and drug developer, on how he serendipitously discovered the drug that would come to be known as Viagra.[22] Since then, Viagra has come full circle back to the heart and is in fact used in patients with high pressures in the lungs, called *pulmonary hypertension,* a life-threatening condition that can result in heart failure and cause difficult breathing.

While they were being used routinely for angina in the early twentieth century, no one really knew how nitrates worked. However, James Herrick was convinced of the "myocardial ischemia" hypothesis, that angina was a consequence of a supply-demand mismatch of oxygenated blood in the heart through the coronary arteries. His hypothesis was that either in states of limited supply—such as if there is a blockage in the coronary arteries— or in states of increased demand when the heart is working overtime—such as when it is beating superfast after an infection—the heart muscle is deprived of oxygen, becomes ischemic, and essentially starts to die. This cellular demise releases chemical substances in the blood, which cause angina. Now, all he had to do was actually prove this theory.

On January 16, 1910, the head of a private banking house came back home from the theater and proceeded to have a sandwich and a beer around midnight.[23] That is when he started to have "sudden, excruciating" chest pain. Along with a slew of other physicians, Herrick worked his way through the different things it could be. He even slept at the banker's overnight. Herrick was convinced there was nothing in the belly, that the lungs were fine, leaving but the heart to be worried about. He stayed up discussing the case all night until at 4:00 a.m., when the man died suddenly but peacefully.

Herrick told the doctor performing the autopsy, "Look for a clot in the coronary artery."

The doctor called Herrick back later that day. "The clot was in the coronary artery, all right. But how in God's name did you guess it?" Herrick, however, was not just guessing, for he had previously conceived that perhaps an occlusion in the coronary arteries might lead to such a situation. It wasn't much later that Herrick realized that this was far from a rare occurrence, but rather one of the most prevalent diseases of his time. But after he presented these findings at a conference, "it fell like a dud." Even after his finding was published in *The Journal of the American Medical Association*, it barely elicited any interest.[24] Herrick then did what few other researchers ever do. "I began consciously to do what I called missionary work, preaching the gospel of the pathology and clinical symptoms of acute coronary obstruction. . . . I talked coronary occlusion almost ad nauseam." He feared he was going "nutty"—the very idea of an acute coronary occlusion, what we all now call a heart attack, was considered outlandish. "The attempt was ridiculous because it was impossible," said one critic, but in a particularly cruel twist of fate, almost a decade after, that very critic called up Herrick, actively in the clutches of a heart attack, asking him for his help.

Many things can cause pain in the chest, and these can range from acid reflux after a particularly spicy meal to an aorta that is tearing open or a punctured lung. But perhaps most importantly, it can mean that there is an atherosclerotic plaque erupting, causing heart tissue to start dying off, releasing acid in the blood, causing the entire body to start to become deprived of oxygenated blood. On any given day or night at the hospital, in the intensive care unit or in the emergency room, and at times when I am at home, I get called about patients having chest pain. In moments like these, like any other physician on the line, I have to read the tea leaves, I have to listen to the story, I have to do my best sleuthing but with a guillotine hanging over, with every grain of sand weighing it down, pushing the patient toward tragedy.

While working in the cardiac intensive care unit at Duke University Medical Center, the cardiologist who is on call is not only responsible for all the critically ill patients in the unit, he or she is also helping to triage some of the sickest patients within a few hundred miles. Because of an emergency network developed by researchers and doctors at Duke, emergency medical services staff and emergency rooms around the state of North Carolina have a direct line of communication with cardiologists manning the intensive care units in the few major hospitals in the state. This model has now been replicated across the country.

When the bat phone rings, I try to not topple anyone in my way as I make my way toward it. Time comes to a halt as I pick up the phone having no idea what awaits me on the other end. One time it was a man found under a tractor after his heart had stopped beating and he had collapsed. Another time it was an emergency room doctor, and I could hear someone counting down their CPR thrusts in the background. Most commonly, though, I am asked about a patient having chest pain. Conferencing on the line, there is a helicopter squad waiting to know if they might need to be deployed to pick this patient up. I have to decide within seconds if the patient is having a heart attack and whether I need to activate the cardiac catheterization lab to come in and perform an emergent procedure on the patient. It is commonly said in cardiology that time is muscle, and with every additional second of ischemia, heart muscle dies off from lack of oxygen without any significant ability to come back to life. Ever. Without even the slightest hint of overstatement, it is almost certainly a matter of life or death.

Every day, millions have chest pain. When is it just something to brush off and when does it merit calling 911? Here is what the research tells us.

He was running on the treadmill when his chest started to burn. He thought he was having acid reflux. He didn't really think much of it, but when it persisted long after he stopped running, he told his wife, who immediately rushed him to the hospital, where it was quickly discovered that he was having a massive heart attack.

When I met him in the intensive care unit, I asked him if he had ever had acid reflux before. He told me the only other time he'd had acid reflux was when he'd had his last heart attack. I stopped him immediately. "The next time you think you are having acid reflux, I hope you realize you might be having a heart attack."

In 2014, almost five million Americans came to emergency rooms primarily for chest pain, up from just under four million in 2006.[25] Yet only about one in ten were actually having some form of heart attack.[26] Over time, the number of people presenting to the emergency room with chest pain who have a heart attack is actually going down, making it increasingly difficult to sift through and figure out which was a dud and which was the real deal. Why is that so important? Every year, almost 2,500 Americans die within seven days of being sent home from the emergency room due to a heart attack or atherosclerotic heart disease.[27] You just can't afford to miss it.

Almost always, the first time I find out about a patient with chest pain is after the emergency room pages me to consult on the patient. In the page, usually the length of a 160-character tweet, some of the most important nuggets of information are present, and my mind, like that of almost any other doctor, goes to work. Perhaps the most important prognostic sign of all is age. While it is fashionable to say age is just a number, when it comes to prognosis, study after study shows that it might be the single most important number of all. The next most important nugget is what is quite simply referred to as the eyeball test—*does the patient look like they are having a heart attack?* Certainly, the reason Herrick gave his first patient amyl nitrate was because he totally flunked the eyeball test. In fact, at that time, and for most of history, the eyeball has been the singular and most important diagnostic test available to physicians. Reliance on the eyeball test alone, however, would be disastrous because of how inferior it is in multiple domains to more objective tests.[28]

A physical exam, which includes listening to a patient's heart and lungs and feeling parts of their body for abnormalities, is actually not particularly useful in diagnosing if someone is having a heart attack, given that heart attacks produce very few classic physical signs. Perhaps the most important thing a physical exam can reveal about chest pain is if it is *not* from the heart. Any pain that worsens by either pressing down on the chest or by moving the arms around is unlikely to represent a heart attack.[29]

The patient's story and their description of what the pain feels like is essential in ruling in or out a heart attack.[30] One of the important characteristics of pain from a potential heart attack is that it can radiate to the arms or the neck. While most commonly it radiates into the left arm, which is closer to the heart, and hence the ring finger's persistence in cultural memory, radiation in both arms is actually the characteristic most highly suggestive of pain from a heart attack. Another very important feature, though this is restricted to only the more unfortunate, is if the pain is similar to when they had a prior heart attack.

Even all this information, however, might not be enough to help reliably diagnose a heart attack. Missing a heart attack could lead to death, while overdiagnosing heart attacks will overexpose patients to risky procedures that might end up doing more harm than good. This is where the electrocardiogram, or EKG, comes in and helps sort things out. The EKG is such an important tool that it can help make a diagnosis in a patient even when that is the only piece of information you have. If a picture can tell a thousand words, an EKG can tell the entire life history of the heart— where it's been and where it's bound—in one single snapshot. As it was first demonstrated in a little-known medical journal in 1910 by two Russian researchers in Kiev, the EKG would prove to be the as-yet-unsurpassed mode of diagnosing heart attacks in man.[31] And almost all that action occurs in the 0.1 seconds on the EKG called the ST segment.

—⋀—

Back in the early twentieth century, even after scientists from across the world began to observe that many people who died suddenly after chest pain had blockages from clots in the coronary arteries, few believed that to be true. Russian scientists W. P. Obrastzow and N. D. Straschesko, and Viennese physician Ludolf von Krehl, were some of the first people to show that coronary occlusion caused heart attacks, something observed later by James Herrick in Chicago. Yet despite Herrick's compelling presentation, few believed him. What would it take to convince the world that angina wasn't just fatigue of the heart muscle or dilation of the aorta, which many assumed to be the cause?

It was the EKG that helped turn the tide of opinion. Physicians discovered that changes occurring in patients having heart attacks were similar to those noted in dogs after their coronary arteries were tied off. They noted that a complete blockage of the blood supply to the heart caused the erstwhile flat segment of the EKG between the dramatic QRS wave and the more subtle T wave that followed it, called the ST segment, to rise up almost like the waters of the ocean being pulled up by the moon in a hump-like, concave tide. In fact, it became clear quickly that just knowing which leads of the EKG the ST elevations occurred in could help predict which of the coronary arteries was obstructed.

Why does the ST segment rise in a heart attack? When a part of the heart becomes completely ischemic, meaning that there is no oxygen-carrying blood reaching it through the coronary arteries, chaos ensues. As the heart muscle cells begin to die from suffocation, the pristine electrical balance that exists between the cells and the surrounding milieu becomes upended. The potassium ions that fill most heart cells come gushing out as if they were lava rushing down the slopes of Vesuvius. The Zen-like harmony of electrical charge represented by the normal ST segment means that no electrolytes are being exchanged between the heart muscle cells and the interstitium that surrounds it. However, when disaster strikes, usually in the shape of a blood clot forming after the acute rupture of an atherosclerotic plaque, the dump of potassium from cells causes the generation of an injury current between sick and not-sick heart muscle that manifests as the mark of cell death—the dreaded ST segment elevation.

Patients who experience a heart attack that results in complete occlusion of one of the major coronary arteries of the heart have what is called an ST elevation myocardial infarction (STEMI). It is one of the most dreadful things that can happen to a human being. Within moments of a STEMI occurring, pink and plush heart muscle begins to change its appearance and very, very quickly, ischemic heart muscle becomes scar tissue. This infarcted tissue is no better than dead meat, and "dead meat don't beat."

Detecting a STEMI is one of the core skills for any nurse or physician. Emergency medical staff are very good at diagnosing a STEMI on an EKG. And as soon as they do, the clock starts. If you are even a few hundred miles from Duke, your best bet is to call the cardiologist manning the phone in the cardiac intensive care unit (CICU).

One day, I was sitting in the CICU after having worked overnight. It had been a busy night, and my morning reinforcements had finally arrived so I could breathe again. Another hour or so and my long-awaited union with my bed would occur. My cell phone rang, and I casually picked it up. On the other end was Joseph Rogers, one of the most senior cardiologists in the hospital. I almost reflexively stood up. *What is Joe Rogers calling me for?*

A man in the waiting area of the lung transplant clinic had collapsed to the ground. Nursing staff rushed to him while he lay on the floor. They called for help, and Dr. Rogers just happened to be there. He asked for an EKG, and as soon as it printed out, he knew the man was having a STEMI. He pulled out his phone, and he called the CICU phone, which was in my possession at the time. I immediately had the patient transported to the emergency room, where I saw him. He didn't look good.

From across the room, I could tell that he was in cardiogenic shock, meaning that his heart was struggling to supply his body, which was shutting down. He had white hair and a scraggly beard; I learned later that he played Santa every Christmas. Santa had smoked most of his life and had developed the worst lung disease ever. He quit smoking, but his remaining lungs were nothing but black cobwebs after decades of tobacco abuse. He mended his ways and eventually received a new pair of lungs via transplant. He was looking to a new life, one in which he wouldn't have to lug his oxygen tank around anymore, one in which he could actually play with the kids who were excited to see him dressed in white and crimson, or with his grandkids, for whom he was Santa all year round. Six months into this new life, he was now in the emergency room in front of me with ST elevations as tall as Mount Doom.

In some ways, a STEMI is the simplest of diagnoses—there's always only one right thing to do, one definitive treatment—blood flow has to be restored, and the offender blocking blood flow has to be removed. To do that, and to do that really quickly, one has to activate the cardiac catheterization lab. That's exactly what I did in one of the most well-equipped heart hospitals in the world, and it was exactly what the medical team in Pakistan did when my dad arrived with a STEMI.

As soon as the patient reached the cath lab, the distress left his face, and he suddenly became limp. The EKG had changed, and suddenly the monitors showed a rapidly oscillating pattern called *ventricular tachycardia* (*VT*), a malignant rhythm often caused by an oxygen-starved heart. Immediately, one of the nurses jumped and started to perform CPR. Another activated the defibrillator we had ready, anticipating this dreaded turn for the worse. It charged like a Death Star about to blow up a planet, and as soon as it did, the nurse performing CPR stopped and leaped back. Another person yelled, "All clear!" making sure no one was touching the patient or the bed before delivering a shock to the unconscious patient. As soon as the defibrillator was discharged, Santa's flaccid body contorted before falling back on the gurney. He was still in VT and CPR was resumed. Another time the defibrillator was charged, another time he jumped after receiving 360 joules of electricity zapped through his chest, and yet he remained intractably in VT.

Whatever we were doing wasn't working, and Santa was dying. And this wasn't just about Santa either. It was also about the young person who had died and who had donated his or her lungs so that Santa could live. It was also about the man or woman who could have gotten those lungs but didn't because they were just behind Santa on the transplant wait list. CPR and electric shocks were the end of the road for most. He lay there with his heart effectively at standstill, but for Santa, we knew we had to reach into the beyond. We paged the cardiac surgery team. We wanted them to perform ECMO.

Behind every abbreviation in medicine is an amalgamation of letters. Behind every abbreviation in medicine, every amalgamation of letters, is either a disease you would wish on no one or a procedure you always wish to avoid. I wish we never needed ECMO; I wish we would never have to ask our surgeons for it. But seeing what I have seen, knowing what I know, and having the best possible surgeons to call on and to ask for help from, I am grateful that ECMO exists and we have people trained to be able to do it.

ECMO stands for *extracorporeal membrane oxygenation*. Of course, that is but gibberish. In ECMO, large plastic tubes are placed into a person's femoral vein and femoral artery in the groin. The plastic catheter in the femoral vein, which is almost the size of a water hose, is advanced up the body until it is almost at the level of the heart and it sucks out all the dark, oxygen-less blood returning to the heart from the rest of the body. This means there is very little blood in the heart and lungs. This oxygen-starved blood that has been sucked out is taken to a box where it is infused with oxygen and then pumped into the other catheter in the femoral artery, which is pushed up into the aorta, the great artery emerging from the heart. This supplies bright red blood to the body. ECMO effectively bypasses the heart and lungs fully, taking over both its chief responsibilities: to circulate blood through the body and to enrich it with oxygen.

As the cardiac surgery team stormed the cath lab, carrying briefcases full of ECMO catheters the size of small javelins, I could see the nurses performing CPR begin to tire. I jumped to the front of the line and took over CPR. On top of his naked body, as I compressed his chest, the stethoscope around my neck began to flail around, smacking me in my face before someone thankfully removed it.

If this were theater, it would have been as if I had jumped from the front seat and onto the stage. It took the surgeons fifteen minutes to get the patient hooked up to the ECMO circuit, and as soon as they did, I stopped doing CPR and the whole room paused. Santa was still in VT, but at this point, it didn't matter even if his heart were beating or not. The surgeons stepped back, and the cardiology team took over. They found a big clot blocking his coronary artery, and they opened it with a stent, but his heart was as effective at beating as a rib eye steak. Connected to the ECMO for his heart, a breathing machine for his lungs, and dialysis for his kidneys, he lingered for a month, but all the support in the world could not bring him back, and he eventually passed away.

Few things in life are as dramatic as a STEMI, yet thankfully the number of people having STEMIs is actually going down in the United States and other high-income countries.[32] We have better treatments than ever before for risk factors such as high blood pressure and high cholesterol, and deleterious behaviors such as smoking are waning. Even when people do have a STEMI, timely and effective treatments ensure that many, many more people like my dad survive a STEMI, at times with few lasting consequences.

Another type of heart attack, though, is on the rise. While it can be less dramatic than a STEMI, it can be even more lethal. Not only is it potentially more dangerous, it can be far more insidious, for there may be no changes on a patient's EKG and patients may not even have any symptoms. And while STEMIs are becoming less common, the type of a heart attack called a *non-ST elevation myocardial infraction*, or NSTEMI, occurs three times more frequently.[33]

An NSTEMI occurs in patients with troponin elevations who do not have a STEMI. While STEMIs are caused by the acute rupture of plaques causing complete obstruction of blood flow in one of the coronary arteries, an NSTEMI usually occurs in the absence of such an acute total occlusion. Often, plaque rupture occurs but doesn't lead to complete occlusion of the coronary artery. Erosion of plaques, without frank rupture, is also fairly common, which leads to the activation of factors in the blood that cause the formation of a blood clot, leading to restriction of blood flowing downstream to the heart.

Lucy had the nicest smile. Almost no one I know is ever happy to be in the hospital, but Lucy was a cheerful person as excited watching her favorite musical as she was in the emergency room. She was a very healthy person who exercised every day, didn't take any medications, and was making her first trip to the emergency room.

It all started when she was doing yoga. Lucy felt a tightness in her chest and in her neck and in the back of her head, but she blew it off. It kept happening until one of her friends told her to go to the hospital. The staff in the emergency room performed an EKG that was stone-cold normal. She wasn't having any classic symptoms suggestive of a heart attack. Out of an abundance of caution, the emergency room team tested for troponin elevation in the blood. When the result came back showing that the amount of troponin in her blood was seriously elevated, they called me to come see her and break the news. I didn't want to burst her happy bubble, but I had no choice.

After chatting with Lucy for a while, sharing pleasantries, tiptoeing around the obvious, I finally asked her, "Do you know why you are here?"

"No."

"Well, you have had a heart attack."

Her smile started to melt, but she fought that downward pull and kept grinning. Her friend who had brought her in looked much more concerned. Neither, in their own different ways, could believe Lucy was having a heart attack. This, of course, was not how people had heart attacks on TV. There was no clutching of the chest, no gasping for air, no dramatic EKGs, no hospital alarms going off, no ambulances blaring or emergency medical staff rampaging around. It was quiet. It was very, very quiet.

"What do you mean she had a heart attack?"

Given the opening, I would now have to proceed with a delicate dance. Lucy had been more or less healthy for her entire life. Until now. Very quickly, she had gone from being not-sick to sick, and this was a big deal. Being sick is like being given a new job that you didn't ask for, didn't want anything to do with. And now you are stuck with it. The moment you wake up, you swipe in until you fall asleep and you swipe out. There are no days off. Being sick is even worse when you have a chronic disease, like when you develop heart failure, because there is almost no chance you will ever get to have a retirement party and ride off into the sunset. If anything, as you get older, chronic disease just gives you more work to do: more medications to take, more visits to the hospital, more limitations on your daily life, with a diminishing chance of a return to normalcy.

As awful as assuming the sick role is, the alternative is arguably even worse—for Lucy, it could mean either death or disability. Nothing is a stronger recruitment pitch for this awful occupation than a shock like a heart attack. Therefore, I had to make a compelling case for Lucy to motivate her to change her lifestyle, take medications regularly, follow up regularly with a doctor, and also be prepared for invasive procedures to ensure that her heart didn't suffer lasting damage. Many of these tasks would have to be repeated indefinitely, and if they were effective, they wouldn't just treat the health shock that she had already experienced but prevent those she never would.

My job would be easier if, for example, Lucy had fractured a bone. A broken bone is something that constantly reminds people that they are not well because it hurts like hell. A broken bone is also different because in most cases, being the custodian of a broken bone is more like having an unrewarding summer internship rather than a lifetime position—broken bones can be put back together, allowing the person to go back to being someone who can fully use their limb.

Traditionally, assuming the sick role has come with some benefits; in many historical societies, the sick were provided special privileges.[34] When the American sociologist Talcott Parson came up with the "sick role," he pointed out that the sick were usually exempted from obligations such as work. There are some other benefits: These days, it isn't uncommon for people to fake cancer diagnoses to obtain duped donations. Yet heart disease, much like other chronic diseases, doesn't carry any of those benefits, and something as potentially silent as an NSTEMI can be even less persuasive. Certainly, Lucy and her serious friend weren't fully sold with the program yet.

Other factors determine how people make the transition from well to unwell. Many men don't seek help when having chest pain because that behavior clashes with their views on masculinity.[35] Many women don't seek help when having a heart attack because they might have "atypical" chest pain and therefore not have the classic symptoms of pressure in the chest radiating to the neck and left arm. NSTEMIs, which might not cause as acute an onset of symptoms unlike most STEMIs, lead to further delays in patients seeking medical care.

If I pushed Lucy too deep into the sick role, there was a chance that she might succumb to nihilism. The sick role only helps if patients feel like they have agency, that they can alter the trajectory of their disease, or if their efforts can make them feel better, such as after a person has a feverish flu. Only then is it a job worth keeping for some even with its lifetime commitment of taking medications, seeing doctors, and getting tests and procedures. In fact, patients with heart disease who feel like they have more control are more likely to attend cardiac rehab and control risk factors such as high blood pressure.[36,37]

What many physicians fail to do, myself included, is think of illness beyond biology. Our rigorous training molds us to think in terms of secular data, such as EKGs, troponins, and ejection fractions, when in fact these are the last things that might matter to someone like Lucy. Illness is not only a biological phenomenon, nor is it only a psychological one. It is part of one's social identity, as much as being a physician is part of mine, coming with responsibilities, expectations, and obligations. Illness is as much about its story, of how it finds a place in the narrative arc of a person's life, as it is about electrolyte derangements and myocardial ischemia.

Physicians are very much a part of how a patient's story gets written. We can't do the writing, but certainly we can help the protagonist find the key to the dungeon and, sometimes, defeat the vile beast that entraps the princess in the tower. How can docs help? Listening to patients' stories—*shockingly*—helps. Patients of physicians who are more empathetic are more likely to adhere to the medications they have been prescribed.[38] Patients of surgeons who provided them not only clear instructions but gave them encouragement have lesser pain and are able to leave the hospital sooner.[39]

On a daily basis in the hospital, I find myself in the middle of many people's stories; most people I take care of have lived with chronic diseases for years if not decades. Often I am with patients at the end of their stories. Only rarely do I find myself where I was in Lucy's story with heart disease—at the beginning.

Before I could continue, though, I had to take a step back and address the swirl of questions hiding behind her smile. What exactly was a troponin, what exactly was an NSTEMI, what could have caused it, and what was the best way to manage it?

If a sick heart can steal one's spirit, a mind gone awry can seize one's very being. She was a vibrant woman, a nurse who had helped her patients through the worst that life could throw at them. That's until she had a massive stroke, complicated by a brain bleed, and now she was left trapped all by herself in the prison that until recently was her body, now rigid like a plank. She couldn't speak, couldn't move, couldn't hear, and by all accounts, couldn't feel. And yet her family kept her dressed up with an unhelpfully excessive amount of makeup, making her look like a life-sized-doll version of her former self. As a physician, I walk into tragedies all the time, with the worst ones sticking and others just disappearing into the faded, dusty vaults of the museum of memories, some to never be opened again. This one would make it on to my museum of horrors' brochure.

When I came to her bedside in the emergency room well past midnight, her tiny room was full of family sleeping on sheets they had laid out on the floor. Earlier during the day while she was being moved from a wheelchair to her bed at home, she slipped and fell, bruising her face. Her family had brought her into the emergency room, and while she was not having any chest pain, breathing difficulties, or any other symptoms suggestive of heart issues, the emergency room doctors tested for the presence of troponins. The test came back positive, and therefore they diagnosed her with an NSTEMI. And that's where I was asked to come in.

At the turn of the millennium, troponins were added to the definition of how heart attacks are defined, and this fundamentally changed what even constitutes a heart attack.[40] It allowed many patients who clearly were having ongoing damage to the heart to be diagnosed and then treated with either medications and procedures. This included people like Lucy, who, if it hadn't been for troponins, might never have been diagnosed with a heart attack. In fact, we know that women's symptoms are more likely to be not taken as seriously as men's.

Yet troponins are far from perfect, and in many cases, troponins can be elevated in the absence of a heart attack. There is a long list of conditions in which troponins can be elevated that have nothing to do with the coronary arteries, such as infection or inflammation of the heart.[41] Even patients who have had CPR can have troponin elevations. Not only that, there are conditions where there is extensive breakdown of muscle such as after someone has run a marathon or kidney failure when the body fails to excrete troponins that can cause them to be elevated.

Troponins have made it so easy to detect any amount of heart damage that in many cases the test will be drawn without rhyme or reason.

For some medical staff, sending for a blood test is easier than examining patients, taking detailed history, and making diagnoses with some old-fashioned sleuthing. A blood test like troponin circumvents the entire interaction between doctors and their patients. It is easier and faster to order tests like CAT scans and EKGs than it is to order Chinese takeout.

Like so many patients with elevated troponins that I had seen in the emergency room, it wasn't until the results came back positive that the team that ordered the test even stopped to think about why they had ordered it in the first place. There was no way that a vegetative patient with no cardiac symptoms would benefit from any treatments that we could provide her, nor could we safely administer them in the first place; the major bleed in her brain would only get worse since most of the usual medical and procedural treatments given to patients having a heart attack would increase her likelihood of bleeding.

Troponins, by virtue of their sensitivity, are a classic driver of what has been called *diagnostic creep* in modern medicine. When heart attacks were first diagnosed with EKGs, only STEMIs made the cut. Additional blood and imaging then expanded the pool, until troponins blew the whole situation up. Initially, when the NSTEMI diagnosis was conceived, many patients also were required to have other findings, including changes visible on the EKG, such as ST segment depressions as opposed to elevations. Yet over time, the culture has changed, with only a troponin elevation trumping all else.

Diagnostic creep is not just an issue in heart disease—the overuse of increasingly sensitive technology has led to overdiagnosis in almost every aspect of human disease. Take breast cancer, for example. We know that earlier use of mammograms increases the diagnosis of breast cancer, but we also know that this earlier use of mammograms does not actually improve survival in these patients.[42] Why? Because treating those low-risk cancers after an earlier diagnosis only detected through mammograms doesn't seem to help and rather exposes women to tests and procedures that don't actually change the outcome. The same is true for screening for prostate cancer with the blood test prostate-specific antigen (PSA).[43]

Without being alarmist, we are on the brink of an epidemic of heart attack overdiagnosis. As it stands, troponins are very sensitive at detecting heart attacks, but newer troponin tests are now being rolled out that are much, much more sensitive than conventionally used troponin tests. In fact, these troponins are found to be circulating in most healthy people. These new tests have some advantages, in that by amplifying tiny changes in the troponin levels, they can help rule in or rule out a heart attack sooner than traditional troponin tests. The underlying problem, however, is that many more of the millions of people who come to emergency rooms for not just chest pain but for all sorts of symptoms will have these tests performed, and many will have results come back positive. What does that test mean for them, how will it affect how they think of themselves and their bodies, and what about the stress and anxiety that comes with being diagnosed with heart disease?

Diagnostic creep in heart attacks is just the tip of the iceberg. Before Alzheimer's dementia, you get diagnosed with pre-dementia; before hypertension, there is pre-hypertension; and before diabetes, there is pre-diabetes. The problem is that many patients diagnosed with these pre-diseases never go on to develop the disease they were supposedly predestined to.[44] Even those that do may take years or decades to do so, and interventions such as medications or lifestyle changes for these pre-diseases doesn't necessarily change the eventual outcome. In many cases, they can expose people to unnecessary testing and procedures.[45]

What drives overdiagnosis? The very premise of newer diagnostic tests that can help them stand above conventional tests is that they are able to diagnose disease at earlier and earlier stages. This can help them show efficacy even if the knowledge gained from an earlier diagnosis doesn't actually help make treatments more effective. Physicians don't want to miss one heart attack in a thousand; however, such risk aversion comes at the risk of hundreds being misdiagnosed.[46]

The health system in general seems to have become adept at expanding the pool of the sick, leaving few if any who could be considered healthy. Medical guidelines, a study showed, almost universally expand disease definitions rather than making them more restrictive and exclusive.[47] There are many cynical ways to look at this trend; the majority of those writing these guidelines were also financially supported by the biomedical industry.[48] Also, in economic terms, to the health industry, patients are merely customers, and expanding the catchment of diagnoses only reels in more users.

Heart disease's version of the mammogram and the PSA is the stress test. The stress test is such a ubiquitous test that it is frequently used in lay speak. Each year, hundreds of thousands in the United States alone are subjected to it. Yet as time has passed, even as millions upon millions of these tests have been performed, the actual benefit gained from stress tests remains murky at best.

In September of 2008, the United States entered the greatest and deepest economic crisis in almost a century. Most of the world followed it down a hole initially created by an epidemic of mortgages that had been doled out to borrowers who under normal circumstances would never be granted them. Many homeowners were able to keep up with their mortgage payments, which in turn were being used to fuel much of the investment banking and insurance world. So when the housing bubble burst, too many defaulted on their loans, and the downstream effects of this crisis affected almost every person on earth in one way or another.

While the U.S. government and the Federal Reserve System were able to bail out most of the largest U.S. banks, there was a pressing need to ensure that such a crisis never occurs again. One mechanism mandated by policy makers under the Dodd–Frank Wall Street Reform and Consumer Protection Act was stress testing—a test conducted by the U.S. Federal Reserve System to check if large financial holding companies could withstand future economic downturns. Subsequently, Timothy Geithner, the secretary of the treasury during this cataclysmic time, wrote a memoir titled *Stress Test* (2014), recalling his role in instituting this test to rescue the economy and to ensure that it will not collapse in the face of a future catastrophe.

The concept underlying financial stress tests was borrowed from a test that has become the backbone of detecting heart disease. Between patients who might be perfectly healthy and have never had an odd twinge in their chest and those actively in the clutches of a heart attack, there is a sea of people who either have some risk factor for heart disease, who have any pain in the chest area or who are undergoing surgery from something as simple as getting cataracts removed to having organ transplantation. Stress tests are used for two main reasons: to see if someone's chest pain is really from their heart and to uncover any significant atherosclerosis of the coronary arteries that so far hasn't become apparent.

A stress test usually involves having the person perform exercise on a treadmill or stationary bike, the idea being that the increased work of the heart will uncover a supply-demand mismatch that atherosclerotic plaque might be causing by blocking the coronary arteries that may not be obvious when the heart is working normally. Those who cannot exercise might be administered medications that simulate the effects of exercise by either causing the heart to beat faster or that dilate the arteries supplying the heart, leading to increased blood flow. Ischemia is then detected either with an EKG or with imaging of the heart during the periods of stress.

As far as biological plausibility and common sense go, a stress test is a slam dunk. A stress test can show—either from an EKG that is being recorded as the participant exercises or through either ultrasound or nuclear imaging—if there was a part of the heart that moved less vigorously with exercise, suggesting lack of blood flow. *It just makes sense.* Not too long ago, and to this date, a stress test is performed as routinely for patients as an oil change for a car. If the diseased heart can be considered a ticking time bomb, a land mine just waiting for an errant footstep to go off, a stress test is the beeping land mine detector that could prevent the heart from exploding into bits and pieces.

Over time, though, the more stress tests have been tested rigorously in various settings, the lesser benefit they seem to offer. Diabetics are at high risk for developing atherosclerosis, and stress-testing diabetics older than forty years of age became routine practice. However, randomized controlled trials found that this strategy offered no benefit and could in fact expose patients to procedures they didn't need.[49] Another time when countless people are subjected to stress tests is before getting surgery. Surgeons and anesthesiologists are always interested in knowing if their patients are at high risk of having a heart attack during or after surgery. Stress testing in patients, therefore, became a requirement before any type of surgery. Yet study after study has shown that stress testing before surgery has no impact on improving patients' outcomes or reducing the risk of heart attacks.[50] If anything, such tests can cause delays in surgery as well as lead to further unnecessary tests and procedures. And even though almost all medical organizations recommend against stress testing inappropriately, leading to their use being somewhat dampened in recent years, the test is performed all too frequently in all sorts of unhelpful situations.

The problem with stress tests, similar to many other diagnostic tests, is that while they are very good at identifying a patient who might be at higher risk of a heart attack, they have a much tougher time showing if doing anything about those results actually changes anything.

And while medications have an important role to play, the most iconic therapy in cardiology, an advance that blurs the line between surgery and medicine, is the coronary stent—a tiny metallic structure placed in the coronary artery to prop it open—which has helped many patients avert what would have been certain death or disability before its discovery. Considered one of the greatest breakthroughs of the twentieth century, coronary stents are now under attack. Where do stents stand in this brave new world?

7

〜

A STENT IN TIME

I'm a heart surgeon, sure, but really I'm just a mechanic.

—Raymond Carver, *Beginners*

Any way you cut it, stories are at the heart of everything a doctor does. Whether it is learning a patient's story or retelling a tale of colleagues at odd hours, creating a vivid and inhabitable landscape is part of the job. And while many storytellers have to embark on elaborate journeys in search of their stories—Hemingway had to face off bulls and fight in the Great War—the only thing doctors and nurses have to do is show up at work. Whether it is early in the morning, when we are waking up our patients from their medication-induced slumber or in the afternoon as we overhear family members sobbing in the hallways or when we are editing copied-and-pasted notes in the computer at the end of the day, our patients' stories have a way of reaching us, whether we want them to or not.

Starting from the first day of medical school, doctors spend days, nights, and everything in between learning about an infinite number of things. What we are rarely taught, however, is how to use words well. Most conversations between patients and their doctors or nurses are told through stories and metaphors. And knowing how to use words well is important because the metaphors we employ can have a very powerful effect on patients and those accompanying them. In their classic book *Metaphors We Live By*, George Lakoff and Mark Johnson wrote, "How we think and act are fundamentally metaphorical in nature."[1]

Perhaps no part of medical care is littered with more questionable metaphors than when people are at the end of life. "Pulling the plug" has become such an essential part of the American medical lexicon that, by itself, it has shaped how generations of people have come to view the withdrawal of life-sustaining care. Not only does it dehumanize the person it is intended for, it somehow also makes disconnecting a critically ill patient from artificial life support sound like an active performance of euthanasia, weighing caregivers with unnecessary guilt. On the other hand, in lieu of difficult and time-consuming conversations, doctors and nurses frequently employ euphemisms to talk about death. CPR and breathing with a ventilator are described as "heroic measures" while the words *death* and *dying* are frequently substituted for an ambiguous alternative in conversations with patients and their loved ones.

No other part of the human body is as ripe for metaphorical imaging as the human heart. Almost every time the pathology of the heart is described for patients, it is done so in the incredibly effective framework of plumbing. The heart is described as a pump, and the arteries supplying it are the pipes. When atherosclerotic plaques build up in the pipes, the pipes get blocked. Then what? In the real world, you call the plumber, and in my world, where the stakes are much higher, you call a cardiologist to place one of the most iconic innovations of the past century—the coronary stent.

The stent is widely considered one of the most crucial technological advances of the last few decades. For patients having a heart attack, it is the most effective therapy we have developed, and this technology has likely saved millions of lives, including my dad's. But a stent is perhaps even more effective as a metaphor. The coronary stent is so mighty a metaphor: once you visualize it, it is almost impossible to unsee.

When patients have buildup of cholesterol-filled atherosclerotic plaques in the coronary arteries that supply the heart, they can obstruct the passage of blood flowing through these teeny-tiny vessels, and in some cases, these blockages can get severe enough to cause a heart attack. A stent is a tiny metallic wire frame that can be deployed minimally invasively right into the arteries where the blockages are and then expanded with minuscule balloons until the artery is wide open again. Almost half of cardiologists equate placing stents with plumbing; when pipes get blocked, they go ahead and open them up with stents.[2] To up the ante, the blood vessels are frequently called "widow-makers."[3]

Millions upon millions of people who have had heart attacks, who feared they would never see their families again, who thought they would never be able to work again, are able to be with their families and friends, are able to go back and make a living and do what they love again, because of stents and because of the people who put them there. And yet stents are under fire. The results of a recent, widely publicized study have cast doubt on the benefits of heart stents for a large number of patients with stable chest pain.[4] It has made some skeptical of the benefits of stents in people with stable symptoms not in the grips of a heart attack.

Stents are placed in what's called the *cardiac catheterization lab,* and I must say, I entered that world with a fair degree of trepidation. Expecting a macho and aggressive culture, instead I found it to be a sea of tranquility. Up to that point, most of my medical experience had been hurried, running from patient to patient, checking boxes, keeping up with a veritable flood of information, always seemingly behind. Everything seemed to slow down in the cath lab. More than an education in manipulating catheters, the cath lab is a meditation on life.

If you ever wonder why doctors would take on so much debt, spend so many sleepless nights studying, why they would live a life tethered to their pagers threatening to go off at any moment, then maybe you should visit a cath lab during a procedure. There is no greater teacher of life than the practice of medicine and nowhere does one learn better than at the place where life and death are often most precariously balanced.

On its face, the cath lab is an opaque, windowless cave filled with large plastic catheters, sharp instruments, and a gurney the patient is placed on right in the middle. Right next to the gurney where the patient lies is usually a massive monitor on which the x-ray images captured are projected in real time. It looks like a room that has had its soul scrubbed off with disinfectant. In every cath lab, one of the walls is made of soundproof glass, outside of which there are doctors and nurses usually looking on, offering commentary when things are smooth and scampering for reinforcements when all hell is breaking loose.

For me, the cath lab experience was almost like the culmination of a long pilgrimage. As a medical student, like so many, I was fascinated by the cath lab, and yet no matter how enthusiastic I was, how competent, I could only see; I could never touch. I always found myself sitting in the control room, across from the glass wall behind which the interventional cardiology team was busy at work, always feeling so close and yet so far.

The cath lab is not like surgery in how direct and visceral it is. In cardiac catheterization, long plastic catheters are inserted through the arteries in either the wrist or the leg and snaked all the way up to heart, where they are manipulated by tiny, precise movements and rotations, with the fingers holding the ends of the catheters or wires outside the body. Getting the end of a two-meter-long catheter to move exactly the way you want it to while holding its distant other end is easier said than done, and in the right hands, it is an art form.

When I first entered the cath lab, I was overwhelmed by the instruments that I had to master. It was like I had been given a pack of feral dogs to train who had no intention of listening to anything I had to say. I also had difficulty just getting the catheter into the artery. Often when I was initiating an attempt to get an IV into a patient's femoral artery, their groin intimidated me like a blank page does an author with writer's block. If I stuck the artery with the needle too high, there was a risk of causing bleeding into the back, forming something called a *retroperitoneal hematoma*. If I stuck the artery too low, I could introduce the catheter into a smaller part of the vessel, causing a partial tear of the artery, creating a pseudoaneurysm. Sometimes these complications could be relatively benign, and at other times patients could require emergency surgery and, in extremely rare circumstances, even die. The promised land where the femoral artery can be safely accessed is therefore only a few millimeters across.

During my training in the cath lab, I thought I would learn all there was about how to manipulate catheters and perform these procedures. And yet what I learned was far beyond that. The cath lab taught me that everything we do has consequences. In the lab, an errant movement, a lapse of concentration, a hint of frustration or fatigue, can weigh one down like a lifetime of having to wear the lead suits while doing these procedures. These suits can weigh up to fifteen pounds and are meant to protect the medical staff from the radiation of the x-ray machine.[5]

I remember once I briefly advanced a wire only 0.035 inches in diameter into a coronary artery rather than the safe embrace of the aorta. Rarely, a wire can cause a tear in a coronary artery, resulting in what can be a massive heart attack. While no damage was done, as I immediately pulled back the wire, those were some of the longest, most anxiety-provoking seconds of my life. The attending cardiologist standing next to me took over the procedure. The technician standing next to me knew how I felt beneath the visor, mask, and sterile hat and suit I was wearing. "It's okay," he whispered.

The cath lab teaches us that the time to act is not when there are no consequences but when inaction is the greatest consequence itself. For me, the cath lab was a reminder of what we physicians can achieve for patients in their darkest hour of need. My mind goes back to the night when I was a resident in the cardiac intensive care unit—a woman who had just turned fifty arrived at the emergency room after a cardiac arrest. She had ST segment elevations so tall on her EKG from the heart attack that had caused her heart to stop beating that they resembled the waves painted by Hokusai. Connected to a ventilator, with a mechanical pump keeping her blood flowing because her heart wasn't up to it, an interventional cardiologist relieved her left anterior descending artery of the grim thrombus lodged in its neck. The woman did not live long afterward, but long enough for her son, a Marine serving in Afghanistan, to return for one final goodbye.

The cath lab also taught me the importance of awareness. "The cath lab is like a sea of adrenaline," one of my senior professors, Mitch Krucoff, told me when I was about to start a case with him. My training required me to master the sea, so that I could transform it into a still and ripple-less pond, such that I could instantly detect any errant aberration, any random wrinkle. In the cath lab, one is bombarded with information, and I had to learn to absorb all these things while at the same time devoting the greatest amount of concentration I could muster to the larger task at hand. This awareness also extends to the person performing the procedure with me. "Four hands, one mind," Krucoff frequently would say. During most of my medical training, I had been tacitly hastened under the benign guise of efficiency: present patients faster, write notes faster, and scroll through patient records faster. The cath lab faculty taught me to slow down.

The third lesson that the cath lab taught me was about the importance of forgiveness. One time I was trying to get access to the artery but kept failing. Although the rest of the case went smoothly, Dr. Krucoff sat me down after the procedure. I had to learn to forgive myself, he told me. For almost anyone who ever makes it as a cardiologist, so much has to go right in life. For most, this means having good grades in high school and college, getting admitted to medical school, and working one's way through a challenging residency before matching into cardiology, the most competitive subspecialty in medicine. Anyone who makes it through a journey such as this is not used to failing, struggling, or not knowing.

What is remarkable about the cath lab is its literal transparency. Every wiggle, every movement is there on jumbo screens for all to see and judge. It is one of the few places where doctors cannot hide their deliberations in their opaque minds or veil their thoughts with jargon or shrug away any questions with vigorous hand waving. Far from distancing us from our colleagues and our patients, it is a place where everyone truly undertakes a shared journey, for better or for worse.

With these Zen thoughts in my head, I was speaking to a patient and his wife. He had served in the Second World War, had so many stories to tell, but today he was telling me about the pain that woke him up from sleep and brought him to the hospital. Despite his age, he looked pretty good—there was something about veterans I treated and met at the Veterans Affairs hospital, something about their fortitude that was special. Nothing could break them, least of all age. It was hard not to feel the love the couple shared with each other. The wife was worried, but he wasn't having any chest pain anymore and was as comfortable in the chair across from me as he would be sitting on his patio flying paper planes in the wind. "He will be okay," I told her, looking into her eyes.

Soon the patient was wheeled into the cath lab, and he stood up and lay himself on the table. The cath lab techs cleaned him up and unwrapped the large sterile drape covering most of his body, leaving his face exposed so he could breathe. I walked up to his wrist, but while I was putting the catheter up his radial artery, he started having chest pain. He went totally pale, translucent almost. The ripple-less sea had arisen from its deep sleep, and adrenaline was leaping in torrential waves, reaching all the way up to the sky, falling back down like the monsoon rain.

A tall, lanky cardiologist rushed in from the control room and took over the procedure. I stepped back and started to coordinate the medical treatments the patient was receiving. Otherwise, I knew I would just be in his way. Within moments, the cardiologist had maneuvered the catheter all the way up to the patient's coronary arteries. The first picture he took made my heart stop. Instead of plush, free-flowing arteries that wrap around the heart like fingers holding a grapefruit, there was a stump that ended abruptly almost as soon as it began. The interventionalist guided a wire up the belly of the catheter, hoping to make it past the clot that had closed off all blood going to the heart through the left main coronary artery. He did so with impeccable concentration, guiding the rickety shanty through the gale-force winds. He snaked the wire past the clot, but the patient's sudden struggle abruptly ended, and his writhing body went flaccid—his heart had gone into a standstill.

I jumped on his chest and started doing chest compressions as the interventionalist continued the procedure. Additional staff rushed in to start giving the patient breaths with a face mask. The interventional cardiologist wormed the wire down the left anterior descending artery that wrapped the heart all the way down to its tip and then back up. Even as I performed chest compressions, causing the patient's body to rock violently, he kept working, methodically placing stents as he came back up the artery, adorning it with a full metal jacket. If cardiac catheterization was art, this was Jackson Pollock violently slinging paint at a defenseless canvas. From a purely technical viewpoint, this was one of the most skillful displays of instrumental mastery I had seen. And yet, this was a masterpiece that would never see the light of day—the patient passed away.

As soon as he died, the room fell still. My eyes met those of the interventional cardiologist who had been performing the procedure. As a trainee, I lived by every word of encouragement, collecting every "Good job!" like gold coins. Every nod of approval, every look of trust I could earn was meaningful. And yet right then, I found myself being the one to offer comfort. As the commotion of the code and procedure receded, now came the hardest part: the walk to the patient's awaiting wife.

To this day, I think back about meeting the couple before the procedure. I seemed to have gotten carried away into their world, thought of them more as family, as people I cared for much longer than that being the first time we had ever met. Should I have told her he would be okay? I am still not sure.

—⟋⟍—

I met my friend Sajjad right after I had started research in Boston after graduating from medical school. He was a cardiac surgeon and one of the mildest-mannered people I knew. He was a keen observer and liked nothing better than to be a fly on the wall, far from the spotlight but always within earshot. I felt like I didn't really know him until one day I saw him in the operating room cut open someone's breastbone with a serrated electric saw. The violent sound of the saw cracking through the person's chest filled the entire room. He was staring right at the patient's bone splitting open, knowing full well that the slightest waver could send the saw straight into the patient's heart beating just underneath.

As he cut the patient open right down the middle, Sajjad wasn't about to start some rare, esoteric procedure—he was only performing one of the most commonly performed surgeries in the world.

Every year, hundreds of thousands of Americans, and millions more around the world, undergo coronary artery bypass graft (CABG) surgery. This surgery goes by many names, including bypass surgery, heart bypass, and open-heart surgery, but to those who have to say its name every day, it's simply called "cabbage." Many famous people over time have had this surgery performed. On the last episode of his TV show *Larry King Live*, Larry King told his guest, Bill Clinton, "We're both in the zipper club." Clinton laughed loudly, but several minutes later, King was asked by the "suits" to clarify what he'd meant by the "zipper club"—they had both had CABG surgery—after which "they have to zip you up again." This unfortunate double entendre notwithstanding, CABG is one of the most well-known operations a human being can undergo, and perhaps no one has spoken more loquaciously about being "cracked open like a lobster" than David Letterman.

Heart disease was not a stranger who happened upon Letterman in a dark alley on a rainy night. Heart disease first visited his home decades ago, taking Letterman's dad away for good suddenly when he was still in his fifties. Only five weeks after his surgery, Letterman hosted his first show back and told the audience, "After everything I have been through, I am just happy to be wearing clothing that opens in the front."

Letterman was in as good health as you could imagine and ran six miles at a stretch without issues the day before he had a cardiac catheterization performed on January 14, 2000. As the images of his coronary arteries started to show up on the screens next to him, he told the audience, "In my left main artery, [there was] a hand grenade."

His first guest, Regis Philbin, asked, "Were you shocked when they said you have to have a quintuple [bypass], and did they give you time to think about it or did they just strap you down and do it?"

"I had one of these [coronary] angiograms two years ago, and I was lucky, and they said everything is fine, keep an eye on it. I kinda had a feeling I wasn't gonna be lucky on this one. I just had a feeling you may not be lucky twice on this."

He was immediately scheduled for a CABG, and within days, the surgeons "redid [his] plumbing." Seven years later, Regis himself would have unfavorable results from a stress test and would also need CABG surgery.

When it became clear that heart attacks occurred because of restricted blood flow to the heart, that in some ways it was a matter of the piping gone bad, surgery seemed to be the intuitive way to restore free-flowing blood to the heart. The first stab, no pun intended, was taken by Alexis Carrel (1873–1944), one of the most fascinating men in the history of medicine.[6] When Carrel was but a medical student in Lyon in France in 1894, the then president of France, Sadi Carnot, was stabbed by an anarchist at a parade in front of his very eyes. The president was rushed to the hospital, but the surgeons there could do nothing more than watch him bleed to death because they didn't know how to sew together severed blood vessels. Alexis was distraught but didn't turn to any of the senior professors in his medical school for answers because he knew they didn't have them. Instead, he went to the most famous dressmaker in town and learned the art of suturing from her. And while his career took a downturn, as his early success earned him many enemies, leading to his exile to Canada, he eventually made his way to the United States to become the most accomplished surgeon of his time. Among his myriad accomplishments, in 1910, Alexis was the first surgeon to ever attach a blood vessel to a dog's coronary arteries, though that procedure ended in failure.

Surgeons knew that somehow, if only they could reroute blood to the diseased coronary arteries, all would be well and gay. Over the years, surgeons sutured the chest muscles to the heart, the lining of the intestines, and even the lung in hopes that they could improve the supply of blood to the heart.[7] Others tried to irritate the covering of the heart, the pericardium, with things like talc, sand, asbestos, and even ground beef bone in the hope of having new blood vessels form. Eventually, though, it was discovered that you didn't have to go far looking for the perfect blood vessel to support the diseased coronary arteries. That blood vessel is the left internal mammary artery (LIMA), also called the left internal thoracic artery, a long artery that runs north-south right behind the heart and can easily be sutured onto the main coronary artery of the heart. The LIMA is the autobahn of arteries.

Surgeons were eager to help patients with angina, and they designed a procedure called *internal mammary ligation,* in which the internal mammary arteries were tied off, redirecting blood back toward the heart, which would help patients with chest pain. Turns out that when they did this procedure, they were right; almost everyone who received this procedure had significant improvements in angina. An effusive article in *Reader's Digest* in 1957, "New Surgery for Ailing Hearts," proclaimed the benefits of this procedure, leading many at that time to ask why there were still some people with chest pain who had *not* had their internal mammary artery tied off.[8] This article, in one of the most widely read publications of its time, was far more influential than any research paper could ever hope to be. The procedure was relatively simple, done with only local anesthesia, and needed a small incision over the ribs.

So why doesn't anyone do this ligation procedure anymore? Well, an incredibly forward-thinking trial published in 1959, which involved more than a generous sleight of hand, is why.[9] Patients, enthusiastic about having this ligation to rid themselves of crippling chest pain, were enrolled in a study and "the patients were told only that they were participating in an evaluation of the procedure." What were they not told? Well, they weren't told about the most important aspect of the study. When the surgeons opened up the patient's chest, they were handed an envelope by researchers containing a note telling them whether to ligate or not ligate the artery while the patients were blinded by a curtain and were never told whether they had gotten the ligation or not. After the procedure, the doctors treating these patients were not told either whether their patient received the ligation. In essence, the patients who didn't receive the ligation received a sham procedure. This small trial that only included seventeen patients, nine of whom received nothing but an incision over their chests, would shape not only how we treat chest pain to this day but has had major implications for patients and research ever since. The trial showed no difference in outcomes or symptoms between patients receiving the ligation and those receiving the sham procedure.

Internal mammary artery ligation died a quiet death after this study, but the role of the internal mammary arteries in the surgical treatment of heart disease was only just beginning. In fact, the left internal mammary artery forms the centerpiece of modern CABG surgery.

The idea behind CABG surgery is very simple: provide parts of the heart not receiving enough blood due to atherosclerosis in the coronary arteries an alternate source of oxygenated blood. Surgeons therefore use other blood vessels that directly connect the aorta to the patient's coronary arteries, beyond the blockage, which is essentially bypassed.

So in a CABG procedure, surgeons take the lower end of the LIMA and suture it commonly to the left anterior descending artery past where it is most blocked, and it therefore provides a rich supply of blood to the heart. For other blockages in other coronary arteries, veins are taken from the leg and are used to connect the aorta to the coronary arteries. Compared to these leg veins, the LIMA is an artery that remains wide open way longer because of its almost magical ability to not develop atherosclerosis. The LIMA is such a vital part of this procedure that it is the main reason CABG surgery can prolong lives in patients with severe atherosclerotic heart disease.

CABG surgery has been around for a while, and at least in recent years, the procedure hasn't changed much. Almost always, the surgeons make an incision in the middle of the chest, through the sternum. As you can imagine, performing surgery on microscopic vessels supplying the heart can be challenging when the heart is jumping like a jackrabbit. Therefore, what really allowed all types of heart surgery to take off was the discovery of the heart-lung machine, allowing surgery to be performed on a heart that is perfectly still and completely bloodless.

How does the heart-lung machine make it happen? Clamps are placed across the blood vessels, bringing blood both back to and from the heart, essentially isolating the heart. This blood, taken from the large vein draining into the heart, is rerouted to a machine that adds oxygen to the blood and returns it back to the aorta. At the same time, the heart is bathed in a fluid that basically causes the heart to be paralyzed so that its oxygen requirements can be minimized. Therefore, the heart-lung machine cleans the field for surgeons, allowing them to make magic happen. Yet every second on the heart-lung machine is critical because it is associated with an increasing risk of damage to the brain, the kidneys, and the heart itself. Therefore, the moment the body's circulation is circumvented, the clock starts and surgeons get to work. However, even when modern techniques were developed to perform CABG surgery without use of the heart-lung machine, there was no advantage to performing the surgery on a beating heart.[10]

The good news, though, is that CABG is getting safer and safer every year. With one in ten people never making it out of the hospital when the procedure first became mainstream, nowadays that's down to one or two in one hundred. Stroke is the most dreaded complication, occurring in 1–2 percent of people undergoing the surgery.[11]

CABG surgery reached its peak in the year 2000, when half a million Americans joined the zipper club every year. That number, though, is now down to about two hundred thousand people a year, with CABG now being performed in older and sicker patients. In fact, all cardiac surgery procedures of all sorts have plummeted, and the number of medical students signing up to train in cardiac surgery is nowhere near what it used to be.

What stole cardiac surgery away from its time in the limelight? It all started with a stunt, followed by a serendipitous mistake, and finally, by a contraption literally put together in a kitchen sink. Despite what poets or lovers would have you believe, the only way to ever see another's heart, for most of human history, was usually after they had died. While out on a drunken night with friends, Werner Forssmann, then a young surgical intern in Germany, had other ideas.

In the annals of heart disease and science, littered with misanthropes and megalomaniacs in equal measure, Werner Forssmann stands out. By all accounts, particularly as a young man, he was just a dude. While many academics' biographies and descriptions suffer from an overabundance of descriptions such as *meticulous, rigorous,* and *persistent,* the one word that recurs in accounts of Werner from when he was a young man is *reckless.*

Anyone who gleans their observations about the inner lives of scientists from television or movies might come to the conclusion that some amount of recklessness is an important ingredient for a scientist. In blockbuster films like *Jurassic Park* and *Planet of the Apes,* impassioned scientists go rogue with what can be mildly described as unintended consequences. In real life, though, rogue scientists usually produce rogue findings, one-offs that produce dead ends that are rarely reproduced. In science, rogue scientists are copying-and-pasting figures, fudging their findings, and abusing their research assistants.

Werner Forssmann frequently touched human hearts, but that was mostly with them splayed open on the autopsy table. In his memoir published in 1972 and translated into English in 1974, he recalled one of his mentors once telling him, "People are evil and stink; corpses just stink."[12] However, Forssmann was just a dude not content with merely touching the dead heart but one who boasted to friends that he would be the first man to touch his own heart. How was he gonna do that?

After witnessing veterinarians insert plastic catheters in the neck veins of horses, Forssmann had a slightly more radical idea—he was going to place a catheter in the arm vein of a patient and snake it back to the heart. There were no catheters available for such a procedure, so he told his boss that he would use a urinary catheter. This was an absurd idea given that urinary catheters are much larger than anything that could reasonably be inserted into a small vein. His request was rebuffed, but Forssmann wasn't hearing no for an answer. Needing a witness for his feat, he convinced a nurse to be a guinea pig. While she was getting all set to have the urinary catheter inserted in her arm, right at the elbow, she realized that Forssmann had fooled her, and instead he inserted the catheter up his own vein. Now with about two feet of catheter reaching all the way to the upper chamber of his heart, the right atrium, the rest dangling outside, along with the help of the nurse, he went to the x-ray suite, where he had the bemused radiologists take an x-ray picture. Forssmann was chastised for his subversiveness, and his dream of being a cardiologist died. He was completely ostracized from cardiology and he went on to pursue a career involving much more appropriate placements of urinary catheters: urology. Yet, despite the change in career paths, he published the picture of the catheter going up from his arm and into his heart in *Klinische Wochenschrift*, Germany's most prestigious medical journal, in 1929.[13]

Forssmann's career and life took an obtuse turn after he joined the Nazi Party in 1931 and he became, at least by his own accounts, a reluctant instrument of the Nazi Party's brutal experiments and executions. A few decades passed that pushed him only further out into the margins and beyond until one day, in 1956, he was sitting in a pub when he got a phone call. His wife let him know someone had called and was asking for him, but he blew it off. Only when he went in for work the next day did he realize what that call was about—he had been awarded the Nobel Prize in Medicine.[14]

In the time that Forssmann had fallen far from his childhood ambitions of being a cardiologist, unbeknownst to him the field had moved forward in leaps and beyond, inspired in large part by that solitary x-ray picture of the urinary catheter in Forssmann's arm. Two major advances had been made; first, catheters had been designed to measure pressure in the heart and vessels, which then provided critical insights into how the heart was functioning; and second, catheters had been equipped to deliver dyes that could be used to visualize cardiac structures and blood vessels under x-ray machines. The long-held dream of being able to see the human heart as it was, that boisterous busy bee, without having to maim or kill its proprietor, was finally realized.

There was, however, one part of the heart that remained off limits. André Cournand, the French physiologist who had moved to the United States and had shared the Nobel Prize with Forssmann, reported that almost every animal that had contrast injected into their coronary arteries had died.[15] So even as cardiologists were able to inject contrast into the left ventricle, the aorta, or other large structures, they tried their very best to stay as far away as possible from the coronary arteries. Yet this meant that perhaps the most important part of the heart, the site of life-snatching atherosclerosis plaques and ruptures, remained a mystery. And while it took a goofball stunt to perform the first cardiac catheterization, the first successful coronary angiogram—the visualization of the coronary arteries supplying the heart—occurred because of the other recurring event in scientific history—the serendipitous mistake.

If Werner Forssmann was an anomaly in the history of science—an intern who reached for the unreachable, got lucky, and never struck gold again in his entire life—F. Mason Sones was similar to the mold of many of the acclaimed academics in whose footsteps he was following. An obsessive man whose desire for control made him fatally allergic to delegation, he was described as the "stormy petrel of cardiology."[16] Sones was a cardiologist in the Cleveland Clinic, where he was pioneering the use of cardiac catheterization. Yet even the most exacting investigators need a lucky break.

On October 28, 1958, Sones injected dye into a young man's aorta while simultaneously taking x-ray images in the cath lab. Yet as soon as the contrast was injected, the catheter popped right into the patient's right coronary artery, discharging its load into the coronary artery, which became fully opacified on the large x-ray screen. "We've killed him!" yelled Sones as he leaped for a scalpel, preparing to cut the patient's chest open, as he was expecting that the patient would go into a malignant arrhythmia. The patient wasn't in ventricular fibrillation, but he had flatlined, with his heart completely still. The patient was still conscious and Sones had the presence of mind to ask the patient to cough, which helped restart the heart without any further incident.

Sones was shaken but understood the gravity of what had happened. He reached out to others who had inadvertently pushed contrast into coronary arteries but only heard horror stories. Yet Sones was determined to do it right, because he understood that being able to actually see what's inside the coronary arteries could be an epochal advance, though even he likely didn't foresee what lay ahead. Years later, he wrote in a letter, "With considerable fear and trepidation we embarked on a program to accomplish the objective." Instead of using the 40–50 cc of contrast that he had been using for the aorta, he used a much smaller dose that adequately filled and opacified the coronary arteries without sending the patient into cardiac standstill.

Coronary angiography immediately started to provide an intimate understanding of heart disease in ways that could have only been imagined previously. Suddenly, it became possible to not only visualize atherosclerosis in the coronary arteries—manifested by its buildup in the inner lining of the vessels, leading to narrowing of the blood vessel—these plaques were followed over time to see how they evolved. Furthermore, coronary angiography, even though it would replace much of CABG surgery, actually allowed cardiac surgery to be performed appropriately in the first place. Before coronary angiography, the procedure du jour for chest pain was called the Vineburg procedure, in which the LIMA was implanted directly into the heart's muscular wall.[17] The thought was that the artery would lead to the development of small blood vessels that would help provide oxygen to the ailing heart. Yet Sones's coronary angiograms showed that development of such collateral vessels was nothing more than wishful thinking. The debunking of the Vineburg procedure would make way for modern CABG surgery, in which the LIMA and other grafts are sutured directly into the coronary arteries past the point of the most severe blockage as assessed on a coronary angiogram. All this progress came at a price, as Sones was unable to spend time with his family and was eventually divorced, and over time he became "more irascible."[18]

While coronary angiography had allowed for diagnoses to be made and for CABG to be appropriately performed, there was an inherent sense of helplessness felt by cardiologists who, despite being able to take really pretty pictures, were able to do little else to help patients. At the tail end of his career, Mason Sones attended a presentation by the German physician Andreas Gruentzig at the annual conference of the American Heart Association in 1977. In his kitchen sink, Gruentzig had developed a contraption that could do what Sones had always dreamed of—to not only document atherosclerosis but to treat it. After Gruentzig's presentation ended, Sones rushed to greet him with tears of joy streaming down his cheeks. After taking on the baton from one German, Sones would now pass it back to another. Gruentzig's contribution to heart disease, however, was no fluke and no act of serendipity—it was the result of years and years of meticulous planning and obsessive conviction.

Born in Dresden, Germany, in 1939, Gruentzig was no dude like

Forssmann and was certainly not a grouch like Sones. He was an artist who had the ways of an avant-garde indie filmmaker. He was a charmer, a "master of the moment," a beautiful man who oozed style, perhaps most when he was in the cath lab.[19] While doing cardiac procedures, a colleague described, "his cap was tilted to the side of his head as a signal to the world that he was accustomed to defying life's obstacles."[20] His "magnificent hands," a staff member said, were "big, strong, expressive and beautifully shaped. Even covered with surgical gloves, they conveyed character."

Gruentzig's father, a meteorologist, went missing during the Second World War, and Gruentzig and his brother were raised by their mother by herself.[21] After a brief detour to be close to relatives in Argentina, his mother moved the family back to Leipzig, Germany, before Gruentzig had to leave his mother behind in East Germany right before the communists closed the border along the Berlin Wall.

During a brief detour for public health research in London, Gruentzig's interest in atherosclerosis lit up. At the time, Gruentzig found it "fascinating" when one of his patients wondered if, instead of drug treatments or undergoing complex coronary bypass operations, it would be possible to just "clean" his obstructed arteries, "like a plumber cleans tubes using wire brushes." Inspired in part by work that Charles Dotter, a radiologist, had pioneered in Oregon, Gruentzig was determined to develop means to alleviate blockages occurring in arteries due to atherosclerosis. He began with introducing catheters into diseased blood vessels, literally pushing plaque down the blood vessel to create openings almost exactly like a plumber would. He began by using this procedure for blockages in people's leg arteries, and even as it produced impressive results, Gruentzig's superiors were "upset that someone would try to attack diseased arteries by forcing catheters into areas of narrowing."

However, one day he thought that a better way might be to squeeze the plaque into the vessel walls, like "footprints in the snow." This was a risky endeavor—blood vessels are fragile things and can easily be ruptured; therefore, too much pressure from the inside could tear them open, leading to catastrophic bleeding. But if there wasn't enough pressure pushing the plaque, the procedure would not be useful, as the obstruction would either not be relieved or it would recur. Gruentzig figured that he could achieve this by introducing and then inflating small balloons in atheroscleric vessels. The balloons had to be thin enough to be maneuvered into arteries only about 3 mm wide yet stout enough to be able to pry open the vessel. Gruentzig's daughter, who had food on the same table that he designed his equipment on, considered the balloons her twins.

It took hundreds of experiments and modifications on his kitchen table on nights and weekends, and collaborations with engineers and chemists and other specialists, for Gruentzig to finally come up with a sausage-like balloon that could be inflated at the far end of a thin catheter. Before he took aim at the heart, he began in relatively safer waters. Fritz Ott, a sixty-seven-year-old gentleman, had crippling pain in his leg that was due to a severe obstruction of the large femoral artery in his leg. Gruentzig reportedly spent an hour explaining the procedure to him, and on February 12, 1974, he performed a balloon angioplasty procedure in Ott's leg. He introduced the balloon into his leg artery through an incision in the groin and then blew up the balloon across the part of the artery where the blockage was tightest, and then he repeated this throughout the blocked parts of the artery until it was as close to normal looking as possible on the x-ray images. This was the first time this procedure had ever been performed, one that is done in an almost similar manner to this day more than forty years later. Fritz Ott, who almost certainly would have had his leg amputated, walked out of the hospital on his own two feet.

Gruentzig, spurred by his success, now took aim at the heart. He designed new balloon catheters specifically for the coronary arteries and first tested them in dogs who had their coronaries ligated. He watched the wires pinching the arteries from the outside break with his balloon being inflated on the inside. When he shared these findings at a conference in Miami, of course he wore an ascot while doing so. Spencer King, a professor and cardiologist at Emory University, was presenting his research there, too, when a colleague told him he should go see the research being shown by Gruentzig.

When I spoke to Spencer King, he clearly remembered what he had told Gruentzig many years back: "This will never work."

Gruentzig continued to demonstrate admirable restraint, and after he returned to Zurich, he first started with trying the procedure in anesthetized patients receiving CABG surgery. Having successfully performed this procedure, he finally found a young man who he thought would be the perfect patient to perform this procedure on.[22] Adolf Bachmann was thirty-seven years old, an insurance salesman with crippling angina, and he was going to get a CABG for a solitary tight lesion in the neck of his left anterior descending artery. The evening before his CABG, though, Gruentzig walked into his room and provided a detailed description, which included illustrations, of both CABG and the balloon angioplasty procedure that he hoped to do. "He told me he's never done the procedure in a human being before," Bachmann said in an interview. "I would be the first patient in the world to have this operation!" His description was so thorough and convincing that Bachmann was "100 percent convinced that it [the angioplasty] would be successful!"[23]

When Gruentzig started the procedure, there was an electricity in the air, with throngs in attendance. Through a nick in the right groin, he inserted the long plastic catheter into Bachmann's femoral artery. The catheter moved up the femoral artery until it merged into the aorta, which went up his chest and then arched down to his heart. Every movement was being captured on an x-ray machine. But the most important few seconds would be when Gruentzig would dilate the balloon in the coronary artery, completely filling it and hoping to push the plaque into the vessel wall. He had no idea what would happen with no blood flowing down the coronary artery while the balloon was inflated. There were also many who feared that the balloon dilation would just cause the plaque to shower downstream, resulting in even more blockages. Yet when the balloon was actually dilated, there was no chest pain, no ST elevations, no ventricular fibrillation. The tightening in the coronary artery was relieved, and celebration ensued. Bachmann was so excited he called a newspaper right from the hospital and a reporter showed up, but Gruentzig convinced the reporter to delay the story until the first scientific report was published in *The Lancet* in 1978.[24] Then, of course, all hell broke loose.

Gruentzig soon became one of the most recognized and successful clinician-scientists of his time. He was very generous with distributing credit to those like Dotter and Sones, who had done the foundational work that allowed him to perform the world's first peripheral and coronary balloon angioplasty. He was also enthusiastic about passing his knowledge forward, holding very well-attended courses in which he taught people from around the world his technique. And yet, Gruentzig also accumulated enemies, the most vociferous of whom were actually closest to his home in Zurich. "He told me he was dissatisfied with Zurich," said Spencer King, who pulled off a coup by recruiting Gruentzig to Emory University in Atlanta, Georgia, where he moved in 1980. King's boss was initially hesitant. "Willis [Hurst] said, 'Don't get involved with him; he is a prima donna,'" though his opinion changed quickly. "It probably took Willis Hurst ten minutes to become an enthusiastic supporter."

At Emory, Gruentzig continued to shine, inviting people from all over the world to witness him perform balloon angioplasties in the cath lab, which were transmitted into an auditorium right next door. Not all cases went the way they had been planned. There was a patient with a discrete lesion in his LAD, similar to the one Bachmann had. "After he blew the balloon up, everything went down, CPR was started, and the transmission was closed," said King, going on to joke, "We saved a lot of lives because we convinced half the audience to never do this procedure!"

After the move to America, "he evolved from a guy living in a flat above a bike shop with his psychoanalyst wife" into a flamboyant and extravagant man. He and his first wife got divorced, and he married a medical student at Emory. He bought expensive houses and became very ostentatious yet, according to King, "his commitment to the patients, and his commitment to investigation never changed."

Spencer King has vivid memories of his time with Gruentzig, perhaps none more so than one Monday morning, October 28, 1985, when he got a call from the cath lab—Andreas had five patients waiting for procedures but was nowhere to be found.

"We called his house, but no one got back. We discovered that he had gone to Sea Island, where he had bought a house. He had become a high roller at this time."

Andreas was an instrument-trained pilot, and he and his young wife had flown down to his house on the island. King called the airport down there. "They said you'd better call the FAA. They said that you need to call the sheriff of Jones County, Georgia, just north of Macon."

When he got ahold of the sheriff's office, King received ominous news. "There have been reports of a plane crash. We are trying to reach it with bulldozers—you'd better come down." When King reached the site, there was nothing left. Gruentzig, who was forty-six, and his wife were dead. Stuck in a freak storm, the plane had crashed, and no mechanical problems could be identified. "For those of us who knew him, it wasn't a surprise that he could die in a crash."

In the history of science, there are few who combined the unique qualities of Andreas Gruentzig. He was a brazen pioneer fully invested in his vision, and a committed physician who performed high-risk procedures. At the same time, he was never noted to be particularly aggressive and was a meticulous and careful researcher. He was also someone who loved throwing fancy parties, who would attempt climbing coconut trees in nothing but Speedos only to fail and come crashing down, who would drive up and down the Swiss Alps recklessly and with complete abandon, who even had the procedure performed on himself by his trainee and showed up at a party afterward just to tell people how convenient it was.

While Andreas died, his legacy lives on, and Adolf Bachmann's left anterior descending remains wide open as of its most recent assessment.[25] Balloon angioplasty, the relief of coronary obstruction from the dilation of balloons in the coronary arteries, however, was far from a perfect procedure. Unlike Adolf Bachmann, most patients had a recurrence of their obstruction. Balloon angioplasty was a Band-Aid at best for many patients, that literally pushed plaque aside, only to see it often plow right back. Yet it paved the way for the next great step for the procedural treatment of coronary atherosclerosis—stents.

Stents were the natural next step for coronary angioplasty since the technological road map had already been drawn. Stents are small wire frames that are fitted on to the ends of catheters and are expanded using balloons to help open up narrow parts of blood vessels. While the initial stents were made of bare metal, newer-generation stents starting around the new millennium were coated with drugs that reduced the rate of these stents closing over a long period of time by reducing the buildup of fibrous tissue within them. Stents have been shown to be invaluable and lifesaving in patients coming in with heart attacks and with severe blockages in their coronary arteries. Even as the story of stents is still being written, it has already seen more twists and turns than a John le Carré spy novel.

Every time Gruentzig treated a patient with coronary artery disease, he would use coronary angiography to first take pictures. After he had those pictures, he would look at the obstruction that he wanted to treat. Based on the length of the obstruction and how wide the blood vessel was, Gruentzig would custom build the balloon he would use for the patient on his kitchen table, discard it after use, and then build another one for the next patient who showed up.

This was an unsustainable process and was eventually taken over by large corporations, paving the way for what has today become the medical-industrial complex. Just in the United States, the medical device industry is valued at $140 billion.[26] This allows high-quality medical devices—many of which are lifesaving, such as coronary stents—to be manufactured at scale. What this also means is that the decision-makers are not researchers or clinicians but businesspeople responsible for the welfare of their shareholders. Given that there is only one metric of success—profits—there are only a few means to maximize that—cut costs, sell more stuff, and jack up the prices.

The ability to manufacture devices at industrial scale also required that consensus about their utility be developed at the same level. That has been fairly easy for the device industry to do. Doctors and hospitals are paid on a fee-for-service basis in the United States and most countries—the more devices they implant, the more they can charge patients and insurance companies—therefore, there was little if any resistance there.

Within cardiology, these forces led to a tsunami of procedures. Heart disease is not only the most prevalent disease in the world, it is also the most expensive. And it's getting only more expensive as an epidemic of cardiac imaging and procedures infiltrates every aspect of cardiovascular care. And while there is often great value provided to patients, in many cases, quality research lags far behind the technology. Even when the research arrives, much of it is generated by the industry, skewed to drive utilization of their products.

While coronary stents have been shown to reduce the risk of death in patients with heart attacks, such as those having STEMIs or NSTEMIs, many patients who undergo these procedures have stable chest pain or have a stress test that comes back positive. In the United States, for example, three hundred thousand such patients had stents placed in the hospital for "stable coronary artery disease," with others likely having this procedure as outpatients. Furthermore, there are many patients who are not so sick as to require stenting, but their illness and acuteness are inflated in the medical record, a strategy called *upcoding*, to justify the procedure so that insurance will pay for it.[27,28] "If you read the chart, no patient has stable coronary artery disease," said Spencer King, "because everyone gets coded as acute coronary syndrome [heart attack]." Upcoding by physicians, which is aided by medical billing specialists, doesn't only affect the least-sick cardiac patients who have stable angina but also the sickest patients to adjust for bad outcomes that might occur in these patients after an invasive procedure.[29,30]

To date, cumulative research showed that when compared to patients taking medications, coronary stents did not reduce the risk of heart attacks or death. Most notable of this research was the Clinical Outcomes Utilizing Revascularization and Aggressive Drug Evaluation (COURAGE) trial, funded by the National Institutes of Health and published in *The New England Journal of Medicine*.[31] The trial showed that among patients with stable chest pain but not having a heart attack, even among those with positive stress tests, coronary stents did not reduce the risk of death or a heart attack, but it did show something important: patients receiving stents had improvements in how much or how bad their chest pain was.[32]

There was one catch, though. To date, none of the studies comparing medications to stents had the procedural equivalent of a placebo—the sham procedure. In fact, it took forty years since the development of stents for the first trial comparing stenting to a sham procedure to be completed. When results of the Objective Randomised Blinded Investigation with optimal medical Therapy of Angioplasty (ORBITA) trial were presented in 2017, it rocked the world of cardiology.[33]

Darrel Francis, the British cardiologist and researcher who led the ORBITA trial, still remembers when he first thought about performing this trial—he was in the cath lab putting a stent in a patient with stable angina. While his fellow, Rasha al-Lamalee, was trying to have him help her decide what size of stent to use for the patient, Francis, who calls himself "the ironic interventionalist," had a much more basic concern when I spoke to him over Skype. "I didn't know if putting a bloody stent was going to do anything about this angina." Rasha, however, was determined to not just let this go. "Girls tend to be more questioning, while boys tend to feel like they know everything. . . . So she decided she will do a Ph.D. on it."

ORBITA, a small but rigorously performed trial, included 230 patients who were very well treated with medications and had a very tight blockage in one of the coronary arteries. While one half received a stent, the other group also undergoing cardiac catheterization never received a stent. Neither of the groups knew if they did or did not receive the stent, nor did the teams that followed them. When the results came back, Francis couldn't believe them and had multiple statisticians analyze them.

"Everything turned to utter shit," he said. The trial showed no meaningful difference between patients receiving stents and those that didn't, not even in reducing chest pain. The trial was presented on the last day of a conference for cardiologists, when almost everyone had left. Yet even that inopportune time did not prevent this study from lighting the world of medicine up. Why? Because it attacked the fundamental idea of atherosclerotic blockages causing angina.

What explained the fact that so many patients had felt better after getting their arteries stented? "That is faith healing," said Francis, adding, "About 70–80 percent of the benefit from PCI comes from telling the patient the artery is fixed and any pain they get is some rubbish pain they don't need to worry about."

Francis faced such a backlash from the cardiology community, rooted deeply in placing stents for stable chest pain, and being completely tied both intellectually and financially to that hypothesis, that he formed a Twitter account just to contest disparagement. Instead of being on the defensive, he unleashed biting criticism of those critiquing his trial. "I was ashamed at the core intellectual level of the criticism of ORBITA," said Francis. "We had prepared for very sophisticated criticism, but that never came."

An interesting thing happened after the trial ended and patients were actually told whether they got a stent or not—85 percent went back to the hospital to have a stent placed. What drove patients to get stents even though they were no different from those who got stents? "Fear of missing out on a stent," Francis says drives this, and it all goes away after the procedure because "they now know they have a stent and everything is fine."

While many cardiologists still believe there is value in continuing to place stents for stable coronary artery disease, the data has changed others' minds. Spencer King, one of the grandfathers of coronary interventions, is one of them. "I am not bullish on the surge in interventions for stable angina," he told me over the phone. "I have thought for a long time that there would be a gradual seeping in of the idea that we are not changing these patients' prognosis, and people would be less enchanted with intervention."

In stable chest pain, stents derive their power from the power of the metaphor. We would never tolerate a blockage in our toilets, so why would we ever take a chance with our hearts, our lives? The caveat is that stents cost a lot of money, and even as they have gotten safer over time, risks such as kidney failure, bleeding (particularly when performed from the groin rather than the wrist), stroke, and death still occur, though in about 1 percent of patients.[34]

Stents are the shiny reminders of our march forward as we try to overcome heart disease. And while there are chinks in their armor, like iPhones or MacBooks, with every generation, medical devices get smaller and smarter, and the people placing them get better and better. As our stent arsenal grows more formidable, researchers developed a stent that was almost too good to be true—the stent that disappears. The problem with stents was that so many patients had severe coronary artery disease, again and again and again, that they would need dozens of stents over the years, many of which were layered within each other in the coronary arteries. What if there were a stent that could open up the coronary artery and then over time dissolve into the ether? "Too good to be true" has never stopped researchers from moving forward, and the story of bioresorbable stents has important lessons for the future of interventional cardiology.

—⋀—

The cardiac medical device industry has all the ingredients to continue its onward march—smart doctors, sick patients, and lots of innovators and entrepreneurs invested in pushing the envelope. And yet, one of the most groundbreaking advances in recent years was something perhaps more fitting in science fiction than real life—a stent that dissolves into thin air after three years. These bioresorbable stents promised to overcome some of the persistent downsides of stents, which can be the site of an immune response leading to gradual narrowing of these stents over time and, in rare cases, the formation of an acute blood clot leading to a heart attack. To prevent the formation of an acute blood clot, called *stent thrombosis,* patients have to religiously take blood-thinning drugs for up to a year after having modern stents placed. There were other possible advantages that some foresaw, including allowing the coronary artery to pulse and flex naturally, the potential to reduce future blockages that occur with permanent metallic stents, and allowing easier access to other treatment options should they prove necessary in the patient's future. Therefore, when the first bioresorbable stent was approved for use in the United States by the Food and Drug Administration in July 2016, many in the medical community reacted to the news in a way "similar to the first moon landing in terms of technological achievement."[35] Patients started showing up to clinic demanding bioresorbable stents. It was like having all the benefits of the stent without any of the drawbacks.

However, all this euphoria fizzled out when longer-term studies showed that these new bioresorbable stents were in fact worse than existing stents, resulting in a higher rate of blood clots leading to heart attacks.[36] These disappearing stents, it turned out, were disappearing into clots. Even as some kept defending them, the manufacturers pulled the plug on the entire bioresorbable stent enterprise, which vanished overnight with a poof.

The bioresorbable stent story has an important lesson for the biomedical world and for the patients who will need their products. While many are holding out for the next revolutionary technology, others have a different forecast for what could be the next big thing in cardiac procedures. "The most exciting thing in the interventional field," said Spencer King about the future of interventional cardiology, the field he raised like a child, "is that we might not have to do this if we get really good at medical therapy."

What about those with stable chest pain? Darrel Francis, the cardiologist and researcher who performed the ORBITA trial, reckons that instead of trying to incrementally improve the procedure for patients with stable angina, he wants the scientific community to focus on what he thinks is the real value of the procedure. "The main purpose of stenting is to enable [the physician] to give them [patients] the placebo effect without lying," Francis told me. "We should work more on what colors of clothes we wear, how much magnification we use to show the pictures, what words we use to instill confidence." With Darrell, sometimes I can't tell if he is joking or being serious.

What is concerning about where cardiac procedures are headed is not the technology but the forces driving this technology. Back when medicine was a cottage industry, cardiac devices were mostly developed and refined by researchers who also saw patients. Whatever was done at the bedside had consequences—some good, some bad—and the treating physician had to take ownership of both. Yet many of the men and women who are at the helm of corporations' multibillion-dollar platforms to not only develop devices but to push their agendas, market them to both patients and doctors, and shape policies. The device industry is so influential that they fund almost all the educational activities undertaken by physicians training in interventional cardiology.

Part of the appeal of cardiac procedures and devices is that they are shiny, visceral, graphic, and *sexy*. They hold the promise of instant release. Asking a patient to take statins is less sexy. So is counseling a patient to stop smoking, arranging for cardiac rehab and an exercise program, and connecting patients to financial assistance programs so that they can afford their medical care. That's why when you see a medical show on TV, you don't see anyone doing any of that.

In the future, we will continue to see a battle whose contours were laid out as soon as medical advances moved from universities to business enterprises. There is a side that urges skepticism, that urges restraint, while another promises innovations and advances. The skeptics have criticized the academics among them for having financial conflicts of interest and accused them of putting industry in front of their patients. To counter, the industry coined a new term—*intellectual* conflict of interest. In fact, the pharmaceutical industry has been successful at having prominent researchers removed from FDA advisory panels because they had previously aired doubts about the products being evaluated.[37]

The forces that wish to accelerate the development and approval of drugs and devices in the United States argue that regulations implemented by the Food and Drug Administration inhibit innovation. They frequently point to Europe, where the path to device approval used to be much less stringent. What they don't highlight is the number of harmful devices that European patients have been exposed to because of those lax standards. These devices span the spectrum from deadly and cancerous breast implants and exploding stomach balloons for weight loss to many useless or harmful cardiac devices like bioresorbable stents. Europe, in fact, having been burned so many times, is now stepping back and making their device regulations far more discerning than even those of the United States.

Therefore, as much as the future will surely see technological advances, some of which will fulfill the dream of further blunting the edge of heart disease, and many more of which will land like a damp squib or in some cases even harm patients, it will be defined by the battle of attrition between the medical device and drug industry and their paid and unpaid spokespeople, and those urging a deep breath and the need for due process and evidence of benefit before patients become live guinea pigs. What is guaranteed is the sustained militarization of academia, pitted against each other increasingly on social media.

The greatest error that can be made is in promising unswerving fealty to what is taken for fact today. The reason science was able to differentiate itself from theology in the Renaissance was that it allowed people an out from blind faith. While religion requires faith to be demonstrated before you can join the club and receive all the perks that come with it, science did not ask any such premeditation of its followers; if anything, it was built on challenging the status quo. A few hundred years later, medical science appears to be adopting much of what was characteristic of the oppressive theology it sought to break free of.

One of the core tenets of faith in modern medicine is what can perhaps most appropriately be called *the plumbing hypothesis*—that chest pain happens due to atherosclerotic blockages in blood vessels, manifesting as ischemia on stress tests, and fixed with placing stents that can relieve the obstruction. While such a hypothesis might be valid during a heart attack, there is no compelling reason to worship the plumbing hypothesis for patients with stable chest pain.

The reason people believe in the plumbing hypothesis is because it is "biologically plausible"—why wouldn't an atherosclerotic plaque that narrows the lumen of an artery cause chest pain, since so many patients who have chest pain have atherosclerosis-laden arteries? Bioplausability, however, is the call to prayer of modern medicine—ringing in the ears of both true and lapsed believers, taking them back to the holy textbooks they read in medical school. Too many times, we are too invested in the pilgrimage that bioplausability urges us to make. Take, for example, the mnemonic that is as faithfully remembered by medical students around the world as New Yorkers do Jay-Z lyrics—MONA. Standing for *morphine, oxygen, nitrates, and aspirin,* MONA was coined to help clueless and flustered doctors and nurses remember the essential things they needed to do for patients with heart attacks.

Over time, though, even as evidence for additional treatments has mounted, that for morphine and oxygen has actually gone in the opposite direction.[38,39] Morphine impairs the absorption of medications that prevent platelets from forming clumps that can lead to blood clot formation and actually leads to worse patient outcomes. Oxygen, too, particularly when the patient's oxygen level is normal—which is the case in the vast majority of patients having heart attacks—actually increases mortality. Yet MONA continues to be an integral part of what medical students are taught just because not only is it believable that morphine and oxygen would help patients with heart attacks but because old habits die hard.

The oldest assumption in heart disease, the one that refuses to go away, is that heart disease is a man's disease. One truth is that more women die of heart disease than anything else, but there is another, one that we are now uncovering. The real truth is that even though heart disease is as common among women as men, much of how women experience heart disease is inextricably different at its very core from how men experience heart disease and how they are then treated. But that is changing, and the real facts are being uncovered not just by scientists and doctors but by the very women who have experienced heart disease, who are banding together and daring medicine to unlearn the oldest of its bad habits.

8

—⋀—

THE HEART OF A WOMAN

She had power over the most magnificent forces on Earth,
but she still didn't feel like she had power over the most important
thing of all—her own heart.

—Josephine Angelini, *Goddess*

Katherine Leon had just given birth to her second baby in 2003, and she had one thing to say to almost everyone she met. "I asked my ob-gyn, I asked my primary care physician, I asked my pediatrician, I even asked the lactation consultant why I was so tired." Since giving birth to her second son, she just felt that she had "mosquito netting over [her] eyes," she told me over the phone. Katherine's own theory was that perhaps she was too old when she had her baby, even though she was just in her thirties, but as time passed, she kept feeling "worse and worse and worse."

One day, five weeks after she had the baby, Katherine's husband came back early from work to find her in great distress. "I hate to use the word *panic*, because so many people say if it's a woman she is just having a panic attack, but I was terrified."

She found it difficult to breathe, and it didn't get better even after she used her asthma inhaler. "Something was wrong, and [my husband] was just not understanding it, until I said, 'Please just call the ambulance.'"

When the 911 crew came in, their response was very different from what Katherine had expected. "It was all very lackadaisical." In the emergency room, the staff didn't seem concerned either. For all intents and purposes, they saw a mom being hysterical. The doctors performed a few tests, including an EKG, and told her there was nothing wrong. Far from being reassured, Katherine felt more worried than ever before. "I was just sitting with my piece of tissue paper and bawling my head off."

After going home, she saw her primary care physician, who had her get an ultrasound to see if her gallbladder was angry, but that test came back normal as well. Things reached a head when one day, while bathing her babies, she had "that impending doom feeling." Reluctantly, she went back to the emergency room, but this time there was one huge difference. "I feel fortunate that there was a young woman doctor who took care of me," said Katherine. "Her reaction was totally different from the male doctors'—she knew that there was something definitely wrong." The physician decided to admit Katherine so she could get to the bottom of what was going on.

When her labs came back, her troponins were elevated, but not by much. She was scheduled for a cardiac catheterization, and Katherine was relieved. She told her doctors, "If this is gonna get the answer, we are good to go. I just wanted to get it over with."

When the procedure started, everything seemed pretty hunky-dory. "It was very lighthearted because they thought there was going to be nothing wrong with me." When the interventional cardiologist took the first picture, everything looked fine. He changed the angulation of the cameras to get a different angle. "The whole vibe changed immediately," said Katherine. The cardiologist suddenly froze. "He kind of went gray, and then he backed away from the procedure."

The cardiologist stepped out of the room without explaining anything to Katherine. From the control room, the cardiologist paged in the cardiac surgical team, calling them back in from the parking lot. When he returned, a cardiac surgeon came with him, who told her, "We are gonna fix you up."

The cardiologist told Katherine she had a 90 percent blockage in her left anterior descending artery. At this point, Katherine was more pissed off than upset. "Are you kidding me? I have two babies, and I was going to do the whole mom thing with playgroups and a jog stroller. I tried one cigarette in my life. I didn't have cholesterol issues. I didn't have blood pressure issues."

The truth is that we have almost all heard by this point that heart disease tends to be unrecognized in women. We also know that more women die of heart disease than any other disease process, just like men. But we are only now finding out, in no small part because of brave patients like Katherine, that heart disease in women seems to be at times fundamentally different from that affecting men.

Katherine didn't have atherosclerotic coronary artery disease. She had something else, now called *spontaneous coronary artery dissection* (SCAD)—in which the coronary arteries literally just tear open, causing blood flow to become obstructed. Yet back in the early 2000s, when Katherine had this disease manifest, few even believed that SCAD was a real thing. "You need to move on and enjoy your children," Katherine told me doctors had said to her. "You are never gonna meet anyone else who has this." Other doctors didn't even believe that SCAD was a real entity and told her, "Some guys are jerks—you just had plaque rupture; there is no such thing as SCAD."

Why did so many cardiologists doubt the existence of SCAD? One reason might have been because of who SCAD primarily affects. In most studies, three-quarters of patients with SCAD are women. And in some research reports, all of those affected are women.[1]

That, however, is changing. And like with so many other things where women have previously been serially disbelieved, it is women themselves who are leading the charge.

—◡—

When Martha, who was in her seventies, went to a nearby hospital with difficult breathing, she was found to have pneumonia. She was started on antibiotics and discharged from the hospital to a nursing facility. Martha, though, never really got much better, until things came to a head and she could hardly breathe. This time, she was sent to our hospital, and a quick EKG laid bare exactly what had happened. She had Q-ed out, meaning that there were Q-waves on her EKG, which meant that a few weeks earlier when she went to the other hospital, she didn't have pneumonia; she had actually had a heart attack, and now all that heart muscle had turned to scar tissue. An ultrasound of her heart revealed that her ejection fraction, a measure of how powerfully her heart was able to squeeze, had gone from being normal to being barely compatible with life.

By this point, she was so sick that there was no time to fool around. She was taken to the cardiac catheterization lab, where she was found to have such severe atherosclerotic disease in her coronary arteries that she received nine(!) stents. The stents, however, could do little to stop her from careening down the cliff. If anything, they might have pushed her further down—the contrast material used to take the pictures during the procedure is known to be toxic to the kidneys. The sheer extent of contrast needed to perform this herculean procedure caused her kidneys to fail, making her need dialysis. Her heart, though, was still struggling, and she ended up needing a balloon pump to help offload the pressure her heart was beating against. Even the pump could barely help her breathe better, and the team eventually called palliative care to come see her.

The electronic health record is one of the banes of a practicing physician's existence because most physicians spend an exorbitant amount of time documenting, when they would rather be seeing patients. Despite its ubiquity, many of the notes in the patient record provide little if any real insights into what is actually going on with the patient. Unless, of course, that note is written by a palliative care physician.

Palliative care is a specialty that focuses on symptom relief and improving quality of life in patients with serious illnesses. Often they are involved with patients at the end of life, when the benefits of more procedures, more treatments, and more visits to the hospital begin to fade. If a cardiologist's job is to make a patient's heart beat better, you could say that a palliative care doctor's is to make their soul feel better.

Most doctor notes start with a chief complaint, which is usually something like "chest pain," "SOB" (shortness of breath), or "nausea/vomiting." The chief complaint that the palliative care physician wrote when he went to see Martha was not what you usually see in the patient's note:

CHIEF COMPLAINT: "I WANT TO DIE."

Despite all the assorted interventions that had been thrown her way, Martha could barely breathe. When the palliative care doctor went to her, Martha was surrounded by her family, and yet even their presence could provide her no consolation. All Martha wanted at this point was for her suffering to end. Midway during the conversation, she couldn't even enunciate properly, and her words became garbled. At the same time, part of her body went limp, and instead of talking to Martha about how she would like to live out the rest of her days and what was truly important to her, the palliative care doctor realized that Martha was having a catastrophic stroke right in front of his eyes. Two days after suffering from the stroke, Martha's heart stopped beating—for good.

The risk of heart attacks is similar in women and men, especially at an older age.[2] Heart disease kills more women than any other disease, killing ten times more women than breast cancer does.[3] And yet, even as awareness of heart disease in women has increased, many continue to be ignorant of some of the hard facts. While there has been significant improvement in awareness, only about half of American women know that heart disease is women's greatest killer, and this knowledge is even lower among ethnic and racial minorities.[4]

Martha had a heart attack that was missed, and it is possible that an earlier diagnosis could have prevented her from dying in one of the most awful ways imaginable. Not only are heart attacks in women missed by doctors, they are missed by those who have them, too.[5,6]

Recent years have seen public health campaigns try to change that by emphasizing not only that heart disease occurs commonly in women but that *how* it occurs is different.[7] This knowledge, though, which is still being gathered, didn't just come about by accident. In fact, the history of the female heart is inextricably tied to the greater feminist movement. As women fought for their rights, their voices, they wanted to earn the right to be taken seriously, perhaps most importantly, when they were in the emergency room, telling the doctor that they were having chest pain.

Until just a few decades ago, women were barely the focus of research in heart disease. The vast majority of patients in studies were men, and it was assumed that what worked in men could just as easily be applied to women. There was no policy to ensure women were included in cardiovascular disease trials, and to date, women continue to be underrepresented in these trials.[8] Some large studies had zero women, while another study, even though it collected data from women, did not report those results in the publication.[9,10,11] It wasn't until large population-based cohort studies were performed, which enrolled all the people living in certain areas such as Framingham, Massachusetts, or Tecumseh, Michigan, that heart disease in women started to be studied effectively.[12,13] The underrepresentation of women in clinical research was due in part to fears of causing pregnancy-related complications in women of childbearing age.[14] Yet this aversion also led to generations of medications and interventions being developed that were "designed by men, for men, and perfected on men," while the safety profile in women went untested.[15]

And part of this was because of how heart disease first manifested itself. Women are much less likely to have a heart attack at a younger age than men.[16] In fact, women have heart attacks at an average of about five years after men do.[17] What this means is that when they have heart attacks, they are more likely to be older and also have other diseases. Therefore, men having heart attacks were perhaps more visible, given how many young men were dying.

What wasn't known until recently is that when young women do have heart attacks, they have a higher risk of death than men.[18] Yet as we know, men and women were never treated equally, and though progress has occurred, it has been far from enough.

The early focus on men reflected the values of society at large, which placed a lot of importance on the health of men, given that they formed the majority of the workforce. Heart disease in older people was thought to be a normal consequence of aging, with one researcher writing, "It is really a question as to whether [heart disease] should even be considered a disease."[19] The hearts of older women were even more likely to be overlooked, yet as the human life span began to extend, it became increasingly harder to ignore the growing number of women suffering from heart disease.

As some began to acknowledge that heart disease affected women as well, they also revealed their own biases. The scion of American cardiology of his time, Paul Dudley White, in a lecture in 1942, declared, "Housewives appear to have angina pectoris less frequently than do business and professional women," going on to add that coronary artery disease is "predominantly a man's disease" and "if a woman is under fifty, chest pain is probably not evidence of heart disease."[20] The term *cardiac neurosis* was used to describe women with symptoms of heart disease.[21] Case reports of patients with crippling heart disease were more focused on putting women in their place than on figuring out how to help them get better. "The cardiac housewife must avoid over-exertion," reads a paper published in 1929, though it went on to suggest "electric labor-saving devices such as washing machines, vacuum cleaners, or sewing machines will do much to decrease expenditure of cardiac reserve."[22] Another paper in 1938 on a patient with severe tightness in her mitral valve described her history quite simply: "There are two alternatives in any girl's life—to support herself or to find someone who will do it. She got married." It went on to fat-shame her by saying, "She has never denied herself the pleasures of food, and undoubtedly this injudicious enjoyment has contributed in part at least to her present condition."[23]

The reason these attitudes changed in cardiology actually has nothing to do with cardiology or medicine. The feminist movement sought to build "a worldview that values women and that confronts systematic injustices based on gender," and perhaps nowhere were women more disadvantaged in those times than when they were sitting across from a physician.[24] Not only were they weighed by all the prejudices of society, they were sick and vulnerable.

The women's health movement started, unsurprisingly, with reproductive rights. In the 1960s, almost a million women had illegal abortions performed annually, a third of whom required hospital admission for complications.[25] However, the women's health manifesto expanded far beyond that, although they still continued to experience paternalism from a deeply traditional health system. Yet women didn't wait for doctors to catch up, and instead, self-help groups began to proliferate, allowing women to assume some control over their own health. However, women were continually asked to fulfill their roles as caregivers, rather than focus on self-care. From the 1960s to the 1980s, there was a flurry of articles in magazines with titles like "How to Reduce Your Husband's Risk" and "How to Heart Attack Proof Your Husband" and public forums like "Hearts and Husbands" in which women were increasingly instructed about helping their husband's cardiac health, while totally ignoring their own.[26] Such notions were furthered by talk of the "feminine advantage" that women had in regard to supposedly lower rates of heart disease. And as women started to transition into the workforce, false notions were used to discourage them. A connection was drawn between women entering professional employment and increased mortality from heart disease due to the supposed added strain of balancing professional and domestic obligations. Aggressive and type A women were told to be particularly wary of heart attacks. Yet most of these notions represented lazy stereotypes rather than actual evidence.[27]

Initially, the women's health movement was restricted mostly to reproductive and gynecologic health, and there was at least a two-decade lag before heart health became a point of emphasis. To address the fact that there was very little known about heart disease in women, the National Institutes of Health (NIH) adopted a policy in 1986 to increase enrollment of women in clinical trials.[28] But it took a congressional investigation in 1989, led by female members of the U.S. House of Representatives, to find out that the NIH had not been following its own policy and to subsequently push all NIH-funded studies to assess gender differences. Congresswomen also ensured that NIH funding was directed toward issues particularly important for women's health, including heart disease. The goal was to move beyond thinking of women as a subset of men, but as individuals who needed to be specially studied.

One of the subtlest ways to suppress female voices in research has been the use of quantitative methods—an overreliance on numbers robs women of their unique experiences with disease. Prying our eyes open to how heart disease afflicts women required an entire new approach to research, which involved the application of a distinctly feminist research methodology.

I met a friend of mine at a party who had twins, a boy and a girl.

"How are they different?" I asked.

"Well, she really takes care of him. She will give him food. She will comb his hair."

I am no fan of gendered stereotypes, but the biologist who sees everything through an evolutionary lens will argue that tending and nurturing is wired into the female brain, so as to complement their childbearing functions. In modern society as well, caregiving is a role predominantly occupied, frequently involuntarily, by women.[29] Women outnumber men among informal caregiving by eight to one in the United States.[30] For women, this comes at a price—their own health.[31]

If you just look at the numbers, they tell you that women are less likely to take their medications.[32] Without any context, the data therefore suggests that it might actually be women's fault when they have worse outcomes. Yet an iota of human awareness will reveal that women are less adherent to medications than men not because men are more meticulous but because men often have women attending to their health, while women have no one most of the time.

Therefore, when it comes to women, numbers can provide information, but they may not tell you why that information looks that way. If anything, when used unopposed, numbers can oppress women's voices.

Numbers aren't women's best friend, and the story that numbers tell is not pretty. When women present to the emergency room with a heart attack, they are less likely to receive cardiac catheterization, particularly during off-duty hours.[33] Women referred to CABG surgery are sicker than their male counterparts and experience higher mortality rates after surgery.[34] Even when programs are created to improve the quality of care that patients having heart attacks receive, women benefit less from these programs than men.[35] Distressingly, the risk of black and white women dying within thirty days of a heart attack is 17 percent and 18 percent, while that of black and white men is 15 percent and 16 percent, respectively.[36]

Obscured by these statistics are women like Martha, whose entire life story was turned by the fact that when she had difficulty breathing, no one looked to her heart. The truth, though, is that she didn't either. How women experience illness is fundamentally different from men.

Take, for example, the simple fact that unlike men, most women can barely focus on their recovery. While for men who are discharged from the hospital, home is a sanctuary, that might not be the case for women. "When we send women home to recover," wrote the nurse and scholar Sheila O'Keefe-McCarthy, "we send them to recover in their traditional place of employment."[37] Despite massive changes in modern society, women continue to bear more responsibility for housework and caregiving. Many women feel guilty when they cannot participate in home activities. Therefore, many don't do what is needed for them to get back to good health. Family obligations and lack of time are some of the biggest reasons women give for not participating in activities that improve their health.[38]

Even when heart disease strikes, many women seek to find meaning in their malady. Qualitative research has shown that many women do not associate their heart attacks with traditional risk factors like high blood pressure or cholesterol but rather with events in their life stories.[39]

Women tend to have greater delays between when chest pain starts and when they seek cardiac care.[40,41] What drives this delay? Denial is one of the first few emotions that follow the onset of potentially life-threatening chest pain for both men and women. Even among women with family members who were afflicted with serious heart disease from a young age, many do not consider the fact that they too could be at risk for heart disease until it is perhaps too late.

How symptoms are experienced is perhaps the most powerful determinant of whether women decide to seek medical care. "It woke me slam right up. It was abrupt, heavy chest pain that radiated down my arm and neck," said one woman in a research study. "I knew instantly that I was having a problem; that it was my heart."[42] Yet even severe chest pain is not enough for some women to tell their loved ones or call 911. We know from extensive research that even when women do have chest pain, they are much less likely than men to have severe and obvious blockages in their coronary arteries that can benefit from stents or bypass surgery. One such woman in this study did not want to be "wrong again" like the last few times she had gone to the emergency room with chest pain, even though this time she had a positive stress test. The situation is further complicated by the fact that women are much more likely to have a stress test suggest a severe blockage when in reality there might be none in the large arteries apparent on cardiac catheterization.[43,44]

In reality, though, for a woman with a heart attack, having chest pain might actually be a good thing. Many more women than men having heart attacks have symptoms other than chest pain.[45] These symptoms can include extreme fatigue, nausea, vomiting, weakness, or even sleep disturbances. Women with such atypical symptoms experience much longer delays than men, simply because they don't even know they might be having a heart attack. In fact, such delays in seeking medical care and a subsequent diagnosis are an important reason why women who don't have chest pain before a heart attack do more poorly. While some of these differences may be explained by the fact that women are generally older when they have heart attacks, research shows that many more women than men with chest pain do not inform anyone of their symptoms because they don't want to "trouble others."

While it is clear that women and men don't always behave in a binary feminine or masculine manner, hegemonic gender roles appear to be preventing many women from caring for themselves rather than others.[46] Why did one woman who had severe chest pain for several days not call for help sooner? "I thought I had to make the bed, I had to make the place tidy, loading the dishwasher and stuff," she told researchers. One woman was concerned about her cardiac symptoms, but when her son had a stroke, she put that on hold. "I'm not going to say anything to anybody," she recalled telling researchers. "Let's let him get over his problem first, and then I'll deal with this."[47] Others are held back by a societal emphasis on judging women by their physical appearance. One woman having a heart attack was worried about what she would look like if she died. "[I had] no makeup on, nothing, I think my hair was unbrushed . . . ugh . . . I hadn't brushed my teeth either, that was the thing that really bothered me."[48]

The stories of women with heart disease are harder to find than those of men. While men like David Letterman can go on television and flash the long incision down their breastbones, few if any prominent women ever do. This is in stark contrast to diseases such as breast cancer, whose scars are far more visible in popular culture. This lack of visibility, as demonstrated by both the numbers and stories of women with heart disease, is having a real, human cost.

While it is clear that heart disease remains an untold story—stories on breast cancer outnumber those on heart disease in fitness magazines ten to one—what is even clearer is that the story that does get around is missing important pieces.[49] Many of the same outlets that lament that heart disease is underappreciated among women also are the greatest proponents of the traditional ideas of womanhood and feminine behavior that result in women ignoring their hearts for those of others. What is missing is that not only do many women not have the classic symptoms of heart disease, many women don't have classic atherosclerotic heart disease to begin with.

A story often repeated is that heart disease affects both men and women, and if you simply look at the statistics, that bears out to be true. Yet, and though this amounts to me stating the glaringly obvious, women's bodies are considerably different from men's. An important part of what makes women different is also what makes their hearts so different—female hormones have an immensely layered effect on their hearts. And as the story of hormone replacement therapy to reduce heart attacks in women revealed, the difference between what we think we know and the truth about the female heart could never have been wider.

For almost all of human history, men lived almost as long as women. In Boston in 1812, for example, men lived to an average of twenty-eight compared to women, who only lived to be twenty-five years of age on average.[50] Why was this the case? Well, that's because pregnancy and childbirth were more dangerous than going to war. Infections and bleeding resulted in maternal mortality being sky-high. And then things changed. Improvements in obstetric practices started to reduce the risk of pregnancy, and suddenly women started to live longer than men. And while American women lived only one year longer than men in 1920, this gap widened all the way to eight years in the late 1970s.[51] What conferred women such a stout advantage in life span?

Turned out that women were much less likely to die than men from heart disease at younger ages. And as the scourge of heart disease spread, fomented in no small part by poor diet, poor exercise, and a rise in smoking, the gap only widened. In fact, what caused men to catch up, ironically, was that smoking rates among women started to rise in the second half of the twentieth century, as women were afforded more freedoms to behave like their male counterparts. In fact, cigarettes were widely marketed around the world as the "torch of freedom," and smoking rates among women are a reliable proxy to how emancipated women in society are.[52]

What really protects women from heart disease, then? Research showed that female hormones do. And how did we know that? Because even though young women had much lower rates of heart disease, as soon as they hit menopause, their risk of heart disease quickly reached that of men's. This finding was used to frame menopause as a villain, as a flawed and diseased state, and spurred efforts to reverse the hormonal changes accompanying menopause.[53] While there were some who felt that "hormone or estrogen replacement therapy [was] a way for male-dominated medical researchers and pharmaceutical companies to fix the lack of femaleness in postmenopausal women," there was considerable evidence showing just how female hormones provided a shield against atherosclerosis.[54] More than thirty studies showed that women who used hormone replacement therapy had a lower incidence of heart disease.[55]

The Nurses' Health Study, published in 1991, followed 48,470 postmenopausal nurses for up to ten years and showed that hormone replacement led to a whopping 44 percent reduction in cardiovascular disease.[56] A small randomized controlled trial showed that markers in the blood that were associated with heart disease were lowered with hormone replacement therapy.[57] In another randomized trial, progression of atherosclerotic plaques in the arteries was slowed down with hormone replacement compared to placebo.[58] Female hormones were thought to be opening up the pipes like Drano, shrinking the plaque away. And finally, a more recent study pooling data from more than three hundred thousand women showed that those who had early menopause had a higher risk of heart disease.[59]

Therefore, starting in the 1980s, many, many women were provided long-term prescriptions for hormone replacement therapy lasting for years specifically to lower their risk of heart disease. Hormone replacement not only reduced bad LDL cholesterol but increased good HDL cholesterol; it also improved the health of blood vessels, making them less likely to prune and constrict. People often joke that we don't need a randomized controlled trial to see if a parachute works for someone who has been flung from a plane, and hormone replacement therapy was as close to a parachute as possible.

Everything changed when randomized controlled trials were conducted and published around the turn of the twenty-first century that brought this supposed parachute crashing to the ground. Randomized trials, when they were finally performed, not only showed that hormone replacement therapy provided no benefit in reducing heart disease when tested in extremely large clinical trials—it actually *increased* the risk of heart disease in addition to increasing the risk of some cancers.[60,61] All the prior data were based on either observational studies, which we know cannot assess causation, or were small trials that looked at outcomes other than what matters most to patients, such as changes in lab values.[62] A similar effect of increased cardiovascular disease is also noted in male-to-female transgender individuals receiving female sex hormones.[63] These trials completely upended the conventional thinking of its time and moved the use of hormone replacement therapy to reduce risk of heart disease from routine clinical use to one of the epic fails in modern medicine. As physician-researcher Vinay Prasad has shown, there are few practices in modern medicine that can truly be considered as effective as parachutes.

The demise of hormone replacement therapy moved the focus back from sex-specific risk factors for heart disease to factors relevant to both men and women. Recent research has started to find how even sex-neutral risk factors might have a different effect on men versus women. Take diabetes, for example, which now affects half a billion people around the world. Turns out that even after accounting for all differences, diabetes confers a much higher risk of heart disease for women than men.[64,65] The same is also true for smoking, seen to be consistently more harmful for women.[66] The combination of oral contraceptive use and smoking is particularly toxic, significantly raising the risk of blood clots and strokes.

While hormone replacement therapy to improve heart health is dead, study of the role of female hormones in heart disease hasn't abated. One of the key insights has been that early hormone replacement use in women who have just gone through menopause carries no additional risk of heart disease, as opposed to the use of hormone replacement in women who went through menopause several years earlier. Yet the greatest amount of interest is perhaps now centered on a time of unprecedented hormonal turmoil—pregnancy.

I was working in the hospital late one night when I got a page from a location I didn't recognize. That, of course, never happens; once you spend enough time in the hospital armed with a pager, you realize there are few parts of the hospital where heart disease doesn't strike. When I called the number back, I was surprised, because it was from the children's emergency room. They wanted me to help out with a teenage girl who had heart failure.

When I made my way past the flimsy curtain outside her room, I found myself standing next to a girl sitting up in bed, working hard to breathe. I was petrified—the average age of the patient hospitalized with heart failure is in the eighties—she was one of the youngest patients I had ever taken care of, but she was perhaps a whisker too old for the pediatric cardiologists.

Four weeks earlier, she had given birth to a baby boy, and today, here she was with heart failure. The baby was being rocked by a woman who looked like she was perhaps in her thirties. Elder sister? No, she was the baby's grandma.

I was trying to focus on the medical details but found myself distracted. The girl was in school, she had a baby, the dad was another kid in her school who was nowhere to be found, and now she had heart failure.

Being pregnant and giving birth is one of the hardest things one can do. When it is compounded by heart disease, it can quickly become a tragedy. The fact is that despite its ubiquity through human history, when it comes to the heart and pregnancy, there is much that we still don't know. Back in the day, part of this lack of information was because of a single drug called *thalidomide*.[67] Marketed in 1957 to help with anxiety and morning sickness, thalidomide caused about ten thousand babies around the world to be born with stunted arms and legs. While half of these babies died, the other half lived with life-altering disability. The drug was never approved in the United States because of one Frances Oldham Kelsey, a pharmacologist at the FDA, who refused the information provided by the German manufacturer because it didn't include any test results.[68] Frances rebuffed the American subsidiary six times, until reports of congenital malformations began to arrive from the world over. For her steadfastness, Frances was awarded the President's Award for Distinguished Federal Civilian Service.

Frances Oldham Kelsey's bureaucratic heroism saved thousands of American children, but the thalidomide travesty brought research in pregnant women to a screeching halt; they were excluded in most future trials, particularly early-phase research in which the safety of medications is tested. However, this policy meant that many drugs developed during those times were never tested for safety or efficacy in women, particularly those young enough to be able to have children. This policy continued until 1993, when the FDA required women of childbearing age using adequate contraception to be included in early-phase clinical trials. What this means is that there is very little safety data on pregnant women for some of the most commonly used cardiovascular drugs. Therefore, it is extremely important for women with heart disease taking these medications who are planning on getting pregnant to have discussions with their cardiologist about what medications they should and should not take.

About 1 to 4 percent of pregnant women have heart disease, and this number is creeping up, as not only do women have children at older ages but because the prevalence of risk factors such as diabetes and hypertension continues to rise.[69] Getting pregnant has a profound effect on the body, including the function of the heart. The expansion in blood volume necessitates the heart to beat both harder and faster.

One of the important effects of pregnancy is that it makes blood more likely to clot. At the same time, the risk of bleeding is also very high in pregnant women, and therefore, anytime a pregnant woman needs to take blood thinners, it can be very difficult to know what the right thing to do is.

That is how I came to know Sam. She was born with an abnormal mitral valve, which ended up being very leaky. She kept chugging along with it until she was a teenager and suddenly just couldn't keep up with the rest of the kids in her school. Ever since she was born, she and her parents knew that she would need surgery to replace her valve with a mechanical one, and that time had arrived. She got the surgery in her early teens, and over all seemed well until she got pregnant in her early twenties. She had been taking a medication called warfarin, a common blood thinner to prevent blood clots from forming around the artificial mechanical valve, ever since her surgery. However, warfarin can cause such birth defects as facial disfiguration and physical and mental growth retardation, especially when used at higher doses during the first trimester, so she had to be switched from the pills to an injectable blood thinner.

The pregnancy was unplanned; Sam was not ready to have a baby. Even from a medical point of view, she had been taking warfarin for the first few weeks while she was pregnant, and there was the risk of the fetus being affected. Her boyfriend was certainly not up to taking care of the baby. Even though she was advised against it, Sam decided to keep the pregnancy, but as time passed, she became bogged down and grew increasingly tired and winded.

She worked as an aide at a nursing home but found herself to be in worse shape than the patients she was supposed to be helping. She went to see her family physician, who placed a stethoscope on her chest. Instead of hearing the clean clicking of the mechanical valve, the family physician heard sounds resembling waves crashing into a rocky cliff. An ultrasound revealed that a massive clot had formed around her valve, blocking the flow of blood through it. Somewhere between when she was switched from the warfarin to the injectable thinner, there was enough of a window for a blood clot to form.

Sam was never ready to be a mom until she became pregnant, but the longer it lasted, the more she wanted to keep the pregnancy. She was transferred to our hospital, and we assembled a team of surgeons, high-risk obstetricians, and social workers—all of us knew that the pregnancy was too dangerous to continue, both for the fetus and Sam. Yet Sam told us, "I just want to try." She wanted to see if we could help her make it through the pregnancy.

Our best try fell apart. The obstruction in her artificial valve kept getting worse, and we could not dissolve the clot with medications. Sam's breathing started to get labored as fluid collected in her lungs. She fainted once while she was walking in the ward. Eventually, she could not stave off the difficult decision and had to have an abortion. Sam was devastated, and only a few days after losing the baby, she went back to the operating room, had her chest opened up yet again, and had a new metallic valve replace the mutilated one that was falling apart in her body. The surgeon texted the team a picture of the valve taken after it was removed that showed that it was covered in clot, and I was surprised she had made it this far.

Sam is still young but now has to live with the fact that perhaps bearing children might be something she never gets to experience. She had already had two open-heart surgeries, and there was no guarantee she would be able to make it through a third one.

For some patients, like the teenager I saw in the emergency room, the effects of pregnancy can occur even after it has ended and can last a lifetime. One to four in a thousand women who become pregnant go on to develop a condition called *peripartum cardiomyopathy*.[70] Peripartum cardiomyopathy, which disproportionately affects black women, results in a weakening of the heart and occurs mostly either at the end of pregnancy or after birth. While some women recover, some end up having heart failure for life and needing a heart transplant or a mechanical heart pump to recover.

What causes peripartum cardiomyopathy? Hormones secreted in late pregnancy such as prolactin, which helps with lactation, and FLT3, which is thought to help the placenta involute after giving birth, are thought to be responsible. Clinical trials are under way to see if any treatments that alter these hormones can help women recover from this disease.

Studying heart disease in women has opened our eyes to just how connected the heart is to the rest of the body. After initially spending years just trying to think of women as "defective males," researchers have started making inroads into opening up the myriad connections that exist between the heart and every bit of the body, ever busy producing hormones, electrical signals, and chemicals. The heart speaks to the body, and the body speaks back in a million voices. And what emerging research is only now teaching us is that of those million voices that the heart attends to, the loudest is the one coming from the mind.

If the heart has always been the beating physical force of emotion in our bodies, our minds have resided in the cool confines of the brain. The heart is the butter to the brain's biscuit. Between the heart and the mind resides our entire sense of existence, for they encapsulate our humanity.

Before we knew that the consciousness centers in the brain, though, we found spirits all around us.[71] In the trees, in the mountains, in the sun, in the moon. When we closed our eyes, we saw the spirits of others, friends and enemies in equal measures. Plato was one of the first few who conceived of the soul as we do today and used the word *mind* to represent the part of the soul concerned with reason. In the Western world, it wasn't until the Renaissance that the soul was identified with consciousness and with being. In the years since, just like we haven't been kind to our hearts, we haven't treated our minds well either.

Many believe that we live in the most stressful of times. Technology, which has made our lives easier in so many ways, has perhaps also spurred another crisis of its own. Social networks were supposed to connect us, but it seems at times that they are best designed to spread falsehoods and to create militant tribes. Motor vehicles were supposed to make it easy to move around, and yet those same cars allowed for cities to be designed in malignant ways that trap people in commutes. Medical care has extended lives but increasingly can put people into financial ruin. Cell phones were supposed to help us never get lost, but that constant connectivity means that we are disconnected from our surroundings at all times.

Many call these times *the age of anxiety*, with one scholar commenting, "Unmitigated stress seems to be threatening the health and happiness of Western populations in particular."[72] Almost fifty years ago, Alvin Toffler, an American writer, diagnosed modern society with "future shock," a mental condition we had acquired due to "the shattering stress and disorientation that we induce in individuals by subjecting them to too much change in too short a time." This state of heightened stress occurred because of the "transience of people and places, the speed of technological innovation, and the surfeit of choice in consumables, education, and the media." In his book *Future Shock*, which he coauthored without sharing credit in 1970 with his wife, Toffler predicted some of the many instruments of future shock such as the internet, antidepressants, the disappearance of traditional blue-collar jobs, and the emergence of knowledge workers. *Future Shock* laid down the blueprint of what would come to be the tentacles of modern life's unresolved angst.

Yet if you turn the pages back further, you find that the age of anxiety is not a recent phenomenon but a damningly persistent one. In 1872, an article in the *Times* lamented "the great mental strain and hurried excitement" that humanity experienced from steam engines, electrical power, urbanization, and the sheer weight of life.[73] Far from ours being the age to take hold of that distinction, a British physician had previously declared the nineteenth century the "century of stress."[74] And just as we were crossing the Industrial Revolution and were entering the age of modern ennui so, too, were we entering the era of heart disease. *Is there any chance that the two scourges of modernity—stress and heart disease—might be related?*

That is certainly what most believed—that heart disease was yet another necessary payment for modernity that we had to make. Remember that most physicians in the nineteenth and early twentieth centuries believed that atherosclerosis was a natural part of aging and that high blood pressure was essential. In 1925, a Chicago-based psychiatrist blamed "the incessant drive of American life, the excited strain of the American temperament" for the rising rates of heart attacks—a condition another psychiatrist named *"Americanitis."*[75,76]

The face of modern heart attacks were young men rising up the ranks, in their prime, running businesses, selling cigarette ads on Madison Avenue, now falling like pins clutching their chests. In a lecture presented in 1892, Sir William Osler painted the image of the typical heart patient as a "keen and ambitious man, the indicator of whose engine is always 'full speed ahead . . .' from 45 to 55 years of age, with a military bearing, iron-gray hair, and a florid complexion."[77] So not only was heart disease associated with men, it only affected the most alpha of alpha males. Therefore, the first large-scale study by Ancel Keys, the famous researcher and nutritionist, drew the link between nutrition and heart disease and was performed exclusively in businessmen in Minneapolis.[78] However, studies like the Framingham Heart Study showed that it was things like high blood pressure, smoking, and blood cholesterol that were more strongly related to the risk of heart attacks rather than mental stress.

While modern science mitigated the role of emotions with heart disease, the link has persisted in the minds of everyday people. "Don't upset them; they are a heart patient," was a frequent refrain I heard when I was little and up to no good. A relaxed and non-stimulating environment continues to be considered essential for people who have had heart attacks. What caused this heart-mind relationship to persist? For one, many people have chest pain when they are feeling worried or panicky. Just recently, Tyronn Lue, the young ex-coach of the Cleveland Cavaliers basketball team, began having chest pains due to the rigors of his work, causing him to take a break to cool off. In the emergency room, almost a third of patients presenting with nonspecific chest pain have anxiety and panic attacks, and many more of these patients are women than men.[79,80]

So even as the idea persisted among people that stress can cause heart attacks, the medical community had put this out to pasture. While a lot of patients having heart attacks were in fact very worried and tense, this was almost certainly because who wouldn't be worried if they were having chest pain from having their heart die off due to a heart attack? But before the concept could be embalmed, a new and mysterious disease emerged that filled in the blanks, charting a path all the way back to the origin of the line that connects the mind to the heart.

Life in the hospital can be likened to war, but not the war you see on TV. For doctors and nurses, their time is usually dominated by mundane paperwork, bureaucratic meetings, and helping patients through their hospitalization with hopefully no untoward incident. Sometimes, though, at times out of the blue, all the fury of hell can be unleashed and the intensity of sickness can become overwhelming. When this day arrives, it is only after it has passed that you see it for what it was.

On one such hellacious day, a woman who barely spoke any English came to the emergency room. She was sixty-one years old and had just flown in from Ecuador. Just after landing at the airport, she experienced very difficult breathing. Her family rushed her to the hospital, where an ultrasound showed that her heart looked very abnormal. The tip at the bottom of the heart, called the *apex*, usually narrows to a sliver when the heart beats, but the apex of her heart was barely moving and had ballooned out. On her EKG, she had massive ST elevations, and she was rushed to cardiac catheterization, but instead of finding a blood clot strangulating her left anterior descending, the cardiologists found her coronary arteries were as wide open as a dam after a downpour. Even though her coronaries were clean, she still had severe heart failure. Her EKG now demonstrated a pattern that no one in the hospital had ever seen before, which we later found was called *macroscopic T wave alternans*, that put her at extremely high risk for having a fatal heart arrhythmia at any moment.[81] After the procedure, she spent a few nervous days in the ICU with pads from a defibrillator connected to her chest at all times, petrified that she would have a heart rhythm necessitating those going off. What exactly did she have?

In the 1990s, cardiologists in Japan began to see a string of patients, the vast majority of whom were women, who would come to the hospital with a heart attack—with ST elevations on their EKG and elevations in troponins from heart muscle damage—yet when cardiac catheterization would be performed, there were no atherosclerotic plaques in the coronary arteries to be found.[82] However, the heart's apex seemed to be severely affected. What was causing these women's hearts to blow out? Not hypertension, not cholesterol, but some of the rawest stressors of life—death, divorce, and dislocation. The Japanese likened the appearance of this condition to an octopus trap with a globular shape but a thin neck, and this condition was named Takotsubo cardiomyopathy.

Also called *stress cardiomyopathy*, the condition occurs predominantly in postmenopausal women, and the media loves calling it *broken heart syndrome*, for it occurs frequently after a tragedy. Further investigation has shown that many times, this condition affects those who are under chronic, unrelenting stress rather than people who experience a paroxysm of brutal cosmic injustice.[83] Many patients who were diagnosed with Takotsubo described "a stressful life situation long before the onset . . . characterized by feelings of injustice and powerlessness." Many patients lived their lives constantly expecting a wrong turn, describing "a prolonged process that slowly peeled away [their] resources until they balanced on the verge of illness." One patient told researchers, "I can't fight it anymore."

How did humanity come to a point in time where our hearts are literally failing because of stress? The irony, of course, is that most of us live in times of unparalleled peace. Instead of having to embark on an unpredictable hunt for food every day, all we have to do is reach into our fridge or make a drive-through run on our way back from work. There is pervasive law enforcement and a complex judicial system that ensures that our daily lives are spent largely secure. Violence around the world, believe it or not, is at the lowest rate in history.

In times like these, it can be hard to think about the stress response for what it truly is—an essential ingredient for our successful existence. And to explain why, let me take you back, way, way back, not even to when we weren't walking on two feet but to when we were singular cells, encapsulating our entire universe within us.

A cell knows only two states—it is either active or inactive. For a cell, an active state can mean that it is moving from one part of the tissue to another. A cell's needs change when it's on the move, as opposed to when it is slouching around. Now, nature needed to come up with mechanisms to intelligently optimize cellular functions during these two states—so it came up with a catabolic and anabolic state. In catabolism, molecules are broken down into energy that can be used to *do*, while in anabolism, during times of rest, simpler molecules are turned into more complex energy stores.

For larger, more complex organisms, not all activations are equal. A special response had to be devised to optimize performance during moments when the organism's carefully balanced subsistence, called *homeostasis,* was vulnerable.[84] This included exposure to cold, starvation, pain, bleeding, infection, and/or an existential threat. Therefore, nature developed potent machinery that could activate organisms faced by such threats. Not only has a stress response *evolved* into being, research has shown that stress itself *drives* evolution by causing cells to adapt faster.[85]

Before the Austrian physician Hans Selye's (1907–1982) pioneering work, the word *stress* represented a purely physical force, one felt by the cables of the Golden Gate Bridge as they held up the mile-long suspension bridge.[86] Selye's research opened our eyes to what so many felt but failed to name. Stress, or distress, could be experienced at any time, even in people who were comatose, and elicits a system-wide response. The operators of the stress response in a human being are nerves and hormones such as adrenaline (also called *epinephrine*) and norepinephrine. The stress response increases blood flow to the brain, improves alertness and attention, and increases blood glucose, which can be used as energy.

But how can acute stress blow your heart out?[87] After an acute stressor, parts of the brain are activated that produce stimulating hormones like norepinephrine, which then stimulate glands to make hormones such as cortisol and adrenaline. At the same time, stressors also activate the sympathetic nervous system, which sends nerves down all the way from the brain along the coronary arteries, innervating the heart. These nerve endings produce norepinephrine that directly affects the heart, making it beat harder and faster.

Takotsubo predominantly affects older women because they lack estrogen, which protects against the constriction of vessels that can occur due to aberrant stressful stimulation, reducing blood flow to the heart. This constriction of blood vessels is particularly harmful at a time when the heart is working extra hard due to sympathetic overload, causing a mismatch between how much oxygen is needed and how much can be delivered, causing transient ischemia.

A surge of stress hormones released right into the heart can have a toxic effect, and given that most of these nerves are densely populated in the apex of the heart explains why the apex is routinely affected in patients with Takotsubo. Patients with Takotsubo have far higher levels of stress hormone activation than even patients who have had STEMIs.[88] In most cases, the effect on the heart muscle in Takotsubo is reversible as the stressor abates. However, one in twenty patients with Takotsubo never make it, similar to patients with STEMIs, underlining just how dangerous this condition is.

The fact is that even moments of great joy, such as winning a jackpot at the casino, the birth of a grandchild, or the wedding of a child, have been reported to result in what has been called the *happy heart syndrome*—the Greek tragedy version of Takotsubo.[89] In fact, people are 27 percent more likely to have a heart attack on their birthday than on other days.[90] And while the happy heart syndrome is much rarer than the broken heart syndrome, it points to the underlying link between how we feel and how that touches our hearts.

Takotsubo cardiomyopathy is the most dramatic illustration of the direct effect emotions can have on the heart. And while people have reported to have had this syndrome after being stuck in a bathtub, crashing a plane in a flight simulator, or being stuck in traffic, the most commonly reported cause of Takotsubo is not the death or illness of a close person or a fiery argument, it is something seemingly much more benign—stress at work.[91]

Takotsubo, though, is only the tip of this treacherous iceberg. I believe that we have come full circle and can now see just how the stress of modern life has tentacles throughout the ongoing pandemic of heart disease, particularly among women.

The human stress response prepared us to escape a flash flood and evade a saber-toothed cat, but perhaps in our modern world of cell phones and social media, it might have met its match. An angry email, a passive-aggressive post on social media, and the constant strain of deadlines evoke similar stress reactions, but unlike yesteryears, these stressors never go away. GPS leads us in straight lines from point A to point B, and we never have to look around, to wander, to be lost, all necessary ingredients for knowing where we are, of finding ourselves in the mazes of our own creations entrapping us.

The excessive strain of modern living represents an instrumental failure of the complex tools that maintain our homeostasis.[92] The stress response was never meant to be turned on all the time because it is an expensive undertaking for the organism to devote resources to constant activation. Many of the most significant effects of the stress response gone haywire are the ones most directly responsible for heart disease.

Internship, the first year of clinical training after medical school, was by far the hardest year of my life. For the first time, I was a full-fledged doctor making thousands of micro-decisions a day. How did I respond? I ate. I had so much decision fatigue from my work as an intern that when it came to a cream cheese bagel or a lemon poppy seed muffin, I just didn't have the intestinal fortitude to say no.

While many have focused on rare conditions such as Takotsubo by emphasizing the role of stress in heart disease, such a view, while appealing to romantic notions of heartbreak, misses the really important role stress and anxiety play in the epidemic of heart disease. Turns out stress is a major driver of obesity and overeating, which in no small part are responsible for the spike in heart disease. Not just obesity, almost every major cardiovascular disease risk factor, including hypertension, diabetes, and smoking, is worsened by stress.[93,94,95] All these risk factors lead to heart disease, which leads to further stress. Stress is linked with patients being less likely to take their medications for blood pressure and diabetes, and one can see how this can spiral out of control.[96] The effect of stress on risk factors such as hypertension is even more pronounced among women than men, and disorders such as depression and anxiety are far more prevalent among women than men, suggesting that at least in women, mental strain is a much greater driver of heart disease than among men.[97]

The modern workplace seems to be the spewing center of bubbling tension in our lives. One of the largest global studies to ever look at the risk factors of heart disease—INTERHEART—included about fifteen thousand people with heart disease and fifteen thousand without heart disease spread across fifty-two countries.[98] The odds of patients with heart disease experiencing general and work-related stress was twice that of matched people who didn't have these frustrations. Work factors that exacerbate the link between work stress and heart disease include a high-pressure environment dominated by deadlines, a sense of not having control over one's work, and a lack of recognition for one's efforts. Stress has a particularly deleterious effect on women's hearts, given that women are twice as likely to experience stress-induced myocardial ischemia than men.[99]

The changing social fabric is increasing how isolated people are, even as the volume of social interactions is paradoxically increased because of the internet, and this isolation is leading to poor health. Women who reported having lower levels of social integration had a 50 percent higher risk of heart disease than women who felt well connected socially.[100] This increased risk was driven by behaviors associated with poor social integration such as smoking, a lack of exercise, and poor dietary choices.

Hans Selye defined stress as the nonspecific response to any demand made upon it. Yet perhaps more presciently, he wrote, "Everybody knows what stress is and nobody knows what it is. . . . Is it effort, fatigue, pain, fear, the need for concentration, the humiliation of censure, loss of blood, or even an unexpected success that requires complete reformulation of one's life?"[101] He divided the stress response into three phases—the acute onset of stress, followed by adaptation, and finally leading to burnout.

It appears that the relationship of humanity with stress has reached its final stage. While we are certainly not the first generation of human beings to experience stress, the changing nature of our lives has brought us to a breaking point, increasingly reflected by its most prevalent organic manifestation—heart disease.

The crushing consternation brought about by modernity and its cardiac consequences weigh particularly heavily on women. And yet women are fighting back and by raising their voices are helping to uncover the deepest, darkest secrets about why women get heart disease and how their hearts are different from men's.

—ᴧ—

After Katherine Leon, the mother of two, was diagnosed with SCAD, she wasn't remorseful. She was angry. She was angry because she felt she had done nothing to deserve this. She had taken good care of her body and had been a good person to those around her. People like her didn't get heart disease. Perhaps the only reason she now had a torn coronary artery was that she was a woman.

As I was talking to Katherine on the phone, I was listening to her both as a person absorbed in her lived experience and as a physician interested in some of the technical details. When she told me what happened next, both the person and the clinician inside me shuddered. The team decided to perform bypass surgery and connect her left internal mammary artery past the tear in her coronary artery. As a person, just the thought of a young mom of two who had never had more than a sneeze now suddenly having her chest cut open was distressing. But as a physician, I cringed, because under the circumstances Katherine described from fifteen years earlier, we know today that with SCAD, sometimes the best thing to do is to do nothing at all.

Katherine reminded me of another woman who had come to the hospital with chest pain and was found to have a STEMI. In the cardiac catheterization lab, though, a small tear was noted in the far end of one of her arteries. While she did not have ST elevations anymore and she had free flow of blood past the tear, she was still having chest pain. The interventional cardiologist decided to place a stent, and the next picture he took found that the entire vessel had now collapsed. From having free-flowing blood, the woman went to having no blood flowing through the most important vessel in her body.

Turns out that managing SCAD with stents is far more difficult than atherosclerotic plaque. In SCAD, there is a tear in the blood vessel's wall in which blood can accumulate, causing a blockage of flow. If there is a pressing need to relieve the blockage, such as no flow of blood across the lesion, a stent can be placed to push the tear back into the wall. The trouble is that the entire tear has to be covered, because if it isn't, the tear can propagate along the lining of the blood vessel like sharp scissors cutting through a silken drape. In this patient who got the stent, it seemed like the dissection tear, which had previously been very small, had snaked down the length of the coronary artery, essentially unzipping the vessel open. Most cases of SCAD actually heal spontaneously if they are stable. An intervention like stenting is only considered for the most serious cases. And almost no one should ever get CABG surgery for it.

Why do women get SCAD? Well, one of the reasons might be something we have already dived deeply into. It turns out that there is a link between Takotsubo and SCAD, suggesting perhaps that the same forces that cause Takotsubo through the nerves that travel down the spinal cord and innervate the heart and its vessels also cause disruptions in the coronary artery that can cause them to both constrict and, in rare cases, to tear.[102] Yet back when Katherine had her bypass surgery, far from knowing what caused SCAD, many doctors who Katherine sought help from didn't even believe that it was a real entity. So what changed?

Katherine was told by many cardiologists in the early 2000s that what she had experienced was so rare that she would never meet anyone else who had suffered from SCAD. The experience of being "blown up like a dead frog with all sorts of lines going into you" while getting surgery was traumatic enough, but SCAD brought many other changes into her life. "To have to change your identity overnight was really, really hard." Her search for answers didn't go far. "Just don't get pregnant. That's all you need to know," she recalled doctors telling her. "I was just astounded that they didn't know more than that," Katherine recalls. She ended up having her uterus removed.

Katherine went on internet message boards, trying to find someone who could relate. She searched for terms and phrases like *torn artery, women's heart attack,* and *dissected artery* and eventually started to find a few other women from around the country. "If I can get a bunch of stories together, maybe someone would research it. Do I try to get into NIH and wander my way around, or do I do something strategic? All the doctors kept telling me I was wrong and I should move on."

Katherine didn't move on. She persisted. She decided that she wanted to dedicate her life to advocating for heart disease prevention in women, particularly SCAD. The largest set of SCAD cases at that point consisted of just a few dozen each. That's how she met Sharonne Hayes in 2009, a cardiologist and professor at the Mayo Clinic. "I walked up to her and told her we had seventy people and we wanted research." Katherine told me, "She was like, 'Wow.'"

Katherine began fund-raising for research and founded a nonprofit, SCAD Alliance in 2013. "You can have all the research coming out, but if it doesn't get to the doctor or patient, is it doing anything?" Her efforts in part have culminated in a new study being started that includes thirteen medical centers around the country that will finally start to answer some of the fundamental questions about what causes SCAD and what might be the best way to manage it.

Katherine's story is far from a one-off. Just like women have had to fight for everything, they have also fought for the right to be considered as distinct from men, even as it pertains to their hearts. A pioneering figure in this crusade is Nanette Wenger, a cardiologist at Emory University. After graduating from Harvard Medical School in 1954, Wenger pursued cardiology at a time when few women chose this specialty. "When I was in medical school, it was the golden age of cardiology," she told me. "Every week, every month, there was something new."

Wenger was surprised by how few female patients were enrolled in research studies after she started collaborating with the National Institutes of Health. "I kept on saying, 'Where are the women?' and I was told that it was too complicated and we should just study men." She describes that time as "bikini medicine" because the only organs studied in women were those covered by a two-piece swimsuit. Eventually, though, as she persisted, the National Institutes of Health organized a workshop chaired by Wenger in the 1980s, which was focused on heart disease in women. Along with others, she started to see how women were less likely to get optimal, timely treatments and experienced worse outcomes than men did. "Was it biology or bias or both? I think both." Along with others, she put together "a research agenda for the decades."

Wenger sees her job extending all the way to advocacy. "I have testified before Congress more times than I care to count. We go off to Capitol Hill, and we talk to our elected representatives and their staff, and we write." Her most recent legislative accomplishment was helping the Research for All Act of 2015 pass, which promotes the inclusion of women in clinical trials, the use of female tissues and cells in lab research, and the testing of drugs and devices granted expedited review in sufficient numbers of women to ensure that they are as safe and effective in women as men.

One of the most persistent barriers to furthering our understanding of heart disease in women and the care that these patients receive is one that even Nanette Wenger hasn't been able to sway. Of all medical specialties, cardiology has one of the lowest numbers of women. While half of medical students in the United States are female, only one in ten cardiologists is a woman.[103] The lack of diversity in cardiology can certainly affect patients like Katherine, who was never taken seriously until a female physician treated her. "I don't like to generalize," said Nanette Wenger, who certainly wouldn't want only female cardiologists to care for female patients and vice versa, "but female physicians listen more."

Listening.

It's perhaps the most primitive skill clinicians have possessed. It is the only thing we had before we had any medications, any stents, any surgeries, or any lab tests.

Interestingly, when women come to the emergency room, they rate their experience better if a female physician takes care of them; for men, the doctor's gender doesn't matter.[104] Why might that be? Perhaps female physicians are more likely to listen to female patients. Certainly how the female brain responds to listening is much different from that of men.[105]

Perhaps, both men and women, though men more so, can do better by listening more intently to their patients, particularly if they are women. For too long, women's voices have been muffled down, whether at home, at the workplace, and certainly in the hospital or clinic. The truth is that listening to women has also revealed truths we didn't realize about heart disease in general, such as the link between the brain and the heart and its vessels.

Heart disease affects women both young and old. Too many are taken away from the world, and as we look to the future, what might be the most important thing to help reduce the toll heart disease takes in women may not be the newest type of medication or procedure. It may be perhaps the only thing doctors had at one point and a skill that seems to get overwhelmed by all the shiny new toys we have acquired along the way. The most important thing to help women remain healthy before they get heart disease and to provide them the best possible treatment after they get it is for doctors to just sit down and listen to their stories.

9

—◠—

FIRST TO LIVE, LAST TO DIE

Ah, nothing is too late,
Till the tired heart shall cease to palpitate.

—Henry Wadsworth Longfellow, *Morituri Salutamus*

July is the month everything in a hospital is double-checked. New interns, having just finished medical school, step out of their protective bubbles and man the pagers that serve as their conduits to the rest of the hospital. Most of the time, especially at night, they are asked to prescribe sleeping aids. Yet there are also times when they are told that they need to come see their patients *stat*—medical jargon for *rightnowimmediately*.

It was on one such July night when I was working with the shiny, new interns that a page came in, which at first seemed so bizarre it deserved a triple check. A nurse paged that a patient with a pacemaker just had a really long run of asystole—meaning they didn't have a single heartbeat originating from either their own or from the pacemaker. This was bizarre because frequently when patients become asystolic, meaning they flatline, it is not communicated in a well-articulated and almost-casual page—it is announced overhead as a code blue and CPR is initiated.

I immediately asked an intern to get up and head over to the patient's room. En route, as we zipped across the wards, I asked him to tell me about the patient as he fumbled through the reams of paper notes that listed all the patients that he was covering.

Mr. Smith had been transferred from another hospital because he had a pacemaker that needed to be upgraded. It appeared that he had a new pacemaker placed earlier during the day that had three wires that paced his heart. One wire was for his atrium, and there were two other leads, one for each of his ventricles.

As I approached his room, I found myself bemused. I was expecting there to be a throng of doctors and nurses outside his room gearing up for emergency measures, yet there wasn't anybody there. The patient himself was comfortably lying in bed reading a newspaper. Mr. Smith hadn't felt a thing and wasn't sure what he had done to garner our attention at such an inopportune time of the night.

There must have been a mistake—sometimes the telemonitoring devices that record patients' heart rhythms can misread the situation. I went over to the desk where the heartbeats of all the patients in the ward were being shown in real time in endless loops. I maximized Mr. Smith's tele, and it showed, almost unbelievably, that he went almost twenty seconds without a single heartbeat, neither his own nor, more distressingly, from the brand-new pacemaker that was supposed to stimulate his heart to beat when it was unable to stimulate itself.

Right as I was scratching my head, Mr. Smith's line went flat again, but this time I heard the nurse cry out from his room that he was gone. From sitting in his bed nonchalantly, he had collapsed back in bed, his chin digging into his chest as he stopped breathing.

He had been hanging by a metal thread. Now that thread had broken and he was in free fall.

As CPR was started, I hollered for an external pacemaker to be brought in, which would deliver electric shocks from small patches that we would stick to his chest and left side. As soon as the device arrived, I cranked up the voltage to maximum so that his heart would capture the external stimuli and beat accordingly. Yet even as they caused his body to convulse, his EKG still remained stubbornly unwavering. Soon the anesthesiologists descended upon him and inserted a plastic breathing tube down his throat and connected him to a breathing machine.

As desperate chest compressions continued, I had broken out in a cold sweat but had an idea—instead of inserting another emergency pacemaker, perhaps I could just reprogram and troubleshoot his existing pacemaker to do the job. I asked one of my colleagues to tell me what type of pacemaker he had, because that would determine which console I would need to bring to adjust its programming.

After I found out, I ran over to bring one of the consoles over, which resembled a very large and clunky laptop with a small antenna attached to it by a wire that needed to be placed right on top of Mr. Smith's pacemaker so that it would be connected and subsequently reprogrammed.

I burst back in the room and made my way through the crowd involved in managing the cardiac arrest. I placed the antenna on his chest, though it kept slipping and falling, given that Mr. Smith's chest was rocking wildly with the forceful chest compressions. When I finally connected it, I called one of the senior doctors on the phone, and we troubleshot the pacemaker as if it were a malfunctioning computer. We maxed out the electric output on both of his ventricular leads, and even though the right ventricular lead still didn't cause the heart to beat, the thin beady wire wrapped around his left ventricle kicked in and started to make the heart dance to its tune.

As soon as Mr. Smith's heart started following the pacemaker's rhythmic call, which I set at sixty times a minute, tranquility descended in and around Mr. Smith.

To what do we all owe the calm that grips our hearts from its first beat to its last? On average, the human heart beats two billion times in a lifetime. What is the thread that connects us through it all? Who is the conductor to whose cadence the heart beats? For the heart isn't an automaton— unlike the sands slipping through the waist of an hourglass—how fast the heart beats changes. Step in front of a speeding train and it comes to life, sending powerful ripples through the body while beating as fast as the flapping wings of a hummingbird. Fall asleep at your desk on a lazy afternoon, and the pulse occurs as infrequently as the last drips of water from a leaky faucet. The captain of this crazy train cannot tire, cannot blink, cannot sleep, cannot afford to be distracted at any moment throughout their lifetime. Thankfully, the heart's master conductor, its pacemaker, called the *sinus node,* is more than up to the task.

The sinus node is located where the vena cava, coming from the neck, connects to the top-right corner of the right atrium. Unlike the rest of the heart, the cells in the sinus node have a superpower—the ability to spontaneously generate electrical impulses. Cells in the crescent-shaped sinus node, spread across but a few millimeters, continue to automatically depolarize, sending electrical impulses racing like waves through the heart, causing those tissues to contract.

The sinus node sets the tone, to which the heart beats at between sixty to a hundred times per minute during normal activity. The sinus node can exist completely on its own if it has to, but in most normal people, it receives marching orders from impulses coming down from the brain. These impulses can speed up the heart rate at times of both physical stress such as when you might be running for your life from a pack of rabid werewolves or emotional stress when your phone battery is about to die. Conversely, the heart is asked to slow down by the brain if the body is feeling particularly relaxed after a bubble bath.

The electrical impulse generated spontaneously by the sinus node ripples initially through the right atrium and then moves across to the left atrium. Yet the electrical impulse cannot simply walk across into the ventricles. Separating the atria from the ventricles is a virtual wall and the electrical impulses in the atria have to converge at a singular checkpoint called the *atrioventricular (AV) node,* which is located in the septum dividing the two ventricles. Here the erstwhile speeding electrical impulses come to a brief halt, like airport travelers at a checkpoint or cars slowing down to pass through a toll booth, which allows the atria to complete their contraction, before moving down the interventricular septum, going all the way down to the apex of the heart and then spreading back up the outer walls of the ventricles. The pause in the AV node prevents both the atria and ventricles from contracting at the same time and therefore not slapping blood across each other's face. And the fact that electrical impulses can only emerge from a single point in the ventricular septum allows both ventricles to approximately contract in unison, which also results in a more efficient pumping of the heart. The left ventricle contracts the way one wrings a wet towel in one's hand—it contracts, it spirals, and it pulls the heart down.

So what happens when the sinus node is diseased and doesn't fire, as happened with Mr. Smith? Most of the time, another part of the heart can kick in and pace the heart at a much slower rate than normal—such a rhythm is called an *escape rhythm*—which represents the heart's get-out-of-jail card. Yet for some patients, such an escape may never manifest, and they succumb to pulselessness unless a timely intervention is performed.

The reason we understand so much about the heart, about its rhythm, about when and how it goes too slow, or when and why it goes fast, is because of an advance that is as important today as it was when it was first developed more than a hundred years ago.

Right before I graduated from internal medicine residency and was about to start my fellowship training in heart disease, I asked one of my mentors, Al Buxton, a professor in Harvard Medical School, for the one thing he wished more people knew when they started their cardiology fellowship. He gave me a handout showing the correct way to place EKG patches on a person's chest. He didn't need to say it in words, but it was clear to me what he meant—the EKG is to the heart what the Rosetta stone was to the history of an entire civilization.

While electricity has always been all around and within us, before the lightbulb, the only real demonstration of electrical power was lightning flashing across the sky, setting trees ablaze and shaking the ground with its power. Only serendipity opened the door into the insight that really all beings are electrical in nature. In the late eighteenth century, a visitor to the Italian biologist Luigi Galvani (1737–1798) accidentally knocked a scalpel into a frog leg touching an electrical machine, causing it to contract.[1] This accident, now repeated as an experiment in high school labs the world over, fundamentally changed how we view living beings.

All of a sudden, by providing a face to the impulses traversing our bodies, the frog leg experiment made clear that the core of the human body is an electrical grid, transmitting directives and processing information, always connected and always in control. Not only does electricity control the beating of the heart and every muscle in the body, it dictates the movement of food through one's intestines, every thought that crosses our busy minds, every memory formed, every sensation felt. And electricity doesn't travel through the body in wires and cables but from cell to cell as each turns from its resting negative to positive and then back to negative charge. Neither could I write this book, nor could you read it, without the movement of electrical charges from one point to another. Yet the human body is without doubt the most efficient electrical machine around.[2] The human body uses such little electricity that, even if fully harnessed, it would take seventy hours for it to charge an iPhone.[3]

It was a Dutch physiologist who, in the early twentieth century, provided the foundation for the modern EKG.[4] Willem Einthoven's EKG machine involved the patient sitting in a chair with both their arms and one of their legs dipped in buckets of salt water that served as electrodes. It would then trace out the pattern of electrical activity occurring in the heart onto a piece of paper. Prior to the EKG, the story of the heart, its triumphs and tribulations, were limited to the oral tradition, spoken from one to another, vivid in the minds of a few and unknown to most. In the EKG, the heart had found its scribe. In our bodies, the heart has always had a voice, even before we emerged fully into this world. In the EKG, now it had a quill.

Einthoven named the waves seen on the EKG, representing the activity of the heart as electricity makes its way through it, from the top to its very bottom, in alphabetical order: P-QRS-T, with the small P wave denoting the contraction of the thin-walled atria that push blood into the large muscular ventricles; the large QRS complex, the most prominent wave in the cycle, representing the powerful contraction of the ventricles that pushes the blood out of the heart and into the lungs and the rest of the body; and lastly, the parabolic T wave, which represents the resetting of the electrical state of the ventricles back to their baseline, ready for another round of activity and start back again, with the puny P wave.

Being able to read an EKG is one of the rites of passage of medical school, but I never really understood how important reading an EKG was until the very last day of medical school. I was part of a group of medical students finishing up our cardiology rotation, and we were almost giddy with excitement. We had worked hard for several weeks, and our supervising cardiologist, an exacting mustachioed man, was surprisingly pleased with how we had done. All we had to do was cross the finish line. As we were wrapping up, the cardiologist asked us what initially sounded like a simple question. We all knew that if you saw a pattern on an EKG called an ST elevation, that patient was likely to be having a heart attack. He asked for five conditions *other than* a heart attack that would show up with ST elevations on an EKG. One of us said pericarditis, which is an inflammation of the sac that covers the heart. Another said early repolarization, in which younger patients who are otherwise healthy just happen to have that suggestive pattern on their EKGs. Then we were stumped. And then we were destroyed. The cardiologist made us feel as if all that we had worked for was for naught, for if a sick patient came in with ST elevations, we could potentially miss some other conditions such as a torn coronary artery or a dead aneurysmal part of the heart generating that pattern. It was one of the most important lessons we learned, delivered in the harshest possible way.

While some physicians at that time argued that a "nervous liquor" transmitted dance moves from the brain to the heart, the EKG, among other tools, made it clear that the heart was truly the master of its own destiny.[5] There are many who have dedicated their entire lives to unraveling the intricacies of the human EKG and have found answers to some of the deepest mysteries of the heart through careful observations of minute variations in the patterns it produces. In the most experienced of eyes, the EKG can reveal answers to some of the greatest medical mysteries. In some cases, what is seen on the EKG and how it is interpreted can be the difference between life and death.

The EKG opened up a world of disorders of heart rhythm going too fast or too slow. When the EKG goes out of control, like a Richter scale used for expressing the magnitude of an earthquake on the basis of seismograph oscillations, it represents the heart's version of a natural disaster, usually some sort of malignant heart rhythm that can frequently lead to death. One such rhythm is ventricular tachycardia. In emergent cases, ventricular tachycardia can be fatal unless it is treated with its most effective antidote—the electric shock. Nothing makes more compelling television than a doctor in a white coat pulling out the shock paddles and applying a ground-shaking dropkick of electricity to the chest of a patient, pulling them back from the land of the dead. Nothing is more potent a demonstration of death than the flatlining of an EKG. And yet it was the EKG that helped us find life from the darkness beyond death. And it all started with a freak experiment that could easily have been devised by the dark fantasies of Edgar Allan Poe.

It was late at night, and Louise was waiting for her clothes to dry in the Laundromat in the strip mall close to her house. It was the sleepy part of town, and she was the only one there. A woman walked past the glass front of the Laundromat and saw her standing awkwardly. She was standing upright next to the dryer, but her entire upper body was stiff and motionless. The woman walked inside to check on her and came upon a sight she would never forget. Louise was wedged between the dryer and the washing machine, unconscious and not breathing.

The woman panicked and dislodged Louise's lifeless body from the appliances, lying her flat on the floor. She called 911, and the dispatcher asked her to see if Louise had a pulse. Louise didn't, and the 911 crew instructed the woman to start CPR, walking her through the steps over the phone as they sent in a rescue squad. When the paramedics arrived and connected Louise to the cardiac defibrillator they had brought with them, her EKG was in an erratic and chaotic heart rhythm, like an angry toddler scribbling furiously. Louise was in ventricular fibrillation, and even the defibrillator knew what needed to be done: "shock indicated."

The electric shock, followed by the dramatic resurrection, is one of the most emblematic images of the world we live in and a forceful reminder of how modern medicine has shaped how we have come to see ourselves as essentially electrical beings. While most medical advances are incremental at best, there was never anything subtle about the electric dropkick. Defibrillation is still a relatively recent development, and the first treatment of a human being with electricity occurred under most inauspicious circumstances.

In the eighteenth century, death from drowning had become so pervasive in Europe that researchers throughout the continent became desperate for anything that could help the victims. In fact, this was one of the core missions of an organization called the Humane Society, which had chapters throughout Europe. When in 1774, Catherine Sophia Greenhill, a three-year-old girl, fell from a window in London, one of her neighbors was a member of the Humane Society and went with her to the nearby hospital, where the surgeons declared her to have died. It was then that the neighbor, Mr. Squires, went to work according to a published account. "Mr Squires, tried the effects of electricity. Twenty minutes elapsed before he could apply the shock, which he gave to various parts of the body in vain; but upon transmitting a few shocks through the thorax, he perceived a small palpation."[7] Sophia rose up from the dead and, just a few days after her "death," walked out of the hospital. A physician in the report asked, "why not have recourse to the most potent stimulus in nature, which can instantly pervade the innermost recesses of the animal frame? Why not immediately apply electric shocks to the brain and heart, the grand forces of motion and sensation, the *primum vivens ct ultimum moriens* of the animal machine?" he asked. Another member of the Humane Society, Charles Kite, followed up this advance with the first rudimentary device to apply electric shocks to differentiate the apparently dead from the actually dead in the late eighteenth century.[8]

The heart has long been referred to as the organ that is "first to live and last to die"—*primum vivens ct ultimum moriens*—and yet this startling, little-known report that preceded the routine use of electric shocks to resuscitate patients from malignant heart rhythms by 150 years showed that the heart didn't have to necessarily be *ultimum moriens*. Yet even though the resurrection of Catherine Sophia Greenhill by Mr. Squires occurred in a hospital, the veracity of this account remains shaky at best. Kite's rudimentary defibrillator failed for most patients, and it isn't even clear if it had anything to do with Sophia's resurrection.

In the early half of the twentieth century, the EKG allowed us to finally better understand how a heart beating too fast could be fatal. The epidemic of heart disease led to many people dying suddenly of it, and contrary to what was conventionally thought, most of these deaths didn't occur because the heart came to a standstill. In ventricular fibrillation or ventricular tachycardia, the heart actually goes into overdrive, often beating as fast as about two hundred times a minute. However, the contractions of the fibrillating heart are about as effective as a heart not beating at all. While ventricular tachycardia is regular, ventricular fibrillation is irregular and faster and subsequently more dangerous. But for 150 years after Sophia's resurrection, the role of electricity to revive those in cardiac arrest had been relegated to history books and experiments on animals. The established means of potentially treating ventricular arrhythmias in the first half of the twentieth century was rather grotesque and was performed by Sherwin Nuland, a surgeon and National Book Award winner, on the first patient he ever treated.

Nuland was a medical student in Yale New Haven Hospital in Connecticut in the early 1950s, and the very first patient he saw, James McCarty, "was a powerfully built construction executive whose business success had seduced him into patterns of living that we now know are suicidal."[9] Just as the twenty-two-year-old Nuland sat on his bed, McCarty "threw his head back and bellowed out a wordless roar that seemed to rise up out of his throat from somewhere deep within his stricken heart." Nuland cried for help, but there was no one around. "My fingers felt for the carotid artery in McCarty's neck, but it was pulseless and still."

Incredibly, without having even seen the procedure being performed, Nuland cut open the man's chest and grabbed the man's heart in his right hand. "Under my fingertips could be felt an uncoordinated, irregular squirming that I recognized from its textbook description as the terminal condition called ventricular fibrillation, the agonal act of a heart that is becoming reconciled to its eternal rest." Nuland performed what was then the customary way to attempt to revive the hearts of those in such rhythms— the rhythmic massage of the heart with one's bare hands. Yet, James McCarty's heart did meet its eternal rest, like that of any other heart going into ventricular tachycardia or fibrillation back then, because even if the arrhythmia didn't kill the patient, the opening of the chest almost always would.

Cardiac surgeons often saw themselves face-to-face with ventricular arrhythmias and often resorted to open cardiac massage to help the fibrillating heart pump blood as it withered away. Claude Beck, a surgeon in Cleveland, was wrapping up an uneventful surgery in a young boy when the boy went into ventricular fibrillation in 1947.[10] Beck massaged the boy's heart with his hands for more than a half hour, but the heart continued to fibrillate. It was then that Beck decided to try something that had failed every time he had previously attempted it: he applied electrodes directly to the heart from the wall socket and delivered a high-voltage shock. He tried it once, and the heart kept fibrillating. He tried it a second time, and the heart just stopped beating. Within a few moments, though, he saw what he had only dreamed of witnessing previously as the heart began "feeble, regular and fairly rapid cardiac contractions." This was the first time electricity was demonstrably used to successfully resuscitate a human being, and within a few days, the boy walked out of the hospital alive and well.

The ward in the hospital I trained at in Boston was named after Paul Zoll (1911–1999), one of the pioneers of what was then the budding field of electrophysiology.[11] Zoll had an interest in heart rhythms since early in his career but was reticent to apply therapies to patients in cardiac arrest given that it was felt to be against the spirit of God or the forces of nature.[12] In time, though, he got over his hesitancy and was one of the first few people to develop a device, today referred to as the defibrillator, that could deliver the shock necessary to rescue the heart from ventricular arrhythmias without having to cut open the chest.[13] Simultaneously, a team of scientists in Russia led by Naum Gurvich had developed an even more effective means of defibrillation using direct current rather than alternating current, as was done by Zoll.[14] These pioneering Russian advances, however, were not widely publicized and it took Western researchers decades to come to the realization that direct current was more effective than alternating.

Over time, defibrillators have become smaller and smaller. In fact, millions of men and women now have defibrillators no bigger than a fat Pringle chip implanted just under the clavicle in their chests with a wire screwed right into their hearts. These defibrillators wait for an abnormal heart rhythm to emerge only to zap it back down. One would think that this would take care of ventricular tachycardias once and for all, but these malignant heart rhythms remain very difficult to treat. Even though Louise's heart was shocked back into a normal rhythm, the effect was only transient. She underwent CPR for hours, initially by the paramedics and later with a machine pushing down on her chest while she was being transported in the ambulance. In the hospital, she went into ventricular tachycardia multiple times, and it was clear that her body had been deprived of oxygen for too long—it was estimated that she had been in ventricular fibrillation for almost an hour when she was first found stuck upright between washing machines in the Laundromat. Her family said that she would have wanted none of this, none of the shocks, nor the mechanical breathing machine, nor the CPR. All artificial support was removed, and Louise never woke up.

In ventricular tachycardia or ventricular fibrillation, the normal rules of the heart are broken. No longer is the sinus node sending impulses down the heart that then perpetuate a contraction throughout the ventricles. In fact, the contractions are emerging from the bottom up in the ventricles. The consequences of such an insurrection over the sinus node can be fatal given how fast the ventricles can fibrillate when left to their own devices. Ventricular arrhythmias by themselves are the most common reason people die suddenly.

Medical vernacular usually serves to soften the blow of colloquial terms used to describe disease. A heart attack, therefore, is a *myocardial infarction* or an *acute coronary syndrome*. Yet when patients have not one but multiple and incessant runs of ventricular tachycardia, the actual medical term for that condition does nothing to assuage—it's called *VT storm*.

I remember the first time I saw VT storm, and it was in the last place I had expected. As part of our residency, we worked for a month in a small hospital outside of Boston. In Brockton, the hospital was bare-bones—in fact, when the patient rolled into the emergency room getting shocked incessantly, the team paged the senior-most person present in the hospital back then—me—who could have potentially managed him: a medical resident in the third year of his training. As soon as I saw him from the other end of the emergency room, stripped naked under bright lights and being shocked relentlessly, going back into VT, and being shocked again, and going back into VT again, I knew this hospital was no place for him.

Despite having his bloodstream bathed in the most potent anti-arrhythmic medications, there was almost nothing we could do to keep him clear of the VT storm he found himself mired in. Turned out that for the previous few days, he had been using cocaine, and every time he took a hit, his heart went into VT, and the defibrillator implanted in his chest shocked him out of it. He would feel awful after the defibrillation, use more cocaine to feel better, and then have more VT. He maintained this suicidal cycle until his defibrillator's battery died and he just stayed in VT. A helicopter came to pick up the patient from the emergency room in Brockton and flew him to the big hospital in Boston, but he never made it out.

A ventricular arrhythmia can be a devastating event, yet many fear being shocked by their defibrillators even more so. A patient I recently met has been shocked so many times he developed PTSD; in fact, we helped him join a support group of those who had previously been shocked by their defibrillators. Another man recently heard the ominous sound that his defibrillator makes when it is about to deliver a shock while he was in a grocery store, only to find out the beeping was coming from one of the refrigerators.

"What does it feel like?" I asked one of my patients who had been shocked by his defibrillator.

"Like a bullet," he told me. "Next time I hear that sound, I am gonna duck!" he joked, knowing he couldn't jump far enough to get out of its cross-hairs.

One problem with defibrillators is that they can shock the heart out of a ventricular arrhythmia but they do nothing to prevent the arrhythmias from occurring in the first place. Some patients can benefit from a procedure called *VT ablation,* in which the part of the heart that appears to be the focus of the arrhythmia can be isolated, preventing the arrhythmia from spreading throughout the heart. A new procedure only now being tested holds the promise of reducing the incidence of VT simply by aiming radiation at the arrhythmia-inducing scars in the ventricles completely noninvasively.[15]

For others, though, more drastic measures might be needed. One devastating diagnosis is called *arrhythmogenic right ventricular cardiomyopathy*, in which patients have frequent and often intractable ventricular arrhythmias. In many instances the condition is hereditary, present from birth, and devastates entire families, wiping them out like the plague. The only definitive treatment for patients with this condition is a heart transplant.

Even though clinical trials showed that implantable defibrillators save lives in many patients, their implantation became so common in recent years that the U.S. Department of Justice opened up an investigation into whether they were being placed appropriately, leading to a notable reduction in the number of patients receiving these devices.[16] The good news, however, is that for these patients, most of whom have heart failure, the most effective therapy to reduce the risk of ventricular tachycardia and sudden death is not some fancy surgery or futuristic procedure—it is simply medications that can cost cents and are available in almost every country in the world. These simple medications, such as ACE inhibitors and beta-blockers, have caused the number of patients with heart failure experiencing sudden death to plummet over the last few decades.[17] Even though traditional studies have found implantable defibrillators to reduce mortality in patients with heart failure with reduced ejection fraction, a more recent study in Denmark showed no benefit of defibrillators in patients with heart failure but without significant atherosclerotic disease, presumably because these patients were on a more effective medical therapy than patients in prior trials had available. With newer medications such as sacubitril/valsartan, approved for use after the Danish study, that lower the risk of sudden death even more, it is quite possible that a modern trial of defibrillators may show no benefit from having the procedure performed in patients with heart failure who have never had a major ventricular arrhythmia before.[18] So even as defibrillators have become a rite of passage for many, they may soon become a relic of the past due to the success of medications.

Implantable defibrillators, and what to do with them, become even more controversial as people approach the end of life. For many, defibrillators may in fact prolong suffering when death is near and inevitable. In fact, death from ventricular arrhythmia, which is quick and painless, frequently causing loss of consciousness, may be desirable, unless it is painfully aborted by an electric shock to the chest. While it is recommended that physicians discuss electronically deactivating the shock therapy from the defibrillator in patients with terminal illnesses, few doctors do. A fifth of patients may get shocked in the last few days of life, with about one in ten getting shocked in the last few minutes of life.[19] In fact, in one study, not a single patient actually had even been told that defibrillators can be turned off.[20] Having turned off defibrillators for many patients, often when they are dying in the intensive care unit, I have seen just how relieved many are, knowing that come what may, the sound of the device charging followed by an electric shock to their chest will not be one of their last lived memories.

As we get better and better at understanding how to tame a heart that beats too fast, there are also hearts that go the other way, that beat too slowly. Heart block can occur anywhere within the heart, from affecting the sinus node itself, leading to no effective impulses being emitted, to affecting the AV node, stopping impulses from the sinus node from reaching the ventricles, thereby resulting in no meaningful heartbeats occurring. In such instances, a pacemaker can be considered, and this is one area in which Zoll definitely was the pioneer. Zoll developed the first machine that could pace the heart from the skin, the way I had to pace Mr. Smith with patches.[21] Pacemakers are usually programmed with a minimum heart rate, and if the patient's heart falls below said heart rate, the pacemakers can kick in. Pacemakers look almost exactly like defibrillators, and in fact, all defibrillators can function as pacemakers. The newest types of pacemakers are called *leadless pacemakers*. As big as a large vitamin pill, these can be implanted directly in the heart and do not carry any of the risks that come with having long leads that can get infected or fractured.

As cardiac devices become more common, getting a health checkup is increasingly like taking your car to the shop. The battery is checked to make sure there is enough charge, and the wires and parts are examined to make sure there are no breaks. Information is downloaded to make sure there have been no aberrancies. Even though most people with pacemakers and defibrillators do okay, there are risks with these devices getting infected, in which case they have to be taken out. Increasingly, though, these implantable devices have become targets ripe for hackers. When former U.S. vice president Dick Cheney had a defibrillator in place, there were actually fears that the device could be commandeered by hackers to remotely deliver shocks. Given how simplistic the underlying programmatic architecture of these devices is, such a feat would not be science fiction. In fact, the U.S. Department of Homeland Security offered exactly such a warning about defibrillators being remotely controlled.[22] And just recently, almost a million pacemakers were recalled because their batteries could be drained by hackers.[23]

The EKG, which used to need an apparatus that fit an entire room to be produced, can now be reproduced by a band around one's wrist. Technology such as the Apple Watch 4 and others can now seamlessly and continuously record individuals' EKGs as they go about their daily lives. This allows devices made by companies such as AliveCor to detect life-threatening conditions, including abnormally high levels of potassium in the blood or a familial life-threatening disease called "Long QT Syndrome," simply by monitoring the EKG from a digital watch or an iPhone. Yet, this new technology, which has essentially democratized the EKG for the masses, can have unintended consequences. A medical test is as good at detecting disease as the prevalence of the disease in the people who get the test—meaning that a positive test in a population where the disease is very common is much more likely to be true than if the test is conducted in people who rarely have the disease. And because things like the Apple Watch 4, for example, are going to be bought by people who are by and large not at risk for these conditions, the number of false-positive alerts or incidental findings that could stem from this wave of digital technology could be unprecedented.

Even as we unravel the mysteries of the heart, layer by layer, developing newer technologies to keep it on a leash as a thermostat does the air conditioner, the heart continues to be a thing of wonder. Not too long ago, we had a patient who came to the hospital to be zapped out of atrial fibrillation, a common arrhythmia. The anesthesiologist gave him just enough meds to put him to sleep. I charged the device and delivered 200 joules of direct current to his chest. As soon as the charge was delivered, my eyes moved to his EKG monitor. He had been going at an irregular rate of about 150 per minute just a moment earlier, and the electric current put the kibosh on that. This procedure is very safe—by this time, I had done it more than a hundred times and had never seen anything go awry.

Most people, as soon as they get the current, go back into normal sinus rhythm, but this patient didn't. His EKG was flat as a granite top. I was hoping for something to bob up, but nothing did. Every small fraction of the few seconds that I stared into the EKG monitor, willing some heartbeats into it with my unflinching stare, seemed to last an eternity. Even within those miniscule moments, I could picture the next step—me jumping on his chest to perform chest compressions, which would be a catastrophic thing to happen to someone who had just come to the hospital for a routine procedure. Yet before I could shake off my inertia, the anesthesiologist landed a hard slap right on to the patient's sternum. It was so sudden, so decisive, that I felt that I was the one who had been smacked. And yet as soon as he did, a regular normal sinus resumed, and all the high-pitched beeping sounds now synonymous with mortal ruin playing in my head faded away.

10

—\/\/—

THE MORBID DANCE OF CANCER
AND HEART DISEASE

When the body escaped mutilation,
seldom did the heart go to the grave unscarred.

—Virginia Woolf, *Jacob's Room*

There is no place on earth quite like a hospital at night. Gleam turns to gloom, and bustling hallways transform into eerily quiet corridors. The hospital's previously pulsing passageways dim down to resemble a muted maze. Hospitals teem with people during the day, and it is not always clear why they are all there. At night, though, everyone at the hospital is there for a reason. When Michelle, a middle-aged black woman, showed up at the emergency room, she showed up for a reason. Ostensibly, what was bothering her the most was that her tongue had grown ginormous. She had tried many drugs without relief. Even surgery could not change the fact that her tongue had started to block her airway. However, what was really ailing her was centered in her heart.

For a doctor, working at night in the hospital is very different from working during the day. There are far fewer of us around, and the goalposts are different. Instead of playing the long game, like getting the patient ready for upcoming open-heart surgery or performing a battery of tests to figure out why the patient is having high-grade fevers, or figuring out how we can get a patient strong and well enough for them to be discharged home, at night our goals are much less lofty.

During most overnight shifts, I try to make sure that the sickest patients are able to make it to dawn. I greet almost every patient I meet with, "I am sorry to see you here, but it's nice to meet you." And almost every time I have to leave their bedside, I leave them with, "I wish you have a nice boring night." Boredom is the best thing that can happen for patients, especially during the course of the night.

In HBO's television series *Game of Thrones*, the red priestess Melisandre frequently proclaims, "The night is dark and full of terrors." Every physician has their own personal trove of terrors, and one that is quite unique to the medical profession is the dreaded "OSH bomb." The OSH bomb can strike at any time unbeknownst to its prey, and all too often, it is accompanied by a binder full of incomprehensible documents. *OSH* stands for *outside hospital* in medical parlance and is a moniker attached to any hospital other than one's own. More than a moniker, though, it is a slur, and an OSH bomb is basically a patient who gets transferred to one's hospital with incomplete, incorrect, or inscrutable information. And if you are the big shop in town, the one others look up to when things are getting out of hand, get ready to duck in the trenches because you will be getting your share of OSH bombs.

What is common between every OSH bomb is that to some extent, it is a tragedy. Sometimes an OSH bomb is a person in a wheelchair being rolled into the hospital while they are still receiving electric shocks to keep their heart beating normally. Sometimes the OSH bomb is a young man in a coma who had torn and occluded blood vessels in his neck that no one from the OSH told you about. Sometimes it's a woman who just wants an answer and for someone to just care enough to try to find it.

Michelle had seen her share of pain and tragedy. A corrections officer in Rikers Island for twenty years—New York City's main jail complex—she told me when she first started working there, she realized, *This is where all the young black men are.* I could tell that being there had been difficult for her, especially when she saw the newer inmates enter a world beyond their most horrifying nightmares. "It was just so hard to not show any emotions."

I felt a knot form in the bottom of my throat. There *are* some similarities between being a physician and being a prison guard. Frequently, we have to hold people against their will when they might be a danger to themselves. No one ever wants to be in a hospital by choice. But there is one important difference—sometimes the best thing doctors can do is show their emotions.

It had been a year since Michelle's tongue had started to grow both longer and wider in size. Her doctors thought that it was an allergic reaction to one of the medications she was taking for high blood pressure called *lisinopril.* They discontinued the medication, but her tongue kept growing until it affected how she spoke. They gave her steroids, hoping that the anti-inflammatory effect of the steroids would make the swelling go down, but it never did. Her tongue grew larger to the point that she started having difficulty breathing. She had surgery to remove her tonsils and make space in her throat. A year passed, and while her doctors assured her they knew what was going on, she wasn't so sure. And so, in the middle of the night, she showed up at our hospital, hoping for a new set of eyes, a second opinion, and that's when my pager went off.

As I spoke to her in the emergency room, it was hard to look at anything but her tongue, though I knew I needed to focus to put it all together. It became clear very quickly that the tongue was but the most obvious manifestation of something much more systemic. An ultrasound of her heart revealed that her heart was pumping weakly. I figured that the two processes were likely connected, since there are only a few things that affect both the heart and the tongue. One of those is a disorder of the thyroid called *myxedema,* but Michelle's thyroid function tests came back normal. Even though I requested our surgeons to take a small biopsy from her tongue and run tests on it to determine what had caused her tongue to balloon, those tests could take days to show a final result, so I ordered an MRI of her heart to get to the bottom of what was going on. When the results came back the next day, they left me stunned. On the MRI, we were looking for a finding that would show up as white speckles, indicating infiltration of the heart with a foreign substance. Michelle's heart lit up like a Christmas tree.

A rush of excitement flowed through my body because I knew that we had made a diagnosis; we had an answer. The reason her tongue had grown was not because of some medication side effect but because of an abnormal protein being excessively produced and then being deposited in various parts of her body. Deposition of this abnormal protein was why her tongue was huge, why her heart was so weak. That protein, called *amyloid,* was likely being overproduced because she had multiple myeloma. Multiple myeloma is a type of blood cancer in which one of the blood cells, called plasma cells, which are responsible for producing antibodies that protect the body from infections, start to multiply, overproducing antibodies. Some types of multiple myeloma overproduce antibodies that are much more likely to stick to each other and result in amyloid deposition throughout the body. Amyloid accumulating in the kidneys can cause them to fail and lose excessive amounts of protein. Deposition in the intestines can cause bleeding and malabsorption of nutrients. Other than the brain, amyloid can deposit in almost every other part of the body, including, rarely, in the tongue.

I saw one of the other doctors taking care of Michelle, and both of us were fired up that we had made a diagnosis. I raised my hand, and we exchanged a tepid, nerdy high five, acting like we had deciphered a previously unsolved mystery. But as soon as our hands clapped, what followed felt like a gut punch—the realization that this was as much a diagnosis as it was a death sentence for our patient. The chances that sweet Michelle, despite all that she had braved in life, despite all the comfort she had given those hopeless inmates, would make it through this disease, this morbid dance between cancer and heart disease, were almost nil.

Many think of cancer and heart disease separately, but as we chart new frontiers, what doctors are now realizing is that too commonly, not only can they coexist, their union can turn the best of dreams sour. Not only can cancer, as in this instance, cause heart disease, many times, the very treatments that can effectively treat or even cure cancer can result in debilitating and life-threatening heart disease.

Kati Gardner was eight years old when she was found to have cancer. "I was diagnosed at a good age," she told me. "I was old enough to have learned things from it, but not old enough for it to interrupt any important things in my life." Now in her thirties, she recalled memories of a time when cancer was not a part of her life. "I remember that I had two legs and I lived a very normal life until I broke my leg."

Two years after her diagnosis, when Kati was ten years old, her life changed irreversibly as she lost her leg to the bone cancer. She had to have her cancerous leg amputated and went through several cycles of chemotherapy.

Other than her amputation, Kati, who does not wear a prosthesis, lived as normal a life as possible, which included becoming a teacher and getting married before things changed once again.

"I was chasing middle-school children sixteen weeks into my pregnancy when I suddenly developed chest pains and couldn't breathe." She went to the hospital, and an ultrasound of her heart revealed that it was pumping very feebly. She had developed heart failure from the chemotherapy she was given almost fifteen years earlier.

Even though, to this day, more people die of heart disease than cancer, cancer continues to be considered the greatest disease of our age. The good news is that all the emphasis, all the funds raised, and all the benefits performed for cancer research and treatment have begun to pay off. The age-adjusted rate of death from cancer in the United States, after peaking in 1990 at 216 per 100,000 people, has been declining every year since according to data recorded by the Centers for Disease Control and Prevention. What this means, though, is that there are more people alive who have lived with a diagnosis of cancer today than ever before. According to recent estimates, there were almost fourteen million cancer survivors in the United States in 2014, with this number slated to rise to eighteen million by 2022.[1] With one in twenty Americans surviving cancer, a cancer cure can sometimes come at a steep price. And many times, it is the heart that suffers.

"There is a generation of us that survived cancer but was lost afterward," said Kati.

Decades removed from her chemotherapy and cancer, Kati's heart failure still keeps rearing its ugly head. "When we were moving from my apartment, I started having a lot of irregular and fast heart rhythms." Things got really serious when she became pregnant for the first time. "At thirty weeks, I got a terrible cold. I couldn't breathe well." She was admitted to the hospital where she had an ultrasound to look at how strong her heart was pumping. One way to assess how much blood is being pumped is through a measure called the ejection fraction. As described earlier, a normal ejection fraction is at least 55 percent. "My ejection fraction had dropped to 30 percent," Kati said. "My doctors asked me to not go to work and to rest."

Things turned out well for Kati, though. Her pregnancy was otherwise unremarkable, and her ejection fraction improved to 45 percent. Kati's oncologist had prepared her to watch out for the cardiotoxic effects of chemotherapy ever since she got treated as a child, and when she found out she was pregnant, she called him even before she contacted her gynecologist. Others, though, don't fare so well. "One of my friends was not prepared, and she had a stroke after giving birth," Kati recalled.

Reassuringly, chemotherapies are becoming more targeted. Earlier chemotherapies, called *cytotoxic chemotherapy*, targeted the most rapidly dividing cells in the body. While in many cases, those cells were cancerous, the collateral damage extended to any cells that actively divided, such as the lining of the mouth and intestines, hair cells, blood cells, and so on. Targeted chemotherapies affect mechanisms of growth that are more specific to cancerous cells, but they can still sometimes have devastating complications that affect the heart. There are so many new chemotherapy medications nowadays that many have not even been tested widely enough for doctors to fully understand complications that might occur because of them.

I was in the cardiac intensive care unit when I was called from the emergency room for a patient who had suffered a heart attack. I rushed down to the emergency room, expecting to find the patient clutching her chest in pain or heaving to take a breath, but I found myself in an entirely different scene. She was just sitting there, seemingly without a care in the world. All she told me was that she just felt tired. Really, *really* tired.

I took a step back. The patient had been diagnosed with an NSTEMI after she was found to have elevated troponin levels, indicating ongoing damage to her heart. I looked at her electrocardiogram but found no telltale sign of a heart attack there. However, I asked the emergency room physicians to perform a quick ultrasound of her heart, which showed that her heart was beating very weakly and her ejection fraction was severely reduced. This was a drastic change because until recently, she had a normally functioning heart.

Puzzled, I started asking her more questions. She had enjoyed very good health until she felt a mass in her thigh. That mass ended up being a manifestation of melanoma, an aggressive form of skin cancer that had already metastasized throughout her body. She was started on a novel chemotherapy medication called *pembrolizumab*. At the time that chemo started, she barely had any symptoms. Her sons told us that she had been living at her home and actually was renovating it after a recent fire had damaged parts of it. She was active in the community, which centered around her church. The first cycle of pembrolizumab went well, and so did the second one. Encouragingly, a scan of her body showed that the cancer's spread was starting to reverse.

Even as her cancer responded to the treatment, she began feeling extremely fatigued. She could barely walk across her room at home. She saw her cancer team in clinic, who drew blood tests. When the tests came back, she was immediately directed to go to the emergency room. Her troponin level had come back elevated, and that's when I met her.

My Spidey Sense was tingling—I knew she was in trouble, but I wasn't sure she was having a heart attack. Given that her heart function was abnormal, I suspected that she had myocarditis, an inflammation of the heart muscle. Myocarditis is mostly caused by infections, commonly from viruses, but it can also rarely be caused by exposures to toxic chemicals such as cocaine and autoimmune conditions such as systemic lupus erythematosus. However, the inflammation in her body was not just affecting her heart—it involved every muscle in her body. She grew weak to the extent that she could not even breathe of her own accord and had to be permanently connected to a breathing machine despite our best efforts at giving her medications to dampen the conflagration of inflammation that the chemotherapy had set off. A month later, and despite maximal medical therapy, she died.

The irony was that at the end, her cancer was actually very well controlled, and its spread had actually reversed.

While chemotherapy can have many short-acting complications, it is becoming clearer that many chemotherapy agents leave an imprint that might last a lifetime. In some instances, such as in patients who develop heart failure, the prognosis of the heart failure caused by the medications is even grimmer than the cancer they were used to treat. The incidence of heart failure from chemotherapy, also called *cardiomyopathy*, has been so widespread that it has led to the development of an entire specialty within cardiology called cardio-oncology. "To me, the primary goal of cardio-oncology is to facilitate an uninterrupted fight against cancer," said Michel Khouri, a cardio-oncologist at Duke University Medical Center, "by effectively mitigating any potential cardiac concerns of cancer and cancer treatment."

Traditionally, the chemotherapy agents most commonly responsible for the development of cardiomyopathy are two classes of medications called *anthracyclines* and *trastuzumab,* both used to treat breast cancer. However, while there has been a shift away from anthracyclines, that doesn't mean that the new chemotherapies are harmless. The novel chemotherapy pembrolizumab that my patient had died of was part of a category of new targeted chemotherapies called *checkpoint inhibitors.* These medications help the body's immune system target cancer cells more efficiently.

One of the many challenges facing patients who develop heart failure after getting chemotherapy is the different narratives surrounding the two diseases and the reactions they generate both among patients themselves and their caregivers. A diagnosis of cardiomyopathy or heart failure, even though it may carry an equally grim prognosis, does not elicit the response cancer does. "When you tell someone you have cancer, they immediately think you are dying," says Kati, "but when I tell people I have cardiomyopathy, they usually don't know what I am talking about."

In 1995, Bob Williams, an astronomer and then director of the Space Telescope Science Institute at NASA, had a wild idea.[2] He wanted to point the most expensive telescope in history, humanity's best pair of eyes, Hubble, to stare at nothing. At a time when the Hubble program was still in its early years and was considered by many as a multibillion-dollar bust, Williams knew he would have a hard time convincing anyone else that the best use of Hubble might be to point it at absolutely nothing.

Good thing Williams didn't have to ask permission. His position afforded him dibs on 10 percent of Hubble's time, and so he built a team and put it to work. For one hundred hours spread out over several weeks, Hubble stared into the blackest of voids. After one hundred hours, the team merged all the images together, and in one fell swoop, Hubble cracked the universe wide open. Galaxies came gushing out of the nothingness, some three thousand in just an image 1/30 the size of the moon, some almost twelve billion years old.

What if we pointed Hubble not at the universe but inward? In many ways, over the past few decades, scientists have done just that by training microscopes on the human body. Out of the darkness, we have started to take heed of the galaxies within. One of the mind-blowing things we have only recently learned is how cancerous cells might actually be responsible for causing atherosclerosis, particularly in patients who don't seem to have any of the traditional risk factors for atherosclerosis, such as high blood pressure or cholesterol.

Among the curiosities found by cancer researchers, who were trying to find common defects in patients who developed blood cancers like leukemia or lymphoma, were small colonies of white cells that were all clones of each other and carried mutations that, in some patients, were linked to the development of leukemias. These clones lived longer than normal white blood cells and over time accounted for an increasing proportion of the total number of white blood cells. Not all of these patients developed cancer, but many did have something else—atherosclerosis. When mice were fed stem cells with this mutation, their blood vessels soon became pockmarked with atherosclerotic plaques. In humans, the presence of these clonal cells increases the risk of heart attacks twofold, and fourfold in those who have heart attacks earlier in life.

For now, doctors don't know what to do when they find these mutant clones, a condition called *clonal hematopoiesis of indeterminate potential* (CHIP).[3] Researchers, however, have fired up their engines. In nothing, they have found the promise of one day perhaps being able to treat or prevent a mutation that can both cause cancer and heart disease.

Cancer and heart disease account for two out of every three deaths in the United States, and there is much that is both similar and different between these two maladies. Cardiologists looking at the world of oncology, from the outside in, find much to aspire to. Oncologic treatment is becoming increasingly targeted, and the concept of "precision medicine" has really taken off in cancer diagnosis and treatment while it is only just being explored in heart disease. Cancer is also able to garner a lot more research funding from the United States government, foundations, donations, and pharmaceutical industries. Breast cancer, for example, receives almost ten times as much money per death attributed to it compared to heart disease.[4]

Some of my most meaningful interactions occurred when I was taking care of patients with cancer. It was during my time on the bone marrow transplant unit and the oncology wards at the Beth Israel Deaconess Medical Center and the Dana-Farber Cancer Institute, both in Boston, that I had some of my most moving experiences and developed some of the strongest relationships of my medical training. While taking care of patients with cancer often leaves one eyeball-to-eyeball with gut-wrenching tragedy, it also lets doctors enter the lives of their patients in ways that are unparalleled. Thus, after my internal medicine residency ended, instead of jumping straight into a cardiology training program, I actually worked as an oncology hospitalist, taking care of cancer patients admitted to the hospital. During that time, managing patients who were enrolled in clinical trials, getting experimental therapies after failing multiple prior rounds of chemotherapy, I realized how important these treatments were. It is clear that the path forward should not involve avoiding these drugs. "These are truly lifesaving drugs," says Javid Moslehi, a pioneering cardio-oncologist at Vanderbilt University, "which is why we have to be very smart about identifying who is at risk."

These days, new cancer drugs are being developed at such a fast rate in clinical trials with so few patients that many may or may not have cardiac side effects that might never be detected in clinical trials because of how small the trials are. Vigilance for so-called off-target effects of chemotherapy has therefore never been this vital.

Cancer and heart disease frequently coexist. Cancer survivors are at high risk of heart disease, even if they don't develop toxicity from their treatments. The danger of heart disease increases the longer the patients make it past their cancer diagnosis.[5] At the same time, many of the risk factors for heart disease, such as obesity and lack of physical activity, also increase the risk of cancer recurrence.[6,7] Physical activity not only helps overcome the deconditioning associated with illness but has also been shown to reduce cancer recurrence as well as reduce the chance of dying from both cancer and non-cancer-related causes.[8] On the other hand, it is now well established that obesity is a strong risk factor for the development of cancer. And as this research is beginning to show, just as cancer and heart disease may coexist, they could also both be averted with the same improvements in lifestyle—better nutrition and exercise.

So even as some of the causes of cancer and heart disease are similar, there is one big difference. "Patients see more of a finality to cancer than heart failure. So when a patient is diagnosed with cancer, they feel they will die from cancer if they aren't aggressive about treating it," said Michel Khouri. "Heart failure is more ambiguous to patients because patients may have friends and families with 'heart conditions' who appear to them to have been doing 'fine' for a number of years."

"People automatically assume with cancer that it is a terminal disease," said Kati. In this regard, though, cancer may not be so different from heart failure. Patients older than sixty-five with heart failure in the United States admitted to the hospital live for only an average of two years.

More than anything else in our time, cancer has metastasized into every facet of our everyday vernacular. The metaphors of war are frequently ascribed to cancer. When the late senator John McCain was first diagnosed with a brain tumor, many, including Barack Obama, were quick to draw up a battle scene with John McCain as the warrior, and cancer as his vile nemesis. What that inadvertently implies is that patients who are unable to defeat cancer are weak, having lost to the enemy, while those who choose a palliative approach to treatment have surrendered. Patients can feel pressured to be "brave," which delegitimizes anyone who may not want aggressive or invasive treatments. The very mention of cancer has now become a call to arms—when ductal carcinoma in situ, a condition in which one in five cases will turn cancerous five to forty years after diagnosis, was referred to in a study as "noninvasive cancer" as opposed to a high-risk lesion, far more women opted for aggressive options such as surgery.[9]

The militarization of cancer has gone to such extents, though, that in many cases, the analogies have flipped, with wars being described in oncologic terms. Addressing troops in Iraq in 2016, then United States defense secretary Ash Carter said, "ISIL's a cancer that's threatening to spread . . . you can't cure the disease just by cutting out the tumor. You have to eliminate it wherever it has spread."[10] Even critics of Mr. Carter's analogy resorted to medical parables, with one foreign policy expert retorting, "You have to destroy the bad Shiite government first, and then the inflammation, the side effects, the ISIS, will dissipate."

The narrative of cancer, of the foreign invader running roughshod through one's sovereign body, leads to many beneficial effects for patients. "More than one patient's family has told me that when their loved one has cancer, the 'whole family has cancer,'" said Michel Khouri. A cancer diagnosis activates a patient's support group, their friends and their family, or even strangers on the internet responding to a Kickstarter funding campaign. At the same time, though, too many times I have seen patients with heart disease suffer by themselves. "People associate heart disease with a lifestyle choice," said Kati, a view shared by many, "but few think of cancer the same way." Many also think of heart disease more as a reflection of the aging process, akin to a car just breaking down over time, rather than something that can be averted and that could occur through no fault of the person who has it. While patients with cancer jump through incredible hoops and sometimes uproot their entire families in order to receive experimental therapies they don't even know will work, many heart failure patients are not prescribed or do not take evidence-based medications known to help extend survival that can be picked up from any local pharmacy at minimal to no cost.[11]

I once lamented in an article I wrote for *The New York Times* that if only heart failure were called heart *cancer,* it could mean that patients might no longer be held responsible for their disease.[12] Perhaps they would not have to suffer by themselves and their families would rally around them the way they would if they had cancer and we would be able to raise the types of research funding needed to further the great progress we have seen in reducing the burden of heart disease. I know now that I was wrong. The answer is to not take cancer's story, cancer's language, cancer's metaphors, and co-opt them for heart disease. The answer is to tell heart disease's story, in heart disease's language, using heart disease's metaphors. And that is just one reason I wrote this book.

11

—◠∿—

THE HEART OF THE MATTER

You have to keep breaking your heart,
Until it opens.

—Rumi

Her room was unlike any other I had ever seen in the hospital. While most hospital rooms are as interchangeable as stale patient gowns, hers looked lived in like worn-out jeans. It was lined with T-shirts and potted plants and books. It was also much warmer than other rooms in the hospital, which could be frigid at times. She always had the curtains drawn, so when I stepped in through the sliding glass door into the balmy environs of her room, it felt like I was leaving the hospital. I felt like I was leaving my world and entering hers.

The hospital makes almost all of a patient's choices on their behalf once they are admitted. As a patient, you are expected to leave your life at the front door or in the back of the ambulance and give yourself up. Wear what we make you wear, eat what we make you eat, sleep when we let you sleep. Patients can only go relieve themselves when we doctors and nurses think it is okay for them to do so; if we think they can't walk to the bathroom, we will allow a commode in the room. If even that doesn't make the cut, we offer a bedpan for people to make the otherworldly effort of pooping while lying straight in bed. Some patients unable to comply with a pan have to do so in a tube.

Lydia was, of course, gonna have none of that. She wasn't in the hospital for a quick tune-up—she was here for the long haul. The day she moved into the hospital, she knew that there was only one way she would ever get out again—with someone else's heart beating in her chest.

It all started with a runny nose and a viral infection that never went away. Weeks passed, and several rounds of antibiotics proved to be useless. Feeling crummy, it took a while to figure out that the stuff in her lungs causing her to cough and gasp, and which was showing up on her x-rays, was not an infection; it was fluid.

Almost everyone reading this tale has had a viral infection. Most have it many, *many* times, and those with kids—those little petri dishes of germs—have them even more frequently. A very, *very* small number of all those who get viral infections, less than a fraction of a percent, will go on to develop dilated cardiomyopathy—a form of heart failure in which the heart becomes inexplicably weak and balloons in size. Some people can get by with medications, but for many, the only way out is with the only key that will allow them to escape from a disease that turns their body into an immobile receptacle.

Lydia was not ready to be incarcerated, and knowing her, chances are she never will be. Her skin was bronzed from riding horses and working on her farm. She had kids at home who needed their mom back. She was the glue of her family, she told me, the peacemaker. Yet knowing how much stuff she had brought with her to the hospital, she must have known she was not going back anytime soon.

The first heart transplant operation was performed in Cape Town, South Africa, by Christiaan Barnard in 1967. Being the first person to perform a heart transplant was more important for Barnard than being the best. Only a few days after performing the operation, Barnard embarked on a worldwide high-five tour while his patient died in his absence just a few days after getting the transplant.[1] However, while Barnard became the face of heart transplantation, other surgeons, like Norman Shumway at Stanford University, kept improving their surgical technique as well as the medications used to keep the body's immune system in check to ensure that those receiving heart transplants survived longer and longer. These days, the median survival of patients receiving heart transplants is almost twelve years. The one thing that hasn't changed much, though, is how many hearts are available for donation. In the United States, even though millions of people have heart failure, the number of hearts available for donation is only around three thousand per year, and that is only because so many young people have been dying recently because of the opioid epidemic. Lydia knew that it could be months before she could find a good match.

Lydia's heart was so weak that at this point she could barely get out of bed. She had multiple medications going 24-7 that helped her heart beat just a bit stronger. These medications were dangerous, though, because they also increased her risk of having potentially fatal heart rhythms. Her life was balanced on a knife-edge, and we trod carefully around her—instead of drawing labs daily, we started getting them once every couple of days. We tried to avoid changing any of her medications, wary that the slightest imbalance could throw her into a tailspin.

Slowly but surely, despite our best efforts, Lydia began to unravel. After the first few weeks, her family stopped coming by. She grew sick of having to be in bed most of the time. We took her to the hospital courtyard a few times, but those trips were few and fleeting.

Then one day, the news arrived early around dawn—a heart that was a great match for Lydia had become available. Everyone was excited, most of all Lydia. All this time, she had been anxious about the surgery, about the pain, about having a tube stuck down her throat, but all of that went away. The nurses helped her pack up her room. All her things were stuffed into large plastic bags. The last thing she did before she left was put on her lipstick. As she was rolled in her bed to the operating room, the staff all waved her goodbye as if she were going off to war.

Over the next several hours, as the team was tending to the rest of our patients, we were also virtually checking in on her. She was still in the operating room, but we had no idea what was going on.

All of a sudden, the doors to the intensive care unit opened, and Lydia was on her way back, almost exactly how she had left. Turns out that by the time the heart had been taken out of the donor and brought to our hospital by the surgeons, it had started to undergo degradation. The cardiac surgeons decided that there was more harm than good possible if they used the heart, and they sent Lydia back to us. We were all devastated; Lydia's clock had to be reset, and the wait started all over again. None of us were sure if she would make it to the next one.

Cabin fever really started to set in for Lydia. Her heart got weak to the point that she had to have a pump placed in her aorta through the large artery in her groin. She couldn't even move around in bed any longer because of the risk of the pump moving in her aorta. The only exercise she could do was pull some brightly colored rubber bands tied to her bed railings with her arms. Frequently, she became restless, and we would have to talk her down.

Just before things reached a boiling point, the call came again. A suitable match had become available. Lydia went through the motions—the packing, the lipstick, and the rolling—but with a lot less verve. We were all hopeful that this would be the right time. There was no way lightning would strike twice.

In the operating room, the surgeons looked at the donor heart that had arrived wrapped in ice via a charter plane. It looked great, and the procedure was started instantly. Lydia's chest was cut open, and everything connecting her heart to her body—all the blood vessels and all the nerves and everything else—was cut, and her heart was thrown into a bucket. The donor heart was placed in her chest, and it was connected to each and every one of the blood vessels in her chest. The moment of truth arrived, but the donor heart lay perfectly still in her body. Despite their best efforts, the donor heart never really took, and Lydia experienced what is the single most devastating complication of heart transplantation—primary graft dysfunction—in which the donor heart, for some mysterious and as yet unknown reason, just never really beats in the recipient's body.

At almost any other time, this is where Lydia's story would end. She had received two shots at one of the most prized and rare gifts of all—a new heart. And yet, here she was, with a dead heart in her chest, deader even than her own, which was now in the wastebasket.

Nanette Wenger and Eugene Braunwald, two of cardiology's timeless pioneers, picked this profession in the 1950s because both believed they were living through the golden age in our battle against heart disease. And yet, almost seventy years on, one can argue that the golden age of cardiology is only now being fully realized. Just a few years ago, if Lydia had a dead heart in her chest, the surgeons might have been calling the morgue. But the surgeons didn't pronounce her dead, or call her family to arrange for her funeral, or perform an autopsy. Instead, they implanted mechanical pumps right into her new heart to whir blood throughout her body. Despite the odds, Lydia survived with the mechanical pumps long enough for a third heart to become available for her after a few months. This time, everything went as planned; the heart took to her body like a baby cub takes to her mother. Lydia is no longer in the hospital. She is back in the big country where she was always destined to be.

Left ventricular assist devices (LVADs) haven't just changed how we deal with heart disease. They represent the dawn of a new era in human life—the union of man and machine—and have implications not only for how we treat heart failure but for what it means to be human. Yet how these devices came to be has much to do with perhaps the most human traits of all—the malignancy of ambition and the perpetuation of ingenuity.

LVADs are mechanical pumps that are surgically implanted into patient's left ventricles, the pumping chamber of the heart. Initially, most patients received an LVAD while they waited in a hospital in the hope that they would get a heart transplant. Some got their wish, but many others never did.

Just in the past decade, twenty thousand patients in the United States have received an LVAD.[2] These people rarely have a pulse, and if you do CPR on their chest, they might actually die because of it. They have an LVAD sewn into their practically vestigial heart to do its work. At any moment, if these patients' batteries discharge, they can die, yet they aren't stowed away in hospitals; they are roaming the streets, lifting weights in the gym, and shopping on Black Friday, doing many things they were able to do before their hearts gave up on them. Some of them call themselves LVAD Warriors, and they might represent the future of mankind.

The 1950s and '60s were the golden era of the space age. *Sputnik* was launched into orbit in 1957, shattering what was thought impossible just a few years earlier. The next year, a stray mongrel name Laika was picked up from the streets of Moscow and was shot into space, becoming the first large mammal *ever* in orbit. Back on earth, though, a familiar threat continued to ravage humanity. In the 1950s, a heart attack was an almost certain death sentence; of the people who survived a heart attack, half were left permanently debilitated.

Advances in medical care turned that grim fate around. Not only was the mortality of heart attacks greatly improved, how much it affects a person's ability to get on with their life has also been transformed. Research I performed with my team showed some impressive progress; these days in the United States, 93 percent of people are able to return to work within a year after a heart attack.[3]

Progress against heart attacks, while allowing many people to live through them, means that many live with a damaged heart. Some of these survivors end up developing heart failure, and as the population ages, the number of Americans living with heart failure now exceeds six million. What makes heart failure such a challenging disease is how difficult it can be to take care of sick heart failure patients at home. Heart failure, in fact, is the most common cause of admissions to the hospital for older adults in the United States.

The heart, for all its wonders, has one Achilles' heel: heart muscle is very poor at regenerating. A heart once damaged can rarely, if ever, heal. Therefore, even though there are medications and procedures that can prevent the heart's function from potentially worsening, there is little that can be done about a heart scarred. While heart transplantation can be an option for a few patients, it comes with its own set of challenges. Patients who receive a heart transplant have to take special medications that suppress the immune system. These medications prevent the body's immune system from rejecting the foreign heart. Yet because they dampen the body's immunity, this can lead to the person becoming very susceptible to infections both common and obscure that can practically affect any part of the body. These medications have to be taken religiously, without fail, for years and years, and not taking them can have disastrous consequences.

It had been several years since Peter received a heart transplant. Peter had been living with a new heart for so long that he had reached the state that one wishes for all patients with a crippling disease—blissful forgetfulness. Ever since he received his heart almost six years ago, Peter had never had to return to the hospital. He was doing all that he was supposed to and by all discernable means had won the game.

So I was curious when he came to the emergency room after a few weeks of progressively worsening breathing. I asked him if something had changed, and he told me he couldn't think of anything. I asked him if he had been taking his immune-suppressing meds, and he said he was. He still looked fairly comfortable, but I have learned to be very wary of patients who have received heart transplants—their physiology is so different from normal that they frequently don't exhibit signs and symptoms doctors are used to seeing in the vast majority of heart patients. They may not even feel pain if they have a heart attack because their heart's nervous connections are severed. He had a routine ultrasound a few weeks earlier that showed that his heart function was normal, but I wanted a second look. As soon as the images started being broadcast on the ultrasound machine, though, that was reduced to a distant memory—Peter's heart was barely moving. It certainly seemed like his body was rejecting his heart.

I turned toward Peter and asked him this time with more than a hint of perturbation if he had been taking his medications. He confessed that for the past few weeks, he hadn't taken them. He told me he couldn't afford them.

"I am sorry," he told me over and over again, even as I tried to tell him it was okay.

I gave him a hefty dose of steroids to blast his immune system into submission, but he seemed to only be getting worse. We connected him to a machine that could filter out all the angry antibodies floating around in his system that had awakened in the absence of the protective shield of his immune-suppressing medications so that they might stop rejecting the transplanted heart. All our efforts were in vain—Peter soon lost his pulse, his heart stopped beating, and after an hour of CPR, just a few hours after he had come to the hospital, he was dead.

Even though receiving and then living with a heart transplant is far from a walk in the park, only a select few of the countless who could benefit from it actually end up being able to receive one. And as technology became more advanced and we developed dialysis to support dying kidneys and mechanical ventilators to support sickly lungs, the ideal for many was not a transplanted heart but one that was even better, one that had none of the inconveniences that came with an organ that is impermanent. It was thus that the idea of the total artificial heart was born.

The space age glorified the man-made over the organic. Shiny metallic satellites were taking humans beyond the sky and on the moon, to places that were previously the realm of scripture. Engineered objects could withstand forces that could decimate the human body in a blink and could allow us to perform unimaginable feats, such as breaking the sound barrier.

At the same time, the transplantation of the heart had greatly diminished the mystique the organ was shrouded in. Heart transplantation proved that the heart was merely a pump, nothing more. Far from being the repository of the soul, the archival bank of human emotions, the heart was no different from a motor that could be picked off the shelf and used interchangeably.

After a South African surgeon with little recognition in the field had won the race for the first transplant, the next frontier was a goal even loftier, even more ambitious. "Frankly, I was sorry I had not been the first," wrote Denton Cooley, a surgeon in Houston. "Barnard's feat was my own personal *Sputnik*."[4] Days after his breakthrough, Cooley sent a telegram to Barnard: "Congratulations on your first transplant, Chris. I will be reporting my first hundred soon." Cooley began transplanting hearts but knew that his chance to be the first was gone. Cooley was now ready to do anything to be the first man to implant an artificial heart in a human being. Even if it meant stealing an experimental device from a rival.

Denton Cooley was once asked in court by a lawyer if he was the best heart surgeon in the world.[5]

"Yes," he replied.

"Don't you think that's being rather immodest?"

"Perhaps," Cooley replied. "But remember I'm under oath."

Others, too, shared that impression. In his autobiography, Christiaan Barnard wrote about observing Cooley at work. "It was the most beautiful surgery I had ever seen in my life. . . . It went forward like a broad river— never fast, never in obvious haste, yet never going back."[6]

Denton Cooley was the first person to implant a totally artificial heart in a human being in 1969. Yet that fact alone is perhaps the least interesting part of his story.

After completing his surgical training at Johns Hopkins, Cooley returned to his hometown of Houston to work alongside Michael DeBakey, one of the most famous surgeons of his time. DeBakey was the first person to perform bypass surgery in the United States and was also one of the first surgeons to implant a temporary LVAD, which provides support to the pumping chamber of the heart but doesn't replace the whole thing. DeBakey thought an LVAD, which provides partial support to the heart, rather than an artificial heart, which is implanted in place of the patient's heart, was more promising. Through their partnership, DeBakey and Cooley came up with several advances, including new procedures for damaged aortas and improvements to the bypass machines that supply blood to the body while the heart is being operated upon. Yet their relationship soured over time until it reached a breaking point. In 1960, Cooley left DeBakey's group, joining a neighboring hospital, and their epic rivalry, which would last for decades, began in earnest. In a cover story in *Life* magazine, an administrator was quoted saying, "Denton just got tired of sucking hind tit."[7]

Cooley was taken in by the race to the stars and found parallels in what he was doing with what astronauts and engineers were hoping to achieve. In a memoir, he quoted the astronaut Eugene Cernan: "A common bond between [moonwalkers and heart surgeons] was the nature of the territories we explored: the moon was an 'almost mythical land' that had long been regarded as a religious icon and romantic symbol; likewise, the human heart was traditionally viewed as the seat of the soul and emotions."[8]

Part of what drove Cooley was geopolitics—just like the space race, Russian surgeons had a distinct leg up on their American counterparts, and had beat DeBakey, for example, in performing the first CABG surgery using modern techniques, and they had significant experience implanting mechanical heart pumps in dogs. "It just sounds a bit supercilious," said Cooley in an interview, but "I did not want the Russians to beat us, as they had with *Sputnik*."[9]

Cooley, it appears, though, was competing as much with DeBakey as he was with the Russians. While Cooley was performing a lot of heart surgeries, DeBakey was far ahead in the quest to the total artificial heart. He had received a research grant from the National Institutes of Health, through which DeBakey had made an experimental heart from plastic and artificial graft material.

Cooley wanted his *Sputnik* moment and saw both the Russians and DeBakey ahead of him in line. So, in cahoots with one of DeBakey's assistants, Cooley "commandeered" one of the artificial hearts from De-Bakey's lab.[10] DeBakey had never implanted the device in a human being because his extensive experience in animals had shown that the device didn't work well. Cooley did not consider that a limitation. "I considered myself the most experienced heart surgeon in the world at that time, there was no question about that," he said in a video interview. "I didn't need to go practice on a bunch of dogs and cats in an animal laboratory at Baylor [College of Medicine]."[11]

In Haskell Karp, Cooley found a patient willing to take the plunge with him. A forty-seven-year-old printing estimator from Illinois, he had come down to Houston specifically hoping to have Denton Cooley replace three of the four valves in his severely diseased heart. Cooley told him that if the originally planned procedure failed, then the total artificial heart could bail him out until a donor heart became available for transplantation. Karp knew he would be the first person ever to receive the artificial heart, but he had been sick for too long and saw no other way.

When Karp was wheeled into the operating room, he was pretty much on death's doorstep, and it was only after his heart had been opened that Cooley realized that there was no way Karp would make it through the procedure. "Was I going to let Mr. Karp die on the operating table or try to save his life by whatever means?" wrote Cooley in his memoir, *100,000 Hearts*. "I decided to proceed with our contingency plan."[12]

Cooley cut out Karp's heart from his chest and connected the plastic heart with his blood vessels. As the artificial heart was turned on and began to fill with blood, "my team members and I held our breaths," wrote

Cooley. "We were immediately relieved when it began to pump blood, almost like a natural heart."

Unlike many others, Cooley was fairly dispassionate about the heart. "The heart was nothing more than a pump," he once said in an interview, "and it was a very simple device compared to the liver and kidneys that had multiple functions in the body but the heart has only one purpose, that was to pump blood, and to push the blood through the circulatory system."[13] The heart was nothing more than a servant of the brain. "Once the brain is gone, the heart is unemployed," said Cooley at a conference in South Africa. "Then we must find it employment."[14]

Karp survived with the pump for only three days before it failed and Cooley transplanted a heart into him. Karp died thirty-six hours later. Cooley was censured by both Baylor and the American College of Surgeons. "He wanted to be able to say he was the first one to use an artificial heart in a patient," DeBakey said later in an interview. "I never quite understood it other than his ambition was almost uncontrolled." Cooley, though, never regretted his decision to implant the device, writing decades later in his memoir, "I see [Haskell Karp's] face—framed by the dark-rimmed glasses he always wore—and am reminded of the trust and hope he put in me and in medical science."

Denton Cooley died in 2016, leaving behind an unassailable legacy, which resulted in serial improvements in heart surgery and helped make surgery safer for patients around the world. Close to his death, he described what made the heart unique: "The heart, you can actually see it working." Unlike the brain, the liver, or kidneys, which perform complex tasks with bureaucratic invisibility, the heart is an incessant striver, whose every action is felt and heard in every body that it beats in. It is visceral and charismatic in a way no other part of the human body is.

After Cooley's demise, things have been in turmoil close to home; the hospital that Cooley turned into one of the most prominent heart transplant centers in the world recently has run into serious trouble. Heart transplant recipients there experienced such adverse outcomes that federal funds for the program have been revoked. Heart transplantation is one of the highest-risk, greatest-reward projects that the human race can embark on. This was in fact the impetus behind Cooley's failed efforts to design the total artificial heart.

The total artificial heart, much to Cooley's eventual dismay, has to date never really taken off. What has exploded onto the scene is what DeBakey had originally hypothesized—partial support with the patient's heart still intact: the left ventricular assist device (LVAD).

I consider myself one of the last generation of people who knew of a world before the internet. When my three-year-old daughter grows up, I will tell her of what it was like to not always have GPS, to not always know where you are, to not be able to talk on the phone and surf the internet simultaneously, and to not always be surveilled. I am also the last generation of physicians, perhaps, who saw a world when there were no people with LVADs.

When I was in internal medicine residency, when heart failure progressed to a critical point, either we referred patients for consideration of a heart transplant or we told them to get their affairs in order. Some patients were started on intravenous drips of medications that increased how hard the heart beat—yet they withdrew their very own pound of flesh. Inotropes, as these medications are called, can actually *increase* how quickly patients die, by initiating malignant arrhythmias, even as they might provide comfort for those with debilitating heart failure. On average, though, these patients with advanced heart failure seemed to only live for an average of six months after they became dependent on inotropes to maintain adequate blood flow.

Then suddenly, whispers started to occur among the residents. A row of rooms on one of the wards that were never managed by the residents began to be occupied with patients receiving LVADs. Here's how they work: Blood is sucked into the LVAD, which is directly sutured into the left ventricle, and then fed back into the aorta, bypassing the aortic valve, which is the usual exit door for blood leaving the heart. A plastic-encased wire called the *driveline* connects the LVAD pump to batteries that patients carry, usually in belts around their waists. LVADs effectively take over the pumping function of the heart, and while LVADs have been around for a while, initial ones were too clunky to be durable.

Early LVADs had a problem—they were trying too hard to be like the human heart. Engineers tried devising pulsatile pumps that pumped blood to the heart in beats. The human body, like every other mammal, has been especially designed to see blood flow in waves, with the heart beating like the wings of a bird rather than the continuous churn of a blender.

Yet as researchers tried to replicate the heart, they realized that an equivalent machine would have to be very large, have tons of moving parts, with chafing and turbulent blood flow, be very technically difficult to implant, and even harder to run. So after a few iterations, they changed their designs from pulsatile pumps to ones more resembling a continuously running turbine that can pump almost eight to ten liters of blood per minute.[15] LVADs finally became good enough that they were able to expand their role beyond just being a bridge to transplantation. In 2010, the FDA approved the first LVAD for destination therapy, meaning that the LVAD by itself was now the destination, the constant companion of the patient until he or she met their eventual end. It was this change that helped exponentially increase the number of patients receiving LVADs.

People who receive LVADs experience a life unlike any other. They are tethered to their devices and their remaining power. If you feel anxious when your cell phone is dangerously low on battery and there is no charging socket in sight, imagine what might happen if you are a patient whose very life depends on remaining fully charged and close to a power source. For many, a power outage is an inconvenience—for an LVAD patient, it can be a close encounter with the celestial plane. Recently, when Hurricanes Florence and Michael hit North Carolina, we were worried sick for all our LVAD patients who might not have access to power. Yet even in these circumstances, one of our LVAD patients, instead of worrying about himself, was busy rescuing elderly men and women stuck in their flooded homes.

The most seemingly benign things can be a challenge for LVAD patients. Every eleven seconds, an older American is treated in an emergency room for a fall. I remember a patient with an LVAD who had a fall and lost consciousness. He didn't hit his head or suffer any major injury but was knocked out long enough for his LVAD to become completely discharged, leading to permanent brain injury. He never woke up again.

LVADs are very effective at improving heart failure, yet they come with a serious set of complications. LVAD patients have very high rates of bleeding since the pumps chew up clotting factors. These patients also need to religiously take blood thinners to prevent the formation of blood clots within the pump, another complication that can lead to stroke. The driveline remains the Achilles' heel of LVAD technology given that it represents a permanent conduit between the sterile inside of the body and the rampaging cacophony of germs in the outside world. This leads to a very high risk of infections.

If you turn on the TV or go to the cinema, watching shows like HBO's *Westworld,* science fiction writers keep returning to the question about what the future of human life looks like. LVADs, however, reveal that the distant fusion of man and machine is already here. Patients with LVADs are literally dependent on their devices for their lives. As LVADs get smaller and smaller and the technology gets more efficient, LVADs might become even more durable and long-lasting than a transplanted heart.

By taking over the function of the body's hardest-working organ, one that beats a hundred thousand times a day, LVADs might represent our first foray into successfully producing artificial organs that can sustain us long past our expiration date. The lived experience of LVAD recipients not only gives us a window into a world where the human heart is redundant but suggests what being human might mean in the future.

Perhaps fittingly, what gave me a window into their lives was not seeing and talking to patients with LVADs in the clinics and wards but joining a Facebook group where patients with LVADs gather for community, for shared experiences both joyous and tragic, where birthdays and deaths are announced in equal measure. It wasn't until I joined Facebook groups for LVAD patients that I knew what the future of mankind might look like.

Doctors and nurses sometimes treat patients unfairly. "As a former fat person who lost more than 120 pounds," a colleague told me, "I hated going to my primary care physician because she judged me."

Like their patients, clinicians also hide behind a thin, depersonalizing veil, and it can take a while before that comes off. So where can patients turn to talk about things that some doctors might dismiss and share experiences that only a select few in the world will ever relate to?

If you step into the world of patients with LVADs, through several Facebook groups such as LVAD Warriors or LVAD Friends, you will realize that these virtual groups give LVAD patients something that neither doctors nor nurses, neither family nor friends can give.

As a fly on the wall in these groups, I catch a vivid window into the realms of people whose lives are marked as much by heroic peaks of joy as spiraling depths of despair. Every member has this sense that they have somehow cheated death, that they are alive because of a technology only a few in the world can access and one that didn't exist until just a few years ago. LVADs let them have babies, get married, be around for their children's and grandchildren's graduations, and so forth. When they dress up to go to a party, they post pictures, letting everyone know they haven't quite given up on life yet.

All this comes at a toll that can be too much for some to withstand. Having an LVAD requires constant and incessant care of the device, the driveline coming out of the skin, the dressings used to cover it, the batteries that always need to be charged, monitoring of the pump at all times to make sure that it is functioning right, and on and on and on. No one person alone can ever take care of an LVAD, and having robust social support is a prerequisite to getting an LVAD.

The need for almost 24-7 caregiver support can place a heavy burden on family members, many of whom I have seen relocating and changing or leaving jobs to be able to make the commitment needed to take on this monumental task. All sorts of family dynamics spill out into the open after an LVAD comes into the picture. Too many patients post stories of painful divorces given how stressful the care and maintenance of an LVAD can be.

Having an LVAD can make some people feel like they are trapped. "I sometimes wake up and remember that this is my life and for a second I have to convince myself," posted a woman. "This life isn't for the weak . . . but it's hard to be a warrior every day." Another woman described walking into a rural hotel bar with her LVAD and everyone stopped talking. "When we got outside I said to my husband that I think these farmers thought I might be [wearing] a suicide belt or special weapons," she wrote. "If they had asked I would have told them I was from the future."

Some, within the same sentence, expressed a dueling sense of deep gratitude and gloom. "The LVAD made me feel as if I was half robot . . . lol . . . it is a journey that I would not wish upon my worst enemy . . . yet I am so grateful that this option was there for me . . . you can do this, LVAD warrior." When a patient was depressed, asking the group if they could just be truthful and say they all hated their LVAD, another replied, "Don't fight the VAD. Kick its butt and make it your bitch."

Even in this closed group, there is a hierarchy, a caste system almost. The upper caste belongs to those who received an LVAD as a bridge to transplantation. For them, there is hope that one day it will be over, that they will receive the "gift," that gift being a heart transplant. After someone gets a heart transplant, there are pictures that are posted, congratulations are offered, and there is a sense that the patient can now graduate from the group. Many will actually donate the supplies that they needed to maintain upkeep of their LVAD as a final act of their absolution.

For those with an LVAD as destination therapy, their outlook on life and their LVAD is very different. For them, there is no out, so they have to accept the LVAD in a way that patients holding out for a transplant never do. I have met people who have had their LVADs for eight years—most enjoy a quality of life unlike anything they experienced when their hearts were failing. Some people do so well with their LVADs that they even give up the opportunity to be listed for a transplant. For many patients with LVADs, the greatest inconvenience is having to wear their batteries around their waist, yet one of my senior mentors, who has witnessed the transformation of heart failure care with his own eyes, put things into perspective for a patient.

"We never thought people would live long enough to complain about the size of the batteries," said Dr. Joe Rogers to me in clinic one day.

A very small number of patients with LVADs actually do experience something quite unusual—recovery of the function of their native hearts. A small percentage of patients will have recovery to the point that they have their LVADs explanted.[16] A patient declared freedom from his LVAD by simply posting an x-ray image of his chest with no large pump to be seen. For some, the only token left behind is a small ruby bearing from the LVAD, which they will wear as a necklace as a constant reminder of what they overcame.

LVADs are the most visible and dramatic piece in a movement that will change what it means to be human, and it starts with the commodification of human organs. Cardiologists are at the forefront of finding a home for devices to live in the human body. Not just LVADs, patients can receive pacemakers and defibrillators that monitor every single heartbeat that we emit. We can have monitors placed in our arteries that constantly measure how much pressure is in the heart, how fast is blood flowing, and if we are experiencing worsening symptoms of heart failure. Unlike a smartwatch that measures your heart rate, these devices require invasive procedures to be placed and surgery to be taken out, and they are vulnerable in the same way as any computerized device is to hacking and sabotage.

Such technology has changed a doctor visit to a tune-up. And sometimes when people are in real trouble, they don't really need a doctor; they
need an engineer. Durable implanted cardiovascular technology is only the
start, and technologies that are housed within our bodies that can take over
the function of other organs are no longer something conceived by Isaac
Asimov or Arthur C. Clarke but by living, breathing scientists in the lab
across town.

Ancient humans imagined the heart as the organ that was the first to
live and the last to die. No longer. The human body can live long past the
failure of the heart. As LVADs change our concept of life, they may have
an even more dramatic effect on what the lack of life is. I learned this, like I
have learned so many important lessons in my training, at three o' clock
in the morning. The heart has for almost all of time been the determinant
of life or death. Yet a patient with an LVAD can die even as their LVAD is
running at full sprint, even as they have a normal rhythm on their EKG.
Living with an LVAD can be really hard, and sometimes, dying with one
can be even harder.

As his LVAD broke down, so did his life. As he became moodier and an-
grier, his care network—a ragtag collection of friends and ex-girlfriends—
started to dissipate until all he had for company was the doctors and nurses
in the hospital. Along the way, he had also contracted a serious infection
around his driveline. Multiple visits back to the operating room to clean
out the infected tissue around his driveline couldn't fully get rid of the colony of bacteria that had now found a home in his body. Every few days,
that colony would seed his blood with bacteria, causing a septic reaction
throughout his body. By this time, antibiotics were keeping him alive as
much as the LVAD was.

The infection just ate him away until he was barely recognizable. He
appeared shriveled like a dried date, and yet despite our best efforts, we
could not slow his descent. He fought it but eventually decided that he didn't

want any breathing machines or additional trips to the intensive care unit—
if it was his time, he wanted us to let him go.

Then one day, I got the call. It was the nurse; she wanted me to come
see him.

No one spends more time with LVAD patients and understands the
patients as well as the nurses do. So imagine my surprise when I reached
his room and found the nursing staff just standing around as if they were
frozen in time, appearing flabbergasted. They thought he had died, but
they weren't sure.

He had stopped breathing or moving, but the question was, how does
one die when they still have blood pumping furiously through their bodies
with an LVAD? Because the room was otherwise oppressively silent, the
hum of the LVAD was faintly audible.

When most people die, it is usually the heart that dies first, starving
the brain of oxygen, which follows inevitably. At other times, the brain dies
first, as it might after someone has a massive bleed in the brain, or someone overdoses on heroin and stops breathing for a while, and the patient is
declared brain-dead, but the heart continues to beat.

The nurses had seen everything that could happen to an LVAD patient,
yet they hadn't seen someone die, and neither had I. I turned on the EKG
monitor, hoping a flat line would bail me out, but there was a regular
rhythm there.

Fact was that I had to think of him as if he were heartless, so I focused
on the brain and what it does. He was not breathing, and when I poked
the corner of his eye with my gloved finger, he didn't blink, meaning that
his brain wasn't performing its most basic functions. I declared that he had
indeed died, but when I scanned the room, it was clear to me that everyone knew that they were entering a new era and had seen a face of death
they had never seen before. Disconcertingly, the LVAD was still running,
so I dialed the number of one of our senior LVAD nurses, who had been
managing LVADs for years.

Like an IT support staffer guiding me over the phone, she walked me through the drop-down menus of the LVAD until I reached the prompt to stop the LVAD. I looked around, still unsure of what exactly I was doing, and then pressed the button, and after a loud and stark countdown, which sounded as if the LVAD was announcing the end of time, it stopped. I had effectively turned a human being off.

More than one in ten cardiologists, in fact, consider turning off an LVAD as equivalent to euthanasia, and almost two-thirds think that an LVAD should only be deactivated if a patient is imminently dying, essentially saying that once one has an LVAD, they are essentially a prisoner of technology, with the only out being death itself.[17]

It can be hard to know what to do with a heart that will not stop until it is asked to. Not only does it change how we doctors think, it changes how patients think. I once took care of a patient who had such a bad infection of his chest from when the LVAD was implanted that his breastbone never really healed and one could actually see a bit of his LVAD at all times whirring away in his chest. Naturally, this window just meant that infections incessantly kept entering his body, and this time, they were severe enough to require him to breathe from a breathing machine under anesthesia.

While he was anesthetized, our team wasn't sure that this was a road he could keep going down. His chest was so intractably infected that there was no way we could clear it. I was hoping to talk to him after he woke up, if possible, about whether perhaps we should deescalate and help him spend some time at home with his family.

When he eventually woke up, he told me with a straight face, "Doc, I want to live forever. And when the end comes, I want to live some more."

Too often when our best efforts fail to improve patients' quality of life, we do not have important conversations with them about not just how they would like to live but how they would like to die.

I met a man in his midseventies who was one of the earliest recipients of a destination therapy LVAD. Clyde had an LVAD implanted seven years earlier, and he had perhaps outlived most people who had received an LVAD. Yet despite the years that he had gained, it had been far from smooth sailing. He had been admitted to the hospital about a dozen times, at times for bleeding from his intestines, at others because he had received electric shocks to get his heart out of dangerous fast rhythms like ventricular tachycardia.

This time around, he was sicker than ever before. After he'd endured a rocky course in the intensive care unit, and when he was a bit more stable, I remember asking him what we could do to help him.

"I want to go home."

Clyde lived on a farm and missed not being able to spend enough time there. All he wanted, he told me, was to ride his tractor one more time. He knew that his time on earth was close to an end but was surprised no one had asked him about these things in the many years that he had been this ill. We called our palliative care team to help us transition our care to a treatment pathway that focused solely on making Clyde feel better and honoring his wishes. Contrary to what many might think, palliative care can actually prolong life in some patients who might otherwise have received procedures or therapies that can have serious complications, bringing an abrupt end to a patient's life.[18]

Clyde's LVAD was unable to provide him the support he needed by itself, so we had to start a continuously running IV medication to help his native heart beat stronger and to help him maintain enough blood pressure so that blood could reach all his vital organs. He wanted to go home, so we made arrangements to enroll him in hospice, a program offered for patients at the end of life that provides them additional resources to be able to spend time at home. The hospice, however, was uncomfortable managing the drip medication and asked us to see if we could turn it off.

It was important for Clyde to be able to go home. At this point, it was the only thing he wanted, the only hope he had left to cling to. We turned off the medication, but his blood pressure dropped, and he died within hours. It had been more than two thousand days since he had received the LVAD and only four days since one of the most important conversations of his life. He died in the last place he wanted to be in.

Clyde is far from the only patient with heart disease to experience what many would consider a bad death. Over the course of the last century, we have made great strides in helping patients with heart disease live both better and longer.[19] And yet the inevitability of death remains the only certain thing in human existence. As we anticipate the next big thing in heart disease that could help patients live better—like a new medication that could dissolve atherosclerotic plaques or the next LVAD that could be wirelessly charged and obviate the need for a driveline—we must also figure out how we can help them in their greatest moment of need.[20]

After I wrote my last book, *Modern Death*, I received the opportunity of a lifetime, an interview with my hero Terry Gross on her NPR radio show. The interview was scheduled for early in the morning, and the night before, I was working in the hospital. I could have rescheduled my shift and gone into the interview nice and fresh, but I decided that the sleep deprivation might help me be more honest and less rehearsed.

The night leading into the interview, one of my friends, also a cardiology fellow, called me. "Haider, I need your help. I have a patient that we are doing CPR on," he told me, so I walked over to the intensive care unit.[21] When I reached the room, there was a throng of people administering medications, performing chest compressions, barking orders. They had been performing CPR on this middle-aged woman for almost an hour and a half, which is way longer than almost any effort I had witnessed.

The fact is that my colleague had done everything right and thought about all the things that could have caused the cardiac arrest. He didn't need me because I carried a secret nugget of knowledge only privy to me. He needed me to tell him if it was okay to stop.

To me, this story, which I narrated to Terry in a hypnotic trance induced by her voice and my lack of sleep, captured the entire arc of modern cardiovascular care. Over the past century, we have made progress that seems unimaginable to those who have lived through it, and if you look at developments like LVADs, that golden age is very much still upon us. The progress of technology is not going to slow down anytime soon, and, with the emergence of big data and ubiquitous connectivity and the globalization of biomedical innovation, progress could further accelerate.

In patients with heart disease, we know when to start things. *No pulse?* Start CPR! *ST elevations on the EKG?* Take 'em to the cath lab! *Lungs full of fluid?* Unleash the diuretics and inotropes! *Cholesterol levels sky-high despite a good diet?* Here are some statins for you!

In patients with heart disease, it is hard to know when to stop. Patients rarely reach an inflection point—the pull of such chronic diseases as heart failure, hypertension, diabetes, and the like draws them closer to the end at all times, sometimes with violent yanks and at others with gentle nudges. What does all this mean for patients?

It means that patients with heart disease are much more likely to die in a hospital than at home—and to die at home is what the vast majority of patients want—than are patients with diseases such as cancer.[22] It means that palliative care, known to improve quality of life in terminally ill patients, is grossly underused in patients with heart disease.

Even when patients with heart disease get sent to receive hospice care at home, hospice nurses visiting them can often do nothing but watch their patients suffer. In a survey I published in the *Journal of Palliative Medicine,* a hospice nurse recalled how she had to see a patient drowning in his own secretion for days before he died. Some patients have to get readmitted to the hospital from hospice, which defeats the whole point of hospice. I took care of a patient in the hospital recently who was on hospice but had to come back to the hospital. He was suffering so much that despite our best efforts, he frequently yelled out, hoping for God to take him away. Just a day before he died in the hospital, he asked for a pastor to come see him in the middle of the night because he couldn't sit, couldn't stand, couldn't breathe.

Many patients have defibrillators implanted to prevent a dangerous heart rhythm from going for too long. However, for terminally ill patients, heart rhythms can represent an easy way out, since they cause people to fall unconscious suddenly and then pass away painlessly. This can also occur when someone is sleeping. Yet if a patient has a defibrillator implanted, the defibrillator will deliver an electric jolt described by those who have felt it as being similar to being dropkicked in the chest by a horse. While shocks from defibrillators can potentially save lives in some patients, for those at the end of life, they only serve to torment. Many patients are never even told that an implanted defibrillator can, in fact, be deactivated because it may not even cross the minds of the doctors to talk about it.[23]

The inevitability of death is what makes life beautiful, what makes life precious, and what makes everything doctors and nurses do on a daily basis worth it. Our mortal spans are juxtaposed with a consciousness to which not existing is a fate worse than hellfire.

Our modern lifestyles are particularly harsh on the heart—our diets, our lack of exercise, and the stress we expose ourselves to are an affront to the evolutionary mechanisms designed over millions of years to help preserve us in a world full of assorted threats.

And yet even an indestructible and everlasting heart cannot grant us immortality. The heart is but one part of a body full of interlocking parts. Perhaps there might come a time when engineers can build a heart that beats forever, chugging on long after everything else comes to a halt. That vision, though, just makes me think of that LVAD patient who had died with his pump still going, pushing blood through dead blood vessels to deader organs.

As we look to the future, we have to contend with the fact that the next big thing in our ceaseless battle with heart disease, the innovation that might save millions of lives and improve countless others, might not be decades away—it might already be here. It might be the very medications that we already have, the dietary interventions we know work, the exercise we know is necessary to remain healthy. If the last century was about developing this foundation of science, the next has to be about getting these to not only every remote corner of the world but to each urban neighborhood and rural outpost in high-income countries such as the United States.

These disparities are widening and at this rate will continue to widen, with the rich getting richer and the poor suffering disproportionately.[24] As health care gets more expensive, cost is becoming one of the most serious adverse effects of medical care. Too many can't afford care, like the patient with a heart transplant who could not pay for his immune-suppressing medications, and many do end up with significant bills. Device and drug-makers will always keep making new things at escalating costs that they will assure us are better than things we already have. Like iPhones and PlayStations, there will be new toys that have more bells and whistles than the previous generation of stuff. Yet the way I see it, in the next century, we will need to invest as much in our schools as we do in our hospitals, to shrink the differences that exist between the most affluent and educated people and the most destitute and poorly educated ones.

Instead of spending an exorbitant amount of money on adding days to the lives of those at the end, we can easily push that investment toward making sure people never develop serious heart disease in the first place, potentially adding years of disease-free time to their lives. Procedures and other invasive therapies are shiny and sexy—it's the stuff you see TV doctors doing—but we need more real doctors to focus on drab and boring activities like preventing disease before it manifests.

The fact is that even as there is such a dramatic focus on treating heart disease, the future may be more about making sure a heart never gets diseased to begin with. As we have learned, once the heart is damaged and muscle turns to scar, there is no way back. Yet not only do we have a myriad of means to minimize the risk of heart disease already available, we have reinforcements on the way. There are medications called *PCSK9 inhibitors* now available that can annihilate bad cholesterol in our bodies.[25] Yet PCSK9 inhibitors can cost tens of thousands of dollars and are unaffordable for the vast majority. There are other medications in development that patients only need to take once or twice a year that could serve as a virtual vaccine against atherosclerosis.[26] The question is whether we can ensure that everyone can afford and have access to these medications that can make heart disease a vestige of history much like smallpox. Unless we make treatments for heart disease universally available, both in rich countries such as the United States and in poorer countries around the world, heart disease will increasingly come to be seen as an economic condition like malnutrition. Inequality is not just rising financially; it is seen in differences in outcomes from heart disease getting worse over time between the rich and the poor.[27] In the next century, heart health needs to be viewed as a right rather than a privilege.

Not only is heart disease going to be increasingly divided along financial lines, it will be increasingly divided by racial and ethnic lines as well. While African Americans, for example, are much more likely to not only have a higher prevalence of hypertension, diabetes, stroke, cardiomyopathy, and atherosclerotic cardiovascular disease, they are also less likely to get appropriate medical care for these conditions. One reason for this disparity is socioeconomic: so many African Americans in the United States are also economically disadvantaged. Yet, differences in biology and the environment that African Americans find themselves in is probably as important. Biology is perhaps even more important for South Asians, such as myself, who are likely to account for half of all people with heart disease in the near future. Unless the underlying biological and genetic differences are better understood, and the effect treatments have on reducing the risk of heart disease in ethnic and racial subgroups are specifically tested, these differences are only going to get wider.

As our efforts at culling heart disease before it ensnares unsuspecting individuals in its clutches gather steam, the war on facts and on science is only going to intensify, particularly as it pertains to heart disease. The number of people having heart attacks is already much lower than it ever has been, and better preventive and diagnostic strategies will mean that fewer people will have life-threatening heart attacks and other dramatic manifestations of heart disease. While heart disease is likely to continue to be displaced from view, the war against conventional and proven therapies such as statins is going to become weaponized similar to how the war on vaccines has been. Therefore, to win the war of the heart, we will have to win over the mind first.

We have already seen the complete arc of the heart, rising for most of human history to being considered the most important organ of all and then falling back to earth as effective medical and surgical treatments have rendered it potentially replaceable for many. Yet as we struggle to get therapies to all those who need them, what will be needed is a full-throated defense of the scientific process represented by the journey captured in these pages. Too many times, people focus on the outcomes, whether stents are good or bad, which type of diet is best for the heart, without focusing on the veracity of the science at the heart of producing these findings. We will have to take into account that there are few things in science that are static, few things that more research will not prove wrong. This means that if science continues to advance, perhaps half of this book will one day be proven false. Perhaps one day, a historian will cite these words snidely to reflect how ignorant we were and how far we have come since. That thought gives me a lot of joy, and the sooner we can break the untouchable idols of today, the sooner we can strip the masters of dogma, the sooner we can focus on the sum of our organs.

Notes

1. Darkness Before Dawn

1. Roth GA, Forouzanfar MH, Moran AE, et al. Demographic and Epidemiologic Drivers of Global Cardiovascular Mortality. *New England Journal of Medicine*. 2015;372:1333–41.

2. Benjamin EJ, Virani SS, Callaway CW, et al. Heart Disease and Stroke Statistics—2018 Update: A Report from the American Heart Association. *Circulation*. 2018;137:e67–e492.

3. Van Norman GA. Overcoming the Declining Trends in Innovation and Investment in Cardiovascular Therapeutics: Beyond EROOM's Law. *JACC: Basic to Translational Science*. 2017;2:613–25.

4. Fordyce CB, Roe MT, Ahmad T, et al. Cardiovascular Drug Development: Is It Dead or Just Hibernating? *Journal of the American College of Cardiology*. 2015;65:1567–82.

5. Stockmann C, Hersh AL, Sherwin CM, Spigarelli MG. Alignment of United States Funding for Cardiovascular Disease Research with Deaths, Years of Life Lost, and Hospitalizations. *International Journal of Cardiology*. 2014;172:e19–21.

6. Berry TR, Stearns JA, Courneya KS, et al. Women's Perceptions of Heart Disease and Breast Cancer and the Association with Media Representations of the Diseases. *Journal of Public Health* (Oxford). 2016;38:e496–e503.

7. Gunderman R. Illness as Failure. Blaming Patients. *Hastings Center Report*. 2000;30:7–11.

8. Vaughan AS, Ritchey MD, Hannan J, Kramer MR, Casper M. Widespread Recent Increases in County-Level Heart Disease Mortality Across Age Groups. *Annals of Epidemiology*. 2017;27:796–800.

9. van der Linde D, Konings EE, Slager MA, et al. Birth Prevalence of Congenital Heart Disease Worldwide: A Systematic Review and Meta-Analysis. *Journal of the American College of Cardiology.* 2011;58:2241–7.

10. Hoffman JI, Kaplan S. The Incidence of Congenital Heart Disease. *Journal of the American College of Cardiology.* 2002;39:1890–900.

11. National Wildlife Foundation. Animals Really Do Have Heart. http://blog.nwf .org/2013/02/amazing-animal-hearts/.

12. Woods HA, Lane SJ, Shishido C, Tobalske BW, Arango CP, Moran AL. Respiratory Gut Peristalsis by Sea Spiders. *Current Biology.* 2017;27:R638–9.

13. Ross J, Jr., Braunwald E. Aortic Stenosis. *Circulation.* 1968;38:61–7.

14. Cribier A, Savin T, Saoudi N, Rocha P, Berland J, Letac B. Percutaneous Transluminal Valvuloplasty of Acquired Aortic Stenosis in Elderly Patients: An Alternative to Valve Replacement? *Lancet.* 1986;1:63–7.

15. Cribier A, Eltchaninoff H, Bash A, et al. Percutaneous Transcatheter Implantation of an Aortic Valve Prosthesis for Calcific Aortic Stenosis: First Human Case Description. *Circulation.* 2002;106:3006–8.

2. The Heart—A Love Story

1. Osler W. *The Evolution of Modern Medicine.* New Haven: Yale University Press; 1921.

2. Sprunt WH. Imhotep. *New England Journal of Medicine.* 1955;253:778–80.

3. Haas LF. Papyrus of Ebers and Smith. *Journal of Neurology, Neurosurgery, and Psychiatry.* 1999;67:578.

4. Sprunt. Imhotep.

5. Willerson JT, Teaff R. Egyptian Contributions to Cardiovascular Medicine. *Texas Heart Institute Journal.* 1996;23:191–200.

6. Boisaubin EV. Cardiology in Ancient Egypt. *Texas Heart Institute Journal.* 1988;15: 80–5.

7. Saba MM, Ventura HO, Saleh M, Mehra MR. Ancient Egyptian Medicine and the Concept of Heart Failure. *Journal of Cardiac Failure.* 2006;12:416–21.

8. Heberden W. Some Account of Disorder of the Breast. *Medical Transactions. The Royal College of Physicians of London.* 1772;2:59–67.

9. Hajar R. Coronary Heart Disease: From Mummies to 21st Century. *Heart Views.* 2017;18:68–74.

10. Saba, Ventura, Saleh, Mehra. Ancient Egyptian Medicine.

11. Ritner RK. The Cardiovascular System in Ancient Egyptian Thought. *Journal of Near Eastern Studies.* 2006;65:99–109.

12. Arikha N. *Passion and Tempers: A History of the Humors.* New York: Ecco; 2007.

13. Ranhel AS, Mesquita ET. The Middle Ages Contributions to Cardiovascular Medicine. *Brazilian Journal of Cardiovascular Surgery.* 2016;31:163–70.

14. Masic I. On Occasion of 800th Anniversary of Birth of Ibn al-Nafis—Discoverer of Cardiac and Pulmonary Circulation. *Medical Archives*. 2010;64:309–13.

15. Abdel-Halim RE. The Role of Ibn Sina (Avicenna)'s Medical Poem in the Transmission of Medical Knowledge to Medieval Europe. *Urology Annals*. 2014;6: 1–12.

16. Loukas M, Lam R, Tubbs RS, Shoja MM, Apaydin N. Ibn al-Nafis (1210–1288): The First Description of the Pulmonary Circulation. *American Surgeon*. 2008; 74:440–2.

17. West JB. Ibn al-Nafis, the Pulmonary Circulation, and the Islamic Golden Age. *Journal of Applied Physiology*. 2008;105:1877–80.

18. Aird WC. Discovery of the Cardiovascular System: From Galen to William Harvey. *Journal of Thrombosis and Haemostasis*. 2011;9 Suppl 1:118–29.

19. Ibid.

20. Osler W. Tercentenary of the Death of William Harvey 1. The Growth of Truth. *British Medical Journal*. 1957;1:8 1–1263.

21. Lubitz SA. Early Reactions to Harvey's Circulation Theory: The Impact on Medicine. *Mount Sinai Journal of Medicine*. 2004;71:274–80.

22. French R. *William Harvey's Natural Philosophy*. Cambridge, UK: Cambridge University Press; 1994.

23. Lubitz. Early Reactions.

24. Erickson R. *The Language of the Heart, 1600–1750*. Philadelphia, PA: University of Pennsylvania Press 1997.

3. The Elephant in the Room (Sitting on the Chest)

1. Benjamin EJ, Virani SS, Callaway CW, et al. Heart Disease and Stroke Statistics—2018 Update: A Report from the American Heart Association. *Circulation*. 2018;137:e67–e492.

2. President Eisenhower's $14 Billion Heart Attack. 2016. www.ozy.com/flashback /president-eisenhowers-14-billion-heart-attack/65157.

3. Lasby CG. *Eisenhower's Heart Attack: How Ike Beat Heart Disease and Held On to the Presidency*. Lawrence, KS: University Press of Kansas, 1997.

4. Bentzon JF, Otsuka F, Virmani R, Falk E. Mechanisms of Plaque Formation and Rupture. *Circulation Research*. 2014;114:1852–66.

5. Strong JP, Malcom GT, McMahan CA, et al. Prevalence and Extent of Atherosclerosis in Adolescents and Young Adults: Implications for Prevention from the Pathobiological Determinants of Atherosclerosis in Youth Study. *Journal of the American Medical Association*. 1999;281:727–35.

6. Giuseppe Zoccai, Mariangela Peruzzi, Enrico Romagnoli. Is the Pathophysiology of Plaque Injury in Acute MI Changing? Revisiting Plaque Erosion vs. Rupture.

2016. www.acc.org/latest-in-cardiology/articles/2016/02/26/09/34/is-the-patho
physiology-of-plaque-injury-in-acute-mi-changing.

7. Stefanadis C, Antoniou CK, Tsiachris D, Pietri P. Coronary Atherosclerotic Vul-
    nerable Plaque: Current Perspectives. *Journal of the American Heart Association*.
    2017;6.

8. Milton K. Back to Basics: Why Foods of Wild Primates Have Relevance for Modern
    Human Health. *Nutrition*. 2000;16:480–3.

9. Pijl H. Obesity: Evolution of a Symptom of Affluence. *Netherlands Journal of Medicine*.
    2011;69:159–66.

10. Fish JL, Lockwood CA. Dietary Constraints on Encephalization in Primates.
    American Journal of Physical Anthropology. 2003;120:171–81.

11. The Oldest Homo Sapiens Yet. *Economist*. June 10, 2017.

12. Neel JV. Diabetes Mellitus: a "Thrifty" Genotype Rendered Detrimental by
    "Progress"? *American Journal of Human Genetics*. 1962;14:353–62.

13. Stern MP. Diabetes and Cardiovascular Disease. The "Common Soil" Hypothesis.
    Diabetes. 1995;44:369–74.

14. Fernandez-Real JM, Ricart W. Insulin Resistance and Inflammation in an Evolu-
    tionary Perspective: The Contribution of Cytokine Genotype/Phenotype to Thrift-
    iness. *Diabetologia*. 1999;42:1367–74.

15. Wells JC. Ethnic Variability in Adiposity and Cardiovascular Risk: The Variable
    Disease Selection Hypothesis. *International Journal of Epidemiology*. 2009;38:63–71.

16. Warraich HJ, Javed F, Faraz-Ul-Haq M, Khawaja FB, Saleem S. Prevalence of
    Obesity in School-Going Children of Karachi. *PLOS ONE*. 2009;4:e4816.

17. Thomas GS, Wann LS, Allam AH, et al. Why Did Ancient People Have Athero-
    sclerosis?: From Autopsies to Computed Tomography to Potential Causes. *Global
    Heart*. 2014;9:229–37.

18. Keller A, Graefen A, Ball M, et al. New Insights into the Tyrolean Iceman's Ori-
    gin and Phenotype as Inferred by Whole-Genome Sequencing. *Nature Communica-
    tions*. 2012;3:698.

19. Ruffer MA. On Arterial Lesions Found in Egyptian Mummies (1580 BC–525 AD).
    Journal of Pathology and Bacteriology. 1911;15.

20. Thompson RC, Allam AH, Lombardi GP, et al. Atherosclerosis Across 4000 Years
    of Human History: The Horus Study of Four Ancient Populations. *Lancet*.
    2013;381:1211–22.

21. Death Rates for 1911 in the United States and Its Large Cities. *Boston Medical and
    Surgical Journal*. 1912;CLXVI:63–4.

22. Gurven M, Stieglitz J, Trumble B, et al. The Tsimane Health and Life History
    Project: Integrating Anthropology and Biomedicine. *Evolutionary Anthropology*.
    2017;26:54–73.

23. Packard RR, Libby P. Inflammation in Atherosclerosis: From Vascular Biology to Biomarker Discovery and Risk Prediction. *Clinical Chemistry*. 2008;54:24–38.

24. Shaharyar S, Warraich H, McEvoy JW, et al. Subclinical Cardiovascular Disease in Plaque Psoriasis: Association or Causal Link? *Atherosclerosis*. 2014;232:72–8.

25. Hemkens LG, Ewald H, Gloy VL, et al. Colchicine for Prevention of Cardiovascular Events. *Cochrane Database of Systematic Reviews*. 2016:CD011047.

26. De Vecchis R, Baldi C, Palmisani L. Protective Effects of Methotrexate Against Ischemic Cardiovascular Disorders in Patients Treated for Rheumatoid Arthritis or Psoriasis: Novel Therapeutic Insights Coming from a Meta-Analysis of the Literature Data. *Anatolian Journal of Cardiology*. 2016;16:2–9.

27. Ridker PM, Everett BM, Thuren T, et al. Antiinflammatory Therapy with Canakinumab for Atherosclerotic Disease. *New England Journal of Medicine*. 2017;377:1119–31.

28. Lerner BH. Crafting Medical History: Revisiting the "Definitive" Account of Franklin D. Roosevelt's Terminal Illness. *Bulletin of the History of Medicine*. 2007;81:386–406.

29. Bruenn HG. Clinical Notes on the Illness and Death of President Franklin D. Roosevelt. *Annals of Internal Medicine*. 1970;72:579–91.

30. Pinals RS, Smulyan H. The Death of President Warren G. Harding. *American Journal of the Medical Sciences*. 2014;348:232–7.

31. Chen G, Levy D. Contributions of the Framingham Heart Study to the Epidemiology of Coronary Heart Disease. *JAMA Cardiology*. 2016;1:825–30.

32. Mahmood SS, Levy D, Vasan RS, Wang TJ. The Framingham Heart Study and the Epidemiology of Cardiovascular Disease: A Historical Perspective. *Lancet*. 2014;383:999–1008.

33. Dawber TR, Moore FE, Mann GV. Coronary Heart Disease in the Framingham Study. *American Journal of Public Health and the Nation's Health*. 1957;47:4–24.

34. Kannel WB, Dawber TR, Kagan A, Revotskie N, Stokes J, 3rd. Factors of Risk in the Development of Coronary Heart Disease—Six Year Follow-Up Experience. The Framingham Study. *Annals of Internal Medicine*. 1961;55:33–50.

35. Rakotz MK, Townsend RR, Yang J, et al. Medical Students and Measuring Blood Pressure: Results from the American Medical Association Blood Pressure Check Challenge. *Journal of Clinical Hypertension* (Greenwich), 2017;19:614–9.

36. Frieden TR. Shattuck Lecture: The Future of Public Health. *New England Journal of Medicine*. 2015;373:1748–54.

37. Sotos JG. President Taft's Blood Pressure. *Mayo Clinic Proceedings*. 2006;81:1507–8.

38. Menger RP, Storey CM, Guthikonda B, Missios S, Nanda A, Cooper JM. Woodrow Wilson's Hidden Stroke of 1919: The Impact of Patient-Physician Confidentiality on United States Foreign Policy. *Neurosurgical Focus*. 2015;39:E6.

39. Steinberg D. President Franklin D Roosevelt (1882–1945) and Doctor Frank Howard Lahey's (1880–1953) Dilemma: The Complexities of Medical Confidentiality with World Leaders. *Journal of Medical Biography*. 2016;24:50–60.

40. Osler W. An Address on High Blood Pressure: Its Associations, Advantages, and Disadvantages: Delivered at the Glasgow Southern Medical Society. *British Medical Journal*. 1912;2:1173–7.

41. White PD. *Heart Disease*. 2nd ed. New York: MacMillan Co; 1937:326.

42. Hay J. A British Medical Association Lecture on the Significance of a Raised Blood Pressure. *British Medical Journal*. 1931;2:43–7.

43. Fisher JW. The Diagnostic Value of the Sphygmomanometer in Examinations for Life Insurance. *Journal of the American Medical Association*. 1914;63:1752–54.

44. Society of Actuaries. *Blood Pressure: Report of the Joint Committee on Mortality of the Association of Life Insurance Medical Directors and the Actuarial Society of America*. New York: 1925.

45. Dawber, Moore, Mann. Coronary Heart Disease.

46. Kannel WB, Dawber TR, Cohen ME, McNamara PM. Vascular Disease of the Brain—Epidemiologic Aspects: The Framingham Study. *American Journal of Public Health and the Nation's Health*. 1965;55:1355–66.

47. Kannel WB. Bishop Lecture. Contribution of the Framingham Study to Preventive Cardiology. *Journal of the American College of Cardiology*. 1990;15:206–11.

48. Kolata G. Lower Blood Pressure Guidelines Could Be "Lifesaving," Federal Study Says. *New York Times*. September 11, 2015.

49. Muntner P, Carey RM, Gidding S, et al. Potential US Population Impact of the 2017 ACC/AHA High Blood Pressure Guideline. *Circulation*. 2018;137:109–18.

50. Frieden. Shattuck Lecture.

51. Bruenn. Clinical Notes.

52. Morris MJ, Na ES, Johnson AK. Salt Craving: The Psychobiology of Pathogenic Sodium Intake. *Physiology & Behavior*. 2008;94:709–21.

53. Tekol Y. Salt Addiction: A Different Kind of Drug Addiction. *Medical Hypotheses*. 2006;67:1233–4.

54. Mozaffarian D, Fahimi S, Singh GM, et al. Global Sodium Consumption and Death from Cardiovascular Causes. *New England Journal of Medicine*. 2014;371:624–34.

55. United Nations Office on Drugs and Crime, World Drug Report 2017 (ISBN: 978-92-1-148291-1, eISBN: 978-92-1-060623-3, United Nations publication, Sales No. E.17.XI.6).

56. Campbell NRC, Train EJ. A Systematic Review of Fatalities Related to Acute Ingestion of Salt. A Need for Warning Labels? *Nutrients*. 2017;9.

57. Hedouin V, Revuelta E, Becart A, Tournel G, Deveaux M, Gosset D. A Case of

Fatal Salt Water Intoxication Following an Exorcism Session. *Forensic Science International.* 1999;99:1–4.

58. Ofran Y, Lavi D, Opher D, Weiss TA, Elinav E. Fatal Voluntary Salt Intake Resulting in the Highest Ever Documented Sodium Plasma Level in Adults (255 mmol L-1): A Disorder Linked to Female Gender and Psychiatric Disorders. *Journal of Internal Medicine.* 2004;256:525–8.

59. Draft Guidance for Industry: Voluntary Sodium Reduction Goals: Target Mean and Upper Bound Concentrations for Sodium in Commercially Processed, Packaged, and Prepared Foods. June 2016. www.fda.gov/Food/GuidanceRegulation /GuidanceDocumentsRegulatoryInformation/ucm494732.htm.

60. Jackson SL, King SM, Zhao L, Cogswell ME. Prevalence of Excess Sodium Intake in the United States-NHANES, 2009–2012. *Morbidity and Mortality Weekly Report.* 2016;64:1393–7.

61. American Heart Association Sodium Reduction Initiative Team. The Salty Six— Surprising Foods That Add the Most Sodium to Our Diets. 2014. https://sodium breakup.heart.org/salty-six-surprising-foods-add-sodium-diets/.

62. Mente A, O'Donnell M, Rangarajan S, et al. Associations of Urinary Sodium Excretion with Cardiovascular Events in Individuals with and without Hypertension: A Pooled Analysis of Data from Four Studies. *Lancet.* 2016;388:465–75.

63. Has Salt Gotten an Unfair Shake? September 3, 2017. www.npr.org/sections/health shots/2017/09/03/547827356/has-salt-gotten-an-unfair-shake-sodium-parti sans-say-yes.

64. Jerusalem Talmud, Horeyot 3:5.

65. Berman LB. Harry Goldblatt: 1891–1977. *Journal of the American Medical Association.* 1977;238:1846.

66. Downey P. Profile of Sérgio Ferreira. *Proceedings of the National Academy of Sciences of the United States of America.* 2008;105:19035–7.

67. Patlak M. From Viper's Venom to Drug Design: Treating Hypertension. *FASEB Journal.* 2004;18:421.

68. Johns EJ, Kopp UC, DiBona GF. Neural Control of Renal Function. *Comprehensive Physiology.* 2011;1:731–67.

69. Barnett HJ, Jackson MV, Spaulding WB. Thiocyanate Psychosis. *Journal of the American Medical Association.* 1951;147:1554–8.

70. Newcombe CP, Shucksmith HS, Suffern WS. Sympathectomy for Hypertension; Follow-Up of 212 Patients. *British Medical Journal.* 1959;1:142–4.

71. Symplicity HTNI, Esler MD, Krum H, et al. Renal Sympathetic Denervation in Patients with Treatment-Resistant Hypertension (The Symplicity HTN-2 Trial): A Randomised Controlled Trial. *Lancet.* 2010;376:1903–9.

72. Bhatt DL, Kandzari DE, O'Neill WW, et al. A Controlled Trial of Renal Denervation for Resistant Hypertension. *New England Journal of Medicine.* 2014;370:1393–
401.

4. You Are What You Eat

1. Nes WD. Biosynthesis of Cholesterol and Other Sterols. *Chemical Reviews.*
2011;111:6423–51.

2. Rifkind B. *Drug Treatment of Hyperlipidemia.* Boca Raton, FL: CRC Press; 1991.

3. *Thoraco-Abdominal Aorta: Surgical and Anesthetic Management.* Edited by Roberto Chiesa,
Germano Melissano, Alberto Zangrillo. Milan: Springer Science & Business Media, 2011.

4. Stamler J. *Lectures on Preventive Cardiology.* New York: Grune & Stratton, Inc.; 1967.

5. Virchow R. *Cellular Pathology as Based upon Physiological and Pathological Histology.* Philadelphia: JB Lippincott; 1863.

6. Benlian P. *Genetics of Dyslipidemia.* Milan: Springer Science & Business Media; 2001.

7. Konstantinov IE, Mejevoi N, Anichkov NM. Nikolai N. Anichkov and His Theory of Atherosclerosis. *Texas Heart Institute Journal.* 2006;33:417–23.

8. Vanitallie TB. Ancel Keys: A Tribute. *Nutrition & Metabolism* (London). 2005;2:4.

9. Brozek J. Bibliographical Note on Behavioral Aspects: On the Margin of the
50th Anniversary of the Minnesota Starvation-Nutritional Rehabilitation Experiment. *Perceptual Motor Skills.* 1995;81:395–400.

10. Keys A. Human Atherosclerosis and the Diet. *Circulation.* 1952;5:115–8.

11. Keys A. Coronary Heart Disease in Seven Countries. 1970. *Nutrition.* 1997;13:250–
2; discussion 49, 3.

12. Marmot MG, Syme SL. Acculturation and Coronary Heart Disease in Japanese-
Americans. *American Journal of Epidemiology.* 1976;104:225–47.

13. Dayton S, Pearce ML, Goldman H, et al. Controlled Trial of a Diet High in
Unsaturated Fat for Prevention of Atherosclerotic Complications. *Lancet.* 1968;2:
1060–2.

14. Miettinen M, Turpeinen O, Karvonen MJ, Elosuo R, Paavilainen E. Effect of Cholesterol-Lowering Diet on Mortality from Coronary Heart-Disease and Other
Causes. A Twelve-Year Clinical Trial in Men and Women. *Lancet.* 1972;2:835–8.

15. Demaret K, Weinraub, J. Dr. George Mann Says Low Cholesterol Diets Are Useless, but the "Heart Mafia" Disagrees. *People.* January 22, 1979.

16. Mann GV. Diet-Heart: End of an Era. *New England Journal of Medicine.* 1977;297:644–
50.

17. Dietary Fat and Its Relation to Heart Attacks and Strokes. Report by the Central
Committee for Medical and Community Program of the American Heart Association. *Journal of the American Medical Association.* 1961;175:389–91.

18. McMichael J. Fats and Atheroma: An Inquest. *British Medical Journal.* 1979;1: 173–5.

19. Steinberg D. The Pathogenesis of Atherosclerosis. An Interpretive History of the Cholesterol Controversy, Part IV: The 1984 Coronary Primary Prevention Trial Ends It—Almost. *Journal of Lipid Research.* 2006;47:1–14.

20. The Lipid Research Clinics Coronary Primary Prevention Trial Results. II. The Relationship of Reduction in Incidence of Coronary Heart Disease to Cholesterol Lowering. *Journal of the American Medical Association.* 1984;251:365–74.

21. Mann G. Coronary Heart Disease—"Doing the Wrong Thing." *Nutrition Today.* 1985;12–4.

22. Endo A. A Historical Perspective on the Discovery of Statins. *Proceedings of the Japan Academy Series B—Physical and Biological Sciences.* 2010;86:484–93.

23. Ibid.

24. Stossel TP. The Discovery of Statins. *Cell.* 2008;134:903–5.

25. Pedersen TR, Kjekshus J, Berg K, et al. Randomized Trial of Cholesterol-Lowering in 4444 Patients with Coronary Heart Disease: The Scandinavian Simvastatin Survival Study (4S). *Lancet.* 1994;344:1383–9.

26. Tang JL, Armitage JM, Lancaster T, Silagy CA, Fowler GH, Neil HAW. Systematic Review of Dietary Intervention Trials to Lower Blood Total Cholesterol in Free-Living Subjects. *British Medical Journal.* 1998;316:1213–9.

27. Bhattarai N, Prevost AT, Wright AJ, Charlton J, Rudisill C, Gulliford MC. Effectiveness of Interventions to Promote Healthy Diet in Primary Care: Systematic Review and Meta-Analysis of Randomised Controlled Trials. *BMC Public Health.* 2013;13.

28. Collins R, Reith C, Emberson J, et al. Interpretation of the Evidence for the Efficacy and Safety of Statin Therapy. *Lancet.* 2016;388:2532–61.

29. Salami JA, Warraich H, Valero-Elizondo J, et al. National Trends in Statin Use and Expenditures in the US Adult Population From 2002 to 2013 Insights from the Medical Expenditure Panel Survey. *JAMA Cardiology.* 2017;2:56–65.

30. Warraich HJ, Salami JA, Khera R, Valero-Elizondo J, Okunrintemi V, Nasir K. Trends in Use and Expenditures of Brand-Name Atorvastatin After Introduction of Generic Atorvastatin. *JAMA Internal Medicine.* 2018;178:719–21.

31. Warraich H. The Measles Outbreak Coming Near You. *Wall Street Journal.* December 3, 2014.

32. Collins, Reith, Emberson, et al. Interpretation of the Evidence.

33. Cohen JD, Brinton EA, Ito MK, Jacobson TA. Understanding Statin Use in America and Gaps in Patient Education (USAGE): An Internet-Based Survey of 10,138 Current and Former Statin Users. *Journal of Clinical Lipidology.* 2012;6: 208–15.

34. Bruckert E, Hayem G, Dejager S, Yau C, Begaud B. Mild to Moderate Muscular Symptoms with High-Dosage Statin Therapy in Hyperlipidemic Patients—The PRIMO Study. *Cardiovascular Drugs Therapy.* 2005;19:403–14.

35. Finegold JA, Manisty CH, Goldacre B, Barron AJ, Francis DP. What Proportion of Symptomatic Side Effects in Patients Taking Statins Are Genuinely Caused by the Drug? Systematic Review of Randomized Placebo-Controlled Trials to Aid Individual Patient Choice. *European Journal of Preventative Cardiology.* 2014;21:464–74.

36. Gupta A, Thompson D, Whitehouse A, et al. Adverse Events Associated with Unblinded, but Not with Blinded, Statin Therapy in the Anglo-Scandinavian Cardiac Outcomes Trial—Lipid-Lowering Arm (ASCOT-LLA): A Randomised Double-Blind Placebo-Controlled Trial and Its Non-Randomised Non-Blind Extension Phase. *Lancet.* 2017;389:2473–81.

37. Price DD, Finniss DG, Benedetti F. A Comprehensive Review of the Placebo Effect: Recent Advances and Current Thought. *Annual Review of Psychology.* 2008;59:565–90.

38. Kaptchuk TJ, Miller FG. Placebo Effects in Medicine. *New England Journal of Medicine.* 2015;373:8–9.

39. Simpson SH, Eurich DT, Majumdar SR, et al. A Meta-Analysis of the Association Between Adherence to Drug Therapy and Mortality. *British Medical Journal.* 2006;333:15.

40. Kam-Hansen S, Jakubowski M, Kelley JM, et al. Altered Placebo and Drug Labeling Changes the Outcome of Episodic Migraine Attacks. *Science Translational Medicine.* 2014;6:218ra5.

41. Colloca L. Nocebo Effects Can Make You Feel Pain. *Science.* 2017;358:44.

42. Barron AJ, Zaman N, Cole GD, Wensel R, Okonko DO, Francis DP. Systematic Review of Genuine versus Spurious Side-Effects of Beta-Blockers in Heart Failure Using Placebo Control: Recommendations for Patient Information. *International Journal of Cardiology.* 2013;168:3572–9.

43. Yusuf S. Why Do People Not Take Life-Saving Medications? The Case of Statins. *Lancet.* 2016;388:943–5.

44. Serban MC, Colantonio LD, Manthripragada AD, et al. Statin Intolerance and Risk of Coronary Heart Events and All-Cause Mortality Following Myocardial Infarction. *Journal of the American College of Cardiology.* 2017;69:1386–95.

45. Selva-O'Callaghan A, Alvarado-Cardenas M, Pinal-Fernandez I, et al. Statin-Induced Myalgia and Myositis: An Update on Pathogenesis and Clinical Recommendations. *Expert Review of Clinical Immunology.* 2018;14:215–24.

46. Levy A. Pill Culture Pops. *New York.* June 9, 2003.

47. Warraich HJ, Schulman KA. Health Care Tax Inversions—Robbing Both Peter and Paul. *New England Journal of Medicine.* 2016;374:1005–7.

48. Warraich, Salami, Khera, Valero-Elizondo, Okunrintemi, Nasir. Trends in Use.

49. Jack JL. *Triumph of the Heart: The Story of Statins.* Oxford, UK: Oxford University Press; 2009.

50. Salami JA, Warraich HJ, Valero-Elizondo J, et al. National Trends in Nonstatin Use and Expenditures Among the U.S. Adult Population From 2002 to 2013: Insights from Medical Expenditure Panel Survey. *Journal of the American Heart Association.* 2018;7.

5. The Method in the Madness

1. Fredrickson DS, Altrocchi, PH, Avioli, LV, Goodman, D, Goodman, HS. Tangier Disease: Combined Clinical Staff Conference at the National Institutes of Health. *Annals of Internal Medicine.* 1961:1016–31.

2. Gordon DJ, Probstfield JL, Garrison RJ, et al. High-Density Lipoprotein Cholesterol and Cardiovascular Disease. Four Prospective American Studies. *Circulation.* 1989;79:8–15.

3. Forey BA, Fry JS, Lee PN, Thornton AJ, Coombs KJ. The Effect of Quitting Smoking on HDL-Cholesterol—A Review Based on Within-Subject Changes. *Biomarker Research.* 2013;1:26.

4. Kodama S, Tanaka S, Saito K, et al. Effect of Aerobic Exercise Training on Serum Levels of High-Density Lipoprotein Cholesterol: A Meta-Analysis. *Archives of Internal Medicine.* 2007;167:999–1008.

5. Berryman CE, Fleming JA, Kris-Etherton PM. Inclusion of Almonds in a Cholesterol-Lowering Diet Improves Plasma HDL Subspecies and Cholesterol Efflux to Serum in Normal-Weight Individuals with Elevated LDL Cholesterol. *Journal of Nutrition.* 2017;147:1517–23.

6. Investigators A-H, Boden WE, Probstfield JL, et al. Niacin in Patients with Low HDL Cholesterol Levels Receiving Intensive Statin Therapy. *New England Journal of Medicine.* 2011;365:2255–67.

7. Group HTC, Landray MJ, Haynes R, et al. Effects of Extended-Release Niacin with Laropiprant in High-Risk Patients. *New England Journal of Medicine.* 2014;371:203–12.

8. Marz W, Kleber ME, Scharnagl H, et al. HDL Cholesterol: Reappraisal of Its Clinical Relevance. *Clinical Research in Cardiology.* 2017;106:663–75.

9. Group HTRC, Bowman L, Hopewell JC, et al. Effects of Anacetrapib in Patients with Atherosclerotic Vascular Disease. *New England Journal of Medicine.* 2017;377:1217–27.

10. Voight BF, Peloso GM, Orho-Melander M, et al. Plasma HDL Cholesterol and Risk of Myocardial Infarction: A Mendelian Randomisation Study. *Lancet.* 2012;380:572–80.

11. Khera AV, Cuchel M, de la Llera-Moya M, et al. Cholesterol Efflux Capacity, High-Density Lipoprotein Function, and Atherosclerosis. *New England Journal of Medicine.* 2011;364:127–35.

12. Pew Research Center. Public Trust in Government Remains Near Historic Lows as Partisan Attitudes Shift. May 2017. www.people-press.org/2017/05/03/public trust-in-government-remains-near-historic-lows-as-partisan-attitudes-shift/.

13. Gallup. Americans' Trust in Mass Media Sinks to New Low. September 2016. https://news.gallup.com/poll/195542/americans-trust-mass-media-sinks-new low.aspx.

14. Pew Research Center. Public Confidence in Scientists Has Remained Stable for Decades. April 2017. www.pewresearch.org/fact-tank/2017/04/06/public-confi-dence-in-scientists-has-remained-stable-for-decades/.

15. *Huffington Post.* People Who Have Sex Four or More Times a Week Make More Money. August 2013. www.huffingtonpost.com/2013/08/14/more-sex-higher wages_n_3755271.html.

16. Moyer MW. It's Not Dementia, It's Your Heart Medication: Cholesterol Drugs and Memory. *Scientific American.* September 2010.

17. Yusuf S. Why Do People Not Take Life-Saving Medications? The Case of Statins. *Lancet.* 2016;388:943–5.

18. Are Statins a Key to Preventing Alzheimer's Disease? December 2016. www.cnn.com/2016/12/12/health/statins-alzheimers-disease/index.html.

19. Canetto SS, Sakinofsky I. The Gender Paradox in Suicide. *Suicide and Life-Threatening Behavior.* 1998;28:1–23.

20. Spurious Correlations. www.tylervigen.com/spurious-correlations.

21. Norton BJ. Karl Pearson and Statistics: The Social Origins of Scientific Innovation. *Social Studies of Science.* 1978;8:3–34.

22. Kalantar-Zadeh K, Block G, Horwich T, Fonarow GC. Reverse Epidemiology of Conventional Cardiovascular Risk Factors in Patients with Chronic Heart Failure. *Journal of the American College of Cardiology.* 2004;43:1439–44.

23. Ravnskov U, Diamond DM, Hama R, et al. Lack of an Association or an Inverse Association Between Low-Density-Lipoprotein Cholesterol and Mortality in the Elderly: A Systematic Review. *British Medical Journal.* Open 2016;6:e010401.

24. Collier R. Legumes, Lemons and Streptomycin: A Short History of the Clinical Trial. *Canadian Medical Association Journal.* 2009;180:23–4.

25. Zetterstrom R. Nobel Prize 1937 to Albert von Szent-Gyorgyi: Identification of Vitamin C as the Anti-Scorbutic Factor. *Acta Paediatrica.* 2009;98:915–9.

26. Moffet HH. Sham Acupuncture May Be as Efficacious as True Acupuncture: A Systematic Review of Clinical Trials. *Journal of Alternative and Complementary Medicine.* 2009;15:213–6.

27. Haygarth J. *Of the Imagination as a Cause and as a Cure of Disorders of the Body*. Bath, UK: R. Cruttwell; 1800.

28. DiMasi JA, Grabowski HG, Hansen RW. Innovation in the Pharmaceutical Industry: New Estimates of R&D Costs. *Journal of Health Economics*. 2016;47:20–33.

29. Spitz V. *Doctors from Hell: The Horrific Account of Nazi Experiments on Humans*. Boulder, CO: Sentient Publications; 2005.

30. Berger RL. Nazi Science—The Dachau Hypothermia Experiments. *New England Journal of Medicine*. 1990;322:1435–40.

31. Bachrach S. In the Name of Public Health—Nazi Racial Hygiene. *New England Journal of Medicine*. 2004;351:417–20.

32. Emanuel EJ. The History of Euthanasia Debates in the United States and Britain. *Annals of Internal Medicine*. 1994;121:793–802.

33. Beecher HK. Ethics and Clinical Research. *New England Journal of Medicine*. 1966;274:1354–60.

34. Ibid.

35. Ibid.

36. Editorial. Sterilization and Its Possible Accomplishments. *New England Journal of Medicine*. 1934;211:379–80.

37. Brandt AM. Racism and Research: The Case of the Tuskegee Syphilis Study. *Hastings Center Report*. 1978;8:21–9.

38. Heller J. Syphilis Victims in U.S. Study Went Untreated for 40 Years. *New York Times*. July 26, 1972.

39. Kaplan S. Dr. Irwin Schatz, the First, Lonely Voice Against Infamous Tuskegee Study, Dies at 83. *Washington Post*. April 20, 2015.

40. Nanna MG, Navar AM, Zakroysky P, et al. Association of Patient Perceptions of Cardiovascular Risk and Beliefs on Statin Drugs with Racial Differences in Statin Use: Insights from the Patient and Provider Assessment of Lipid Management Registry. *JAMA Cardiology*. 2018.

41. Pitt B, Pfeffer MA, Assmann SF, et al. Spironolactone for Heart Failure with Preserved Ejection Fraction. *New England Journal of Medicine*. 2014;370:1383–92.

42. de Denus S, O'Meara E, Desai AS, et al. Spironolactone Metabolites in TOPCAT-New Insights into Regional Variation. *New England Journal of Medicine*. 2017;376:1690–2.

43. Chavalarias D, Wallach JD, Li AH, Ioannidis JP. Evolution of Reporting P Values in the Biomedical Literature, 1990–2015. *Journal of the American Medical Association*. 2016;315:1141–8.

44. The Lipid Research Clinics Coronary Primary Prevention Trial Results. II. The Relationship of Reduction in Incidence of Coronary Heart Disease to Cholesterol Lowering. *Journal of the American Medical Association*. 1984;251:365–74.

45. Sumner P, Vivian-Griffiths S, Boivin J, et al. The Association Between Exaggeration in Health Related Science News and Academic Press Releases: Retrospective Observational Study. *British Medical Journal.* 2014;349:g7015.

46. Benjamin DJ, Berger JO, Johannesson M, et al. Redefine Statistical Significance. *Nature Human Behaviour.* 2018;2:6–10.

47. Baker M. 1,500 Scientists Lift the Lid on Reproducibility. *Nature.* 2016;533:452–4.

48. Ioannidis JP. Contradicted and Initially Stronger Effects in Highly Cited Clinical Research. *Journal of the American Medical Association.* 2005;294:218–28.

49. Is Watching Sports Bad for Your Health? Here's What New Research Says. October 2017. www.reuters.com/article/us-health-sleep-heart/too-little-sleep-or-too -much-linked-to-risk-of-heart-disease-idUSKCN11P2DU.

50. Too Little Sleep, or Too Much, Linked to Risk of Heart Disease. September 2016. www.reuters.com/article/us-health-sleep-heart/too-little-sleep-or-too-much -linked-to-risk-of-heart-disease-idUSKCN11P2DU.

51. Statins "May Be a Waste of Time:" Controversial Report Claims There's NO Link Between "Bad Cholesterol" and Heart Disease. June 2016. www.dailymail.co.uk/ health/article-3638162/Statins-waste-time-60s-Row-controversial-report-says -no-link-bad-cholesterol-heart-disease.html.

52. Phillips DP, Kanter EJ, Bednarczyk B, Tastad PL. Importance of the Lay Press in the Transmission of Medical Knowledge to the Scientific Community. *New England Journal of Medicine.* 1991;325:1180–3.

53. Selvaraj S, Borkar DS, Prasad V. Media Coverage of Medical Journals: Do the Best Articles Make the News? *PLOS ONE.* 2014;9:e85355.

54. Dumas-Mallet E, Smith A, Boraud T, Gonon F. Poor Replication Validity of Biomedical Association Studies Reported by Newspapers. *PLOS ONE.* 2017;12:e0172650.

55. Ibid.

56. Wang MT, Bolland MJ, Grey A. Reporting of Limitations of Observational Research. *JAMA Internal Medicine.* 2015;175:1571–2.

57. Dumas-Mallet, Smith, Boraud, Gonon. Poor Replication Validity.

58. Sumner, Vivian-Griffiths, Boivin, et al. Association Between Exaggeration.

59. Study: Half of the Studies You Read About in the News Are Wrong. March 2017. www.vox.com/science-and-health/2017/3/3/14792174/half-scientific-studies -news-are-wrong.

60. Caspi A, Sugden K, Moffitt TE, et al. Influence of Life Stress on Depression: Moderation by a Polymorphism in the 5-HTT Gene. *Science.* 2003;301:386–9.

61. Blendon RJ, Benson JM, Hero JO. Public Trust in Physicians—U.S. Medicine in International Perspective. *New England Journal of Medicine.* 2014;371:1570–2.

62. Newman D. *Hippocrates' Shadow: Secrets from the House of Medicine.* New York: Scribner; 2009.

63. *Emergency Physicians Monthly*. Practicing Medicine in Hippocrates' Shadow. January 2009. http://epmonthly.com/article/practicing-medicine-in-hippocrates -shadow/.

64. "What I Did Was Awful and Disgusting": Ex-Mt. Sinai Doctor Sentenced to 2 Years for Sexually Abusing Patients. January 2017. http://gothamist.com/2017/01/24 /mt_sinai_doctor_prison.php.

65. Klein M. Officials Find NYC Hospitals Riddled with Shocking Violations. *New York Post*. February 10, 2018.

66. Rosenberg R. Prison for Doctor Who Drugged, Sexually Assaulted Patient. *New York Post.* January 23, 2017.

67. Omer SB, Amin AB, Limaye RJ. Communicating About Vaccines in a Fact-Resistant World. *JAMA Pediatrics*. 2017;171:929–30.

68. Mergler MJ, Omer SB, Pan WK, et al. Are Recent Medical Graduates More Skeptical of Vaccines? *Vaccines* (Basel). 2013;1:154–66.

69. Johnson SB, Park HS, Gross CP, Yu JB. Complementary Medicine, Refusal of Conventional Cancer Therapy, and Survival Among Patients with Curable Cancers. *JAMA Oncology*. 2018.

70. Hyland M, Birrell J. Government Health Warnings and the "Boomerang" Effect. *Psychological Reports*. 1979;44:643–7.

71. Nyhan B, Reifler J, Richey S, Freed GL. Effective Messages in Vaccine Promotion: A Randomized Trial. *Pediatrics*. 2014;133:e835–42.

72. Amin AB, Bednarczyk RA, Ray CE, et al. Association of Moral Values with Vaccine Hesitancy. *Nature Human Behaviour*. 2017;1:873–80.

6. The Passion of the Heart

1. Warraich HJ, Benson CC, Khosa F, Leeman DE. Diagnosis of Acute Myocardial Infarction on Computed Tomography Angiogram. *Circulation*. 2014;129:272–3.

2. Procacci P, Maresca M. Historical Considerations of Cardiac Pain. *Pain*. 1985;22:325–35.

3. Mitchell SW. *Characteristics*. New York: Century; 1891.

4. De Moulin D. A Historical-Phenomenological Study of Bodily Pain in Western Man. *Bulletin of the History of Medicine*. 1974;48:540–70.

5. Caton D. The Secularization of Pain. *Anesthesiology*. 1985;62:493–501.

6. De Moulin. Historical-Phenomenological Study.

7. Buytendijk F. *Over de pijn (About the Pain)*. 3rd ed. Utrecht-Antwerp: Aula Books; 1957.

8. Stephenson J. Veterans' Pain a Vital Sign. *Journal of the American Medical Association*. 1999;281:978.

9. Jackson M. *Pain: The Fifth Vital Sign: The Science and Culture of Why We Hurt*. New York: Crown; 2002.

10. Fauber J. 9 of 19 Experts on Pain Panel Tied to Drug Companies. *Milwaukee-Wisconsin Journal Sentinel.* June 25, 2014.

11. Vila H, Jr., Smith RA, Augustyniak MJ, et al. The Efficacy and Safety of Pain Management Before and After Implementation of Hospital-Wide Pain Management Standards: Is Patient Safety Compromised by Treatment Based Solely on Numerical Pain Ratings? *Anesthesia & Analgesia.* 2005;101:474–80, table of contents.

12. Krebs EE, Gravely A, Nugent S, et al. Effect of Opioid vs Nonopioid Medications on Pain-Related Function in Patients with Chronic Back Pain or Hip or Knee Osteoarthritis Pain: The SPACE Randomized Clinical Trial. *Journal of the American Medical Association.* 2018;319:872–82.

13. Blanchflower DG, Oswald A. Unhappiness and Pain in Modern America: A Review Essay, and Further Evidence, on Carol Graham's Happiness for All? National Bureau of Economic Research Working Paper Series 2017;No. 24087.

14. Harvey W. *The Works of William Harvey Volume 7* (translated from Latin by Robert Willis). London: Sydenham Society; 1847.

15. Haneveld GT. ["A Sad and Painful Heart"—Andreas Vesalius as Cardiologist]. *Verhandelingen—Koninklijke Academie voor Geneeskunde van België.* 1993;55:683–99.

16. Eslick GD. Chest Pain: A Historical Perspective. *International Journal of Cardiology.* 2001;77:5–11.

17. Herrick J. An Intimate Account of My Early Experience with Coronary Thrombosis. *American Heart Journal.* 1944;27:1–18.

18. Pagliaro P, Gattullo D, Penna C. Nitroglycerine and Sodium Trioxodinitrate: From the Discovery to the Preconditioning Effect. *Journal of Cardiovascular Medicine* (Hagerstown). 2013;14:698–704.

19. Fye WB. T. Lauder Brunton and Amyl Nitrite: A Victorian Vasodilator. *Circulation.* 1986;74:222–9.

20. Steinhorn BS, Loscalzo J, Michel T. Nitroglycerin and Nitric Oxide—A Rondo of Themes in Cardiovascular Therapeutics. *New England Journal of Medicine.* 2015;373:277–80.

21. Ghofrani HA, Osterloh IH, Grimminger F. Sildenafil: From Angina to Erectile Dysfunction to Pulmonary Hypertension and Beyond. *Nature Reviews Drug Discovery.* 2006;5:689–702.

22. Osterloh I. How I Discovered Viagra. *Cosmos.* April 2015.

23. Herrick J. Intimate Account.

24. Herrick JB. Landmark Article (*JAMA* 1912). Clinical Features of Sudden Obstruction of the Coronary Arteries. By James B. Herrick. *Journal of the American Medical Association.* 1983;250:1757–65.

25. Moore BJ, Stocks C, Owens PL. Trends in Emergency Department Visits, 2006–2014. HCUP Statistical Brief #227. Agency for Healthcare Research and Quality,

Rockville, MD. www.hcup-us.ahrq.gov/reports/statbriefs/sb227-Emergency
-Department-Visit-Trends.pdf. September 2017.

26. Amsterdam EA, Kirk JD, Bluemke DA, et al. Testing of Low-Risk Patients Presenting to the Emergency Department with Chest Pain: A Scientific Statement from
the American Heart Association. *Circulation*. 2010;122:1756–76.

27. Obermeyer Z, Cohn B, Wilson M, Jena AB, Cutler DM. Early Death After Discharge from Emergency Departments: Analysis of National US Insurance Claims
Data. *British Medical Journal*. 2017;356:j239.

28. Ahmed A, Sorajja P, Pai A, et al. Prospective Evaluation of the Eyeball Test for
Assessing Frailty in Patients with Valvular Heart Disease. *Journal of the American College of Cardiology*. 2016;68:2911–2.

29. Christenson J, Innes G, McKnight D, et al. A Clinical Prediction Rule for Early
Discharge of Patients with Chest Pain. *Annals of Emergency Medicine*. 2006;47:
1–10.

30. Fanaroff AC, Rymer JA, Goldstein SA, Simel DL, Newby LK. Does This Patient
with Chest Pain Have Acute Coronary Syndrome?: The Rational Clinical Examination Systematic Review. *Journal of the American Medical Association*. 2015;314:
1955–65.

31. Obrastzow WP, Straschesko ND. Zur Kenntnis der Thrombose der Koronarar-
terien des Herzens (To Note the Thrombosis of the Coronary Arteries of the Heart).
Zeitschrift für klinische Medizin. 1910;71:116–32.

32. Yeh RW, Sidney S, Chandra M, Sorel M, Selby JV, Go AS. Population Trends in
the Incidence and Outcomes of Acute Myocardial Infarction. *New England Journal
of Medicine*. 2010;362:2155–65.

33. Ibid.

34. Parsons T. The Sick Role and the Role of the Physician Reconsidered. *Milbank Me-
morial Fund Quarterly: Health and Society*. 1975;53:257–78.

35. Galdas P, Cheater F, Marshall P. What Is the Role of Masculinity in White and
South Asian Men's Decisions to Seek Medical Help for Cardiac Chest Pain? *Journal
of Health Services Research & Policy*. 2007;12:223–9.

36. French DP, Cooper A, Weinman J. Illness Perceptions Predict Attendance at Cardiac Rehabilitation Following Acute Myocardial Infarction: A Systematic Review
with Meta-Analysis. *Journal of Psychosomatic Research*. 2006;61:757–67.

37. Chen SL, Tsai JC, Chou KR. Illness Perceptions and Adherence to Therapeutic
Regimens Among Patients with Hypertension: A Structural Modeling Approach.
International Journal of Nursing Studies. 2011;48:235–45.

38. Beck RS, Daughtridge R, Sloane PD. Physician-Patient Communication in the Primary Care Office: A Systematic Review. *Journal of the American Board of Family Practice*. 2002;15:25–38.

39. Egbert LD, Battit GE, Welch CE, Bartlett MK. Reduction of Postoperative Pain by Encouragement and Instruction of Patients. A Study of Doctor-Patient Rapport. *New England Journal of Medicine.* 1964;270:825–7.

40. Alpert JS, Thygesen K, Antman E, Bassand JP. Myocardial Infarction Redefined— A Consensus Document of the Joint European Society of Cardiology/American College of Cardiology Committee for the Redefinition of Myocardial Infarction. *Journal of the American College of Cardiology.* 2000;36:959–69.

41. Rahman A, Broadley SA. Review Article: Elevated Troponin: Diagnostic Gold or Fool's Gold? *Emergency Medicine Australasia.* 2014;26:125–30.

42. Autier P, Boniol M, Koechlin A, Pizot C, Boniol M. Effectiveness of and Overdiagnosis from Mammography Screening in the Netherlands: Population-Based Study. *British Medical Journal.* 2017;359:j5224.

43. Ilic D, Neuberger MM, Djulbegovic M, Dahm P. Screening for Prostate Cancer. *Cochrane Database of Systematic Reviews.* 2013:CD004720.

44. Yudkin JS, Montori VM. The Epidemic of Pre-Diabetes: The Medicine and the Politics. *British Medical Journal.* 2014;349:g4485.

45. Moynihan R. Caution! Diagnosis Creep. *Australian Prescriber.* 2016;39:30–1.

46. Than M, Herbert M, Flaws D, et al. What Is an Acceptable Risk of Major Adverse Cardiac Event in Chest Pain Patients Soon After Discharge from the Emergency Department?: A Clinical Survey. *International Journal of Cardiology.* 2013;166:752–4.

47. Moynihan RN, Cooke GP, Doust JA, Bero L, Hill S, Glasziou PP. Expanding Disease Definitions in Guidelines and Expert Panel Ties to Industry: A Cross-Sectional Study of Common Conditions in the United States. *PLOS Medicine.* 2013;10: e1001500.

48. Ibid.

49. Upchurch CT, Barrett EJ. Clinical Review: Screening for Coronary Artery Disease in Type 2 Diabetes. *Journal of Clinical Endocrinology and Metabolism.* 2012;97:1434–42.

50. Reed S, Pearson S. ICER. Choosing Wisely Recommendation Analysis: Prioritizing Opportunities for Reducing Inappropriate Care. *Preoperative Stress Testing.* 2016.

7. A Stent in Time

1. George Lakoff and Mark Johnson. *Metaphors We Live By.* 1st ed. Chicago, IL: University of Chicago Press; 2003.

2. Goff SL, Mazor KM, Ting HH, Kleppel R, Rothberg MB. How Cardiologists Present the Benefits of Percutaneous Coronary Interventions to Patients with Stable Angina: A Qualitative Analysis. *JAMA Internal Medicine.* 2014;174:1614–21.

3. The Widow Maker Heart Attack. January 2015. https://myheart.net/articles/the -widowmaker/.

4. Al-Lamee R, Thompson D, Dehbi HM, et al. Percutaneous Coronary Intervention in Stable Angina (ORBITA): A Double-Blind, Randomised Controlled Trial. *Lancet*. 2018;391:31–40.

5. Badawy MK, Deb P, Chan R, Farouque O. A Review of Radiation Protection Solutions for the Staff in the Cardiac Catheterisation Laboratory. *Heart, Lung and Circulation*. 2016;25:961–7.

6. Menzoian JO, Koshar AL, Rodrigues N. Alexis Carrel, Rene Leriche, Jean Kunlin, and the History of Bypass Surgery. *Journal of Vascular Surgery*. 2011;54:571–4.

7. Head SJ, Kieser TM, Falk V, Huysmans HA, Kappetein AP. Coronary Artery Bypass Grafting: Part 1—The Evolution over the First 50 Years. *European Heart Journal*. 2013;34:2862–72.

8. JD R. New Surgery for Ailing Hearts. *Reader's Digest*. 71:70 1957.

9. Cobb LA, Thomas GI, Dillard DH, Merendino KA, Bruce RA. An Evaluation of Internal-Mammary-Artery Ligation by a Double-Blind Technic. *New England Journal of Medicine*. 1959;260:1115–8.

10. Shroyer AL, Grover FL, Hattler B, et al. On-Pump versus Off-Pump Coronary-Artery Bypass Surgery. *New England Journal of Medicine*. 2009;361:1827–37.

11. ElBardissi AW, Aranki SF, Sheng S, O'Brien SM, Greenberg CC, Gammie JS. Trends in Isolated Coronary Artery Bypass Grafting: An Analysis of the Society of Thoracic Surgeons Adult Cardiac Surgery Database. *Journal of Thoracic and Cardiovascular Surgery*. 2012;143:273–81.

12. Forssmann W. *Experiments on Myself. Memoirs of a Surgeon in Germany*. New York: St. Martin's; 1974.

13. Forssmann W. Die Sondierung des rechten Herzens. *Klinische Wochenschrift*. 1929;8:2085–7.

14. Heiss HW. Werner Forssmann: A German Problem with the Nobel Prize. *Clinical Cardiology*. 1992;15:547–9.

15. Ryan TJ. The Coronary Angiogram and Its Seminal Contributions to Cardiovascular Medicine over Five Decades. *Circulation*. 2002;106:752–6.

16. Sheldon WC. F. Mason Sones, Jr.—Stormy Petrel of Cardiology. *Clinical Cardiology*. 1994;17:405–7.

17. Shrager JB. The Vineberg Procedure: The Immediate Forerunner of Coronary Artery Bypass Grafting. *Annals of Thoracic Surgery*. 1994;57:1354–64.

18. Sheldon. F. Mason Sones.

19. Hurst JW, King SB, 3rd, Greene L. In Memory of Andreas Roland Gruentzig and Margaret Anne Thornton Gruentzig. *American Journal of Cardiology*. 1986;57:333–6.

20. Ibid.

21. Barton M, Gruntzig J, Husmann M, Rosch J. Balloon Angioplasty—The Legacy of Andreas Gruntzig, M.D. (1939–1985). *Frontiers in Cardiovascular Medicine.* 2014;1:15.

22. Hurst JW. The First Coronary Angioplasty as Described by Andreas Gruentzig. *American Journal of Cardiology.* 1986;57:185–6.

23. Byrne RA, Capodanno D, Mylotte D, Serruys PW. State of the Art: 40 Years of Percutaneous Cardiac Intervention. *EuroIntervention.* 2017;13:621–4.

24. Gruntzig A. Transluminal Dilatation of Coronary-Artery Stenosis. *Lancet.* 1978;1:263.

25. Meier B. The First Patient to Undergo Coronary Angioplasty—23-Year Follow-Up. *New England Journal of Medicine.* 2001;344:144–5.

26. International Trade Administration. Department of Commerce. *2016 Top Markets Report: Medical Devices. Overview and Key Findings.* www.trade.gov/topmarkets/pdf/Medical_Devices_Executive_Summary.pdf.

27. Psaty BM, Boineau R, Kuller LH, Luepker RV. The Potential Costs of Upcoding for Heart Failure in the United States. *American Journal of Cardiology.* 1999;84:108–9, A9.

28. Coding in the Anti-Fraud Era. Skirt the Upcoding Spotlight. *Hospital Peer Review.* 1997;22:141–3.

29. Desai NR, Bradley SM, Parzynski CS, et al. Appropriate Use Criteria for Coronary Revascularization and Trends in Utilization, Patient Selection, and Appropriateness of Percutaneous Coronary Intervention. *Journal of the American Medical Association.* 2015;314:2045–53.

30. Gupta A, Yeh RW, Tamis-Holland JE, et al. Implications of Public Reporting of Risk-Adjusted Mortality Following Percutaneous Coronary Intervention: Misperceptions and Potential Consequences for High-Risk Patients Including Nonsurgical Patients. *JACC Cardiovascular Interventions.* 2016;9:2077–85.

31. Boden WE, O'Rourke RA, Teo KK, et al. Optimal Medical Therapy with or without PCI for Stable Coronary Disease. *New England Journal of Medicine.* 2007;356:1503–16.

32. Sedlis SP, Hartigan PM, Teo KK, et al. Effect of PCI on Long-Term Survival in Patients with Stable Ischemic Heart Disease. *New England Journal of Medicine.* 2015;373:1937–46.

33. Al-Lamee, Thompson, Dehbi, et al. Percutaneous Coronary Intervention.

34. Carrozza JP, Levin T. Periprocedural Complications of Percutaneous Coronary Intervention. UpToDate. Last updated February 8, 2018.

35. Fornell D. Tempering the Bioresorbable Stent Euphoria Following FDA Clearance of the Absorb. August 2016. www.dicardiology.com/content/blogs/tempering-bio-resorbable-stent-euphoria-following-fda-clearance-absorb.

36. De Rosa R, Silverio A, Varricchio A, et al. Meta-Analysis Comparing Outcomes After Everolimus-Eluting Bioresorbable Vascular Scaffolds Versus Everolimus-Eluting Metallic Stents in Patients with Acute Coronary Syndromes. *American Journal of Cardiology*. 2018;122:61–8.

37. Lenzer J. When Is a Point of View a Conflict of Interest? *British Medical Journal*. 2016;355:i6194.

38. de Alencar Neto JN. Morphine, Oxygen, Nitrates, and Mortality Reducing Pharmacological Treatment for Acute Coronary Syndrome: An Evidence-Based Review. *Cureus*. 2018;10:e2114.

39. Gouda P, Bainey K, Welsh R. The Demise of Morphine Oxygen Nitroglycerin Aspirin (MONA). *Canadian Journal of Cardiology*. 2016;32:1578 e7.

8. The Heart of a Woman

1. Hayes SN, Kim ESH, Saw J, et al. Spontaneous Coronary Artery Dissection: Current State of the Science: A Scientific Statement from the American Heart Association. *Circulation*. 2018;137:e523–e57.

2. Lerner DJ, Kannel WB. Patterns of Coronary Heart Disease Morbidity and Mortality in the Sexes: A 26-Year Follow-Up of the Framingham Population. *American Heart Journal*. 1986;111:383–90.

3. Mehta LS, Watson KE, Barac A, et al. Cardiovascular Disease and Breast Cancer: Where These Entities Intersect: A Scientific Statement from the American Heart Association. *Circulation*. 2018;137:e30–e66.

4. Mosca L, Hammond G, Mochari-Greenberger H, et al. Fifteen-Year Trends in Awareness of Heart Disease in Women: Results of a 2012 American Heart Association National Survey. *Circulation*. 2013;127:1254–63, e1–29.

5. Pope JH, Aufderheide TP, Ruthazer R, et al. Missed Diagnoses of Acute Cardiac Ischemia in the Emergency Department. *New England Journal of Medicine*. 2000;342:1163–70.

6. Bugiardini R, Ricci B, Cenko E, et al. Delayed Care and Mortality Among Women and Men with Myocardial Infarction. *Journal of the American Heart Association*. 2017;6.

7. Zwas DR. Redressing the Red Dress: Rethinking the Campaign. *Circulation*. 2018;137:763–5.

8. Kragholm K, Halim SA, Yang Q, et al. Sex-Stratified Trends in Enrollment, Patient Characteristics, Treatment, and Outcomes Among Non-ST-Segment Elevation Acute Coronary Syndrome Patients: Insights from Clinical Trials over 17 Years. *Circulation: Cardiovascular Quality and Outcomes*. 2015;8:357–67.

9. Rosenman RH, Brand RJ, Jenkins D, Friedman M, Straus R, Wurm M. Coronary Heart Disease in Western Collaborative Group Study. Final Follow-Up Experience of 8 1/2 Years. *Journal of the American Medical Association*. 1975;233:872–7.

10. Keys A, Taylor HL, Blackburn H, Brozek J, Anderson JT, Simonson E. Coronary Heart Disease Among Minnesota Business and Professional Men Followed Fifteen Years. *Circulation*. 1963;28:381–95.

11. Chapman JM, Massey FJ, Jr. The Interrelationship of Serum Cholesterol, Hypertension, Body Weight, and Risk of Coronary Disease. Results of the First Ten Years' Follow-Up in the Los Angeles Heart Study. *Journal of Chronic Diseases*. 1964;17:933–49.

12. Chen G, Levy D. Contributions of the Framingham Heart Study to the Epidemiology of Coronary Heart Disease. *JAMA Cardiology*. 2016;1:825–30.

13. Epstein FH, Ostrander LD, Jr., Johnson BC, et al. Epidemiological Studies of Cardiovascular Disease in a Total Community—Tecumseh, Michigan. *Annals of Internal Medicine*. 1965;62:1170–87.

14. Merkatz RB, Temple R, Subel S, Feiden K, Kessler DA. Women in Clinical Trials of New Drugs. A Change in Food and Drug Administration Policy. The Working Group on Women in Clinical Trials. *New England Journal of Medicine*. 1993;329:292–6.

15. McCormick KM, Bunting SM. Application of Feminist Theory in Nursing Research: The Case of Women and Cardiovascular Disease. *Health Care of Women International*. 2002;23:820–34.

16. Albrektsen G, Heuch I, Lochen ML, et al. Lifelong Gender Gap in Risk of Incident Myocardial Infarction: The Tromso Study. *JAMA Internal Medicine*. 2016;176:1673–9.

17. Berg J, Bjorck L, Nielsen S, Lappas G, Rosengren A. Sex Differences in Survival After Myocardial Infarction in Sweden, 1987–2010. *Heart*. 2017;103:1625–30.

18. Ricci B, Cenko E, Vasiljevic Z, et al. Acute Coronary Syndrome: The Risk to Young Women. *Journal of the American Heart Association*. 2017;6.

19. Wyckoff J. Heart Disease: Points Every Nurse Should Know About It. *American Journal of Nursing*. 1924;24:529–32.

20. White PD. Important Clues in Cardiovascular Diagnosis. *New England Journal of Medicine*. 1942;227:980–4.

21. Hamilton BE. The Care of a Cardiac Patient During Pregnancy. *American Journal of Nursing*. 1927;27:173–7.

22. Upton NB. Home Adjustments in Chronic Heart Disease. *New England Journal of Medicine*. 1929;200:5–7.

23. Jones RL. A Case Study: Mitral Stenosis with Auricular Fibrillation. *American Journal of Nursing*. 1938;38:1151–6.

24. Chinn PL, Wheeler CE. Feminism and Nursing. *Nursing Outlook*. 1985;33:74–7.

25. Nichols FH. History of the Women's Health Movement in the 20th Century. *Journal of Obstetric, Gynecologic, & Neonatal Nursing*. 2000;29:56–64.

26. Miller CL, Kollauf CR. Evolution of Information on Women and Heart Disease 1957–2000: A Review of Archival Records and Secular Literature. *Heart & Lung.* 2002;31:253–61.

27. King KM, Paul P. A Historical Review of the Depiction of Women in Cardiovascular Literature. *Western Journal of Nursing Research.* 1996;18:89–101.

28. Thomas JL, Braus PA. Coronary Artery Disease in Women. A Historical Perspective. *Archives of Internal Medicine.* 1998;158:333–7.

29. Pope TP. Maternal Instinct Is Wired into the Brain. March 2008. https://well.blogs.nytimes.com/2008/03/07/maternal-instinct-is-wired-into-the-brain/.

30. AARP. National Alliance for Caregiving and AARP. *Caregiving in the U.S.* www.caregiving.org/wp-content/uploads/2015/05/2015_CaregivingintheUS_Final-Report-June-4_WEB.pdf.2015.

31. Adelman RD, Tmanova LL, Delgado D, Dion S, Lachs MS. Caregiver Burden: A Clinical Review. *Journal of the American Medical Association.* 2014;311:1052–60.

32. Granger BB, Ekman I, Granger CB, et al. Adherence to Medication According to Sex and Age in the CHARM Programme. *European Journal of Heart Failure.* 2009;11:1092–8.

33. Pilgrim T, Heg D, Tal K, et al. Age-and Gender-Related Disparities in Primary Percutaneous Coronary Interventions for Acute ST-Segment Elevation Myocardial Infarction. *PLOS ONE.* 2015;10:e0137047.

34. Swaminathan RV, Feldman DN, Pashun RA, et al. Gender Differences in In-Hospital Outcomes After Coronary Artery Bypass Grafting. *American Journal of Cardiology.* 2016;118:362–8.

35. Hinohara TT, Al-Khalidi HR, Fordyce CB, et al. Impact of Regional Systems of Care on Disparities in Care Among Female and Black Patients Presenting with ST-Segment-Elevation Myocardial Infarction. *Journal of the American Heart Association.* 2017;6.

36. Singh JA, Lu X, Ibrahim S, Cram P. Trends in and Disparities for Acute Myocardial Infarction: An Analysis of Medicare Claims Data from 1992 to 2010. *BMC Medicine.* 2014;12:190.

37. O'Keefe-McCarthy S. Women's Experiences of Cardiac Pain: A Review of the Literature. *Canadian Journal of Cardiovascular Nursing.* 2008;18:18–25.

38. Hart PL. Women's Perceptions of Coronary Heart Disease: An Integrative Review. *Journal of Cardiovascular Nursing.* 2005;20:170–6.

39. Kirchberger I, Heier M, Wende R, von Scheidt W, Meisinger C. The Patient's Interpretation of Myocardial Infarction Symptoms and Its Role in the Decision Process to Seek Treatment: The MONICA/KORA Myocardial Infarction Registry. *Clinical Research in Cardiology.* 2012;101:909–16.

40. Bugiardini, Ricci, Cenko, et al. Delayed Care.

41. Davis LL. A Qualitative Study of Symptom Experiences of Women with Acute Coronary Syndrome. *Journal of Cardiovascular Nursing.* 2017;32:488–95.

42. Ibid.

43. From AM, Prasad A, Pellikka PA, McCully RB. Are Some False-Positive Stress Echocardiograms a Forme Fruste Variety of Apical Ballooning Syndrome? *American Journal of Cardiology.* 2009;103:1434–8.

44. Fitzgerald BT, Scalia WM, Scalia GM. Female False Positive Exercise Stress ECG Testing-Fact Vers[u]s Fiction. *Heart, Lung and Circulation.* 2018.

45. Canto JG, Rogers WJ, Goldberg RJ, et al. Association of Age and Sex with Myocardial Infarction Symptom Presentation and In-Hospital Mortality. *Journal of the American Medical Association.* 2012;307:813–22.

46. Lichtman JH, Leifheit EC, Safdar B, et al. Sex Differences in the Presentation and Perception of Symptoms Among Young Patients with Myocardial Infarction: Evidence from the VIRGO Study (Variation in Recovery: Role of Gender on Outcomes of Young AMI Patients). *Circulation.* 2018;137:781–90.

47. Galdas PM, Johnson JL, Percy ME, Ratner PA. Help Seeking for Cardiac Symptoms: Beyond the Masculine-Feminine Binary. *Social Science & Medicine.* 2010;71:18–24.

48. Ibid.

49. Canto, Rogers, Goldberg, et al. Association of Age and Sex.

50. Abstract of the Bill of Mortality for the Town of Boston. *New England Journal of Medicine and Surgery.* 1812:1:320–1.

51. Arias E, Heron M, Xu J. United States Life Tables, 2014. *National Vital Statistics Reports.* 2017;66:1–64.

52. Amos A, Haglund M. From Social Taboo to "Torch of Freedom": The Marketing of Cigarettes to Women. *Tobacco Control.* 2000;9:3–8.

53. McCormick, Bunting. Application of Feminist Theory.

54. Ibid.

55. Manson JE, Martin KA. Clinical Practice. Postmenopausal Hormone-Replacement Therapy. *New England Journal of Medicine.* 2001;345:34–40.

56. Stampfer MJ, Colditz GA, Willett WC, et al. Postmenopausal Estrogen Therapy and Cardiovascular Disease. Ten-Year Follow-Up from the Nurses' Health Study. *New England Journal of Medicine.* 1991;325:756–62.

57. Effects of Estrogen or Estrogen/Progestin Regimens on Heart Disease Risk Factors in Postmenopausal Women. The Postmenopausal Estrogen/Progestin Interventions (PEPI) Trial. The Writing Group for the PEPI Trial. *Journal of the American Medical Association.* 1995;273:199–208.

58. Hodis HN, Mack WJ, Lobo RA, et al. Estrogen in the Prevention of Atherosclero-

sis. A Randomized, Double-Blind, Placebo-Controlled Trial. *Annals of Internal Medicine.* 2001;135:939–53.

59. Muka T, Oliver-Williams C, Kunutsor S, et al. Association of Age at Onset of Menopause and Time Since Onset of Menopause with Cardiovascular Outcomes, Intermediate Vascular Traits, and All-Cause Mortality: A Systematic Review and Meta-Analysis. *JAMA Cardiology.* 2016;1:767–76.

60. Hulley S, Grady D, Bush T, et al. Randomized Trial of Estrogen Plus Progestin for Secondary Prevention of Coronary Heart Disease in Postmenopausal Women. Heart and Estrogen/Progestin Replacement Study (HERS) Research Group. *Journal of the American Medical Association.* 1998;280:605–13.

61. Rossouw JE, Anderson GL, Prentice RL, et al. Risks and Benefits of Estrogen Plus Progestin in Healthy Postmenopausal Women: Principal Results from the Women's Health Initiative Randomized Controlled Trial. *Journal of the American Medical Association.* 2002;288:321–33.

62. Ioannidis JP. Contradicted and Initially Stronger Effects in Highly Cited Clinical Research. *Journal of the American Medical Association.* 2005;294:218–28.

63. Gooren LJ, Wierckx K, Giltay EJ. Cardiovascular Disease in Transsexual Persons Treated with Cross-Sex Hormones: Reversal of the Traditional Sex Difference in Cardiovascular Disease Pattern. *European Journal of Endocrinology.* 2014;170:809–19.

64. Kannel WB, D'Agostino RB, Wilson PW, Belanger AJ, Gagnon DR. Diabetes, Fibrinogen, and Risk of Cardiovascular Disease: The Framingham Experience. *American Heart Journal.* 1990;120:672–6.

65. Anand SS, Islam S, Rosengren A, et al. Risk Factors for Myocardial Infarction in Women and Men: Insights from the INTERHEART Study. *European Heart Journal.* 2008;29:932–40.

66. Puymirat E, Simon T, Steg PG, et al. Association of Changes in Clinical Characteristics and Management with Improvement in Survival Among Patients with ST-Elevation Myocardial Infarction. *Journal of the American Medical Association.* 2012;308:998–1006.

67. Lenz W. A Short History of Thalidomide Embryopathy. *Teratology.* 1988;38:203–15.

68. Watts G. Frances Oldham Kelsey. *Lancet.* 2015;386:1334.

69. Elkayam U, Goland S, Pieper PG, Silverside CK. High-Risk Cardiac Disease in Pregnancy: Part I. *Journal of the American College of Cardiology.* 2016;68:396–410.

70. Arany Z, Elkayam U. Peripartum Cardiomyopathy. *Circulation.* 2016;133:1397–409.

71. Bennett MR. Development of the Concept of Mind. *Australian and New Zealand Journal of Psychiatry.* 2007;41:943–56.

72. Jackson M. The Stress of Life: A Modern Complaint? *Lancet.* 2014;383:300–1.

73. *English Mechanic and World of Science. No. 366. Increase of Heart-Disease.* London: Mechanics; March 29, 1872.

74. Jackson. The Stress of Life.

75. Beck J. "Americanitis": The Disease of Living Too Fast. *Atlantic.* March 2016.

76. Jackson. The Stress of Life.

77. Osler W. *Lectures on Angina Pectoris and Allied States.* New York: D. Appleton and Company; 1897.

78. Keys, Taylor, Blackburn, Brozek, Anderson, Simonson. Coronary Heart Disease.

79. Huffman JC, Pollack MH, Stern TA. Panic Disorder and Chest Pain: Mechanisms, Morbidity, and Management. *Primary Care Companion to the Journal of Clinical Psychiatry.* 2002;4:54–62.

80. Demiryoguran NS, Karcioglu O, Topacoglu H, et al. Anxiety Disorder in Patients with Non-Specific Chest Pain in the Emergency Setting. *Emergency Medicine Journal.* 2006;23:99–102.

81. Warraich HJ, Buxton AE, Kociol RD. Macroscopic T-Wave Alternans in a Patient with Takotsubo Cardiomyopathy and QT Prolongation. *Heart Rhythm.* 2014;11:1848–9.

82. Sato TH, Uchida T, Dote K, Ishihara M. Takotsubo-Like Left Ventricular Dysfunction Due to Multivessel Coronary Spasm. In: Kodama K, Haze K, Hori M, eds. *Clinical Aspect of Myocardial Injury: From Ischemia to Heart Failure.* Tokyo, Japan: Kagakuhyoronsha Publishing Co:56–64. 1990.

83. Wallstrom S, Ulin K, Maatta S, Omerovic E, Ekman I. Impact of Long-Term Stress in Takotsubo Syndrome: Experience of Patients. *European Journal of Cardiovascular Nursing.* 2016;15:522–8.

84. Nesse RM, Young EA. Evolutionary Origins and Functions of the Stress Response. In: *Encyclopedia of Stress.* Amsterdam: Elsevier; 2000.

85. Kim NH, Lee G, Sherer NA, Martini KM, Goldenfeld N, Kuhlman TE. Real-Time Transposable Element Activity in Individual Live Cells. *Proceedings of the National Academy of Sciences of the United States of America.* 2016;113:7278–83.

86. Koolhaas JM, Bartolomucci A, Buwalda B, et al. Stress Revisited: A Critical Evaluation of the Stress Concept. *Neuroscience & Biobehavioral Reviews.* 2011;35:1291–301.

87. Pelliccia F, Kaski JC, Crea F, Camici PG. Pathophysiology of Takotsubo Syndrome. *Circulation.* 2017;135:2426–41.

88. Wittstein IS, Thiemann DR, Lima JA, et al. Neurohumoral Features of Myocardial Stunning Due to Sudden Emotional Stress. *New England Journal of Medicine.* 2005;352:539–48.

89. Ghadri JR, Sarcon A, Diekmann J, et al. Happy Heart Syndrome: Role of Positive Emotional Stress in Takotsubo Syndrome. *European Heart Journal.* 2016;37:2823–9.

90. Saposnik G, Baibergenova A, Dang J, Hachinski V. Does a Birthday Predispose to Vascular Events? *Neurology*. 2006;67:300–4.

91. Ghadri, Sarcon, Diekmann, et al. Happy Heart Syndrome.

92. Gross M. Chronic Stress Means We're Always on the Hunt. *Current Biology*. 2014;24:R405–8.

93. Foss B, Dyrstad SM. Stress in Obesity: Cause or Consequence? *Medical Hypotheses*. 2011;77:7–10.

94. Hu B, Liu X, Yin S, Fan H, Feng F, Yuan J. Effects of Psychological Stress on Hypertension in Middle-Aged Chinese: A Cross-Sectional Study. *PLOS ONE*. 2015;10:e0129163.

95. Kelly SJ, Ismail M. Stress and Type 2 Diabetes: A Review of How Stress Contributes to the Development of Type 2 Diabetes. *Annual Review of Public Health*. 2015; 36:441–62.

96. Roohafza H, Kabir A, Sadeghi M, et al. Stress as a Risk Factor for Noncompliance with Treatment Regimens in Patients with Diabetes and Hypertension. *ARYA Atherosclerosis*. 2016;12:166–71.

97. Hu, Liu, Yin, Fan, Feng, Yuan. Effects of Psychological Stress.

98. Yusuf S, Hawken S, Ounpuu S, et al. Effect of Potentially Modifiable Risk Factors Associated with Myocardial Infarction in 52 Countries (the INTERHEART Study): Case-Control Study. *Lancet*. 2004;364:937–52.

99. Vaccarino V, Sullivan S, Hammadah M, et al. Mental Stress-Induced-Myocardial Ischemia in Young Patients with Recent Myocardial Infarction: Sex Differences and Mechanisms. *Circulation*. 2018;137:794–805.

100. Chang SC, Glymour M, Cornelis M, et al. Social Integration and Reduced Risk of Coronary Heart Disease in Women: The Role of Lifestyle Behaviors. *Circulation Research*. 2017;120:1927–37.

101. Selye H. The Evolution of the Stress Concept. *American Scientist*. 1973;61:692–9.

102. Buccheri D, Zambelli G. The Link Between Spontaneous Coronary Artery Dissection and Takotsubo Cardiomyopathy: Analysis of the Published Cases. *Journal of Thoracic Disease*. 2017;9:5489–92.

103. Jagsi R, Biga C, Poppas A, et al. Work Activities and Compensation of Male and Female Cardiologists. *Journal of the American College of Cardiology*. 2016;67:529–41.

104. Derose KP, Hays RD, McCaffrey DF, Baker DW. Does Physician Gender Affect Satisfaction of Men and Women Visiting the Emergency Department? *Journal of General Internal Medicine*. 2001;16:218–26.

105. Phillips MD, Lowe MJ, Lurito JT, Dzemidzic M, Mathews VP. Temporal Lobe Activation Demonstrates Sex-Based Differences During Passive Listening. *Radiology*. 2001;220:202–7.

9. First to Live, Last to Die

1. Aloysio Luigi Galvani (1737–1798) Discoverer of Animal Electricity. *Journal of the American Medical Association.* 1967;201:626–7.

2. Sengupta B, Stemmler MB. Power Consumption During Neuronal Computation. Proceedings of the IEEE 2014;102:738–50.

3. Could You Charge an iPhone with the Electricity in Your Brain? August 2015. https://gizmodo.com/could-you-charge-an-iphone-with-the-electricity-in -your-1722569935.

4. Fye WB. A History of the Origin, Evolution, and Impact of Electrocardiography. *American Journal of Cardiology.* 1994;73:937–49.

5. Fye WB. Disorders of the Heartbeat: A Historical Overview from Antiquity to the Mid-20th Century. *American Journal of Cardiology.* 1993;72:1055–70.

6. Goldberger ZD, Whiting SM, Howell JD. The Heartfelt Music of Ludwig van Beethoven. *Perspectives in Biology and Medicine.* 2014;57:285–94.

7. Perman E. Successful Cardiac Resuscitation with Electricity in the 18th Century? *British Medical Journal.* 1978;2:1770–1.

8. Kite C. *An Essay on the Recovery of the Apparently Dead.* London: C. Dilly; 1788.

9. Nuland S. *How We Die: Reflections of Life's Final Chapter.* New York: Knopf; 1994.

10. Beck CS, Pritchard WH, Feil HS. Ventricular Fibrillation of Long Duration Abolished by Electric Shock. *Journal of the American Medical Association.* 1947;135:985.

11. Cohen SI. Resuscitation Great. Paul M. Zoll, M.D.—The Father of "Modern" Electrotherapy and Innovator of Pharmacotherapy for Life-Threatening Cardiac Arrhythmias. *Resuscitation.* 2007;73:178–85.

12. Cohen S. *Paul Zoll, MD: The Pioneer Whose Discoveries Prevent Sudden Death.* Salem, NH: Free People Publishing; 2014.

13. Zoll PM, Linenthal AJ, Gibson W, Paul MH, Norman LR. Termination of Ventricular Fibrillation in Man by Externally Applied Electric Countershock. *New England Journal of Medicine.* 1956;254:727–32.

14. Cakulev I, Efimov IR, Waldo AL. Cardioversion: Past, Present, and Future. *Circulation.* 2009;120:1623–32.

15. Cuculich PS, Schill MR, Kashani R, et al. Noninvasive Cardiac Radiation for Ablation of Ventricular Tachycardia. *New England Journal of Medicine.* 2017;377: 2325–36.

16. Desai NR, Bourdillon PM, Parzynski CS, et al. Association of the U.S. Department of Justice Investigation of Implantable Cardioverter-Defibrillators and Devices Not Meeting the Medicare National Coverage Determination, 2007–2015. *Journal of the American Medical Association.* 2018;320:63–71.

17. Shen L, Jhund PS, Petrie MC, et al. Declining Risk of Sudden Death in Heart Failure. *New England Journal of Medicine.* 2017;377:41–51.

18.   Kober L, Thune JJ, Nielsen JC, et al. Defibrillator Implantation in Patients with Nonischemic Systolic Heart Failure. *New England Journal of Medicine.* 2016;375:1221–30.

19.   Goldstein NE, Lampert R, Bradley E, Lynn J, Krumholz HM. Management of Implantable Cardioverter Defibrillators in End-of-Life Care. *Annals of Internal Medicine.* 2004;141:835–8.

20.   Goldstein NE, Mehta D, Siddiqui S, et al. "That's Like an Act of Suicide" Patients' Attitudes Toward Deactivation of Implantable Defibrillators. *Journal of General Internal Medicine.* 2008;23 Suppl 1:7–12.

21.   Zoll PM. Resuscitation of the Heart in Ventricular Standstill by External Electric Stimulation. *New England Journal of Medicine.* 1952;247:768–71.

22.   Pycroft L, Aziz TZ. Security of Implantable Medical Devices with Wireless Connections: The Dangers of Cyber-Attacks. *Expert Review of Medical Devices.* 2018; 15:403–6.

23.   Dyer O. Abbott Laboratories Offers Fix for 745 000 Pacemakers Vulnerable to Hacking. *British Medical Journal.* 2017;358:j4190.

10. The Morbid Dance of Cancer and Heart Disease

1.   de Moor JS, Mariotto AB, Parry C, et al. Cancer Survivors in the United States: Prevalence Across the Survivorship Trajectory and Implications for Care. *Cancer Epidemiology, Biomarkers & Prevention.* 2013;22:561–70.

2.   Drake N. When Hubble Stared at Nothing for 100 Hours. *National Geographic.* April 2015.

3.   Jaiswal S, Fontanillas P, Flannick J, et al. Age-Related Clonal Hematopoiesis Associated with Adverse Outcomes. *New England Journal of Medicine.* 2014;371:2488–98.

4.   Stockmann C, Hersh AL, Sherwin CM, Spigarelli MG. Alignment of United States Funding for Cardiovascular Disease Research with Deaths, Years of Life Lost, and Hospitalizations. *International Journal of Cardiology.* 2014;172:e19–21.

5.   Okwuosa TM, Anzevino S, Rao R. Cardiovascular Disease in Cancer Survivors. *Postgraduate Medical Journal.* 2017;93:82–90.

6.   Steele CB, Thomas CC, Henley SJ, et al. Vital Signs: Trends in Incidence of Cancers Associated with Overweight and Obesity-United States, 2005–2014. *Morbidity and Mortality Weekly Report.* 2017;66:1052–8.

7.   Friedenreich CM, Shaw E, Neilson HK, Brenner DR. Epidemiology and Biology of Physical Activity and Cancer Recurrence. *Journal of Molecular Medicine.* (Berlin). 2017;95:1029–41.

8.   Holmes MD, Chen WY, Feskanich D, Kroenke CH, Colditz GA. Physical Activity and Survival After Breast Cancer Diagnosis. *Journal of the American Medical Association.* 2005;293:2479–86.

9. Omer ZB, Hwang ES, Esserman LJ, Howe R, Ozanne EM. Impact of Ductal Carcinoma In Situ Terminology on Patient Treatment Preferences. *Journal of the American Medical Association. Internal Medicine*. 2013;173:1830–1.

10. Pentagon Gets ISIS Metaphor Wrong, Critics Say. January 2016. www.npr.org/2016/01/26/464399975/how-to-keep-isis-from-spreading-is-still-up-for-debate.

11. Greene SJ, Butler J, Albert NM, et al. Medical Therapy for Heart Failure with Reduced Ejection Fraction: The CHAMP-HF Registry. *Journal of the American College of Cardiology*. 2018;72:351–66.

12. Warraich H. Failing Heart Failure Patients. *New York Times*. August 2015.

11. The Heart of the Matter

1. Thomson JG. Provisional Report on the Autopsy of L. W. (Louis Washkansky). *South African Medical Journal*. 1967;41:1277–8.

2. Kirklin JK, Pagani FD, Kormos RL, et al. Eighth Annual INTERMACS Report: Special Focus on Framing the Impact of Adverse Events. *Journal of Heart and Lung Transplantation*. 2017;36:1080–6.

3. Warraich HJ, Kaltenbach LA, Fonarow GC, Peterson ED, Wang TY. Adverse Change in Employment Status After Acute Myocardial Infarction: Analysis from the TRANSLATE-ACS Study. *Circulation: Cardiovascular Quality and Outcomes*. 2018;11:e004528.

4. Cooley DA. Some Thoughts About the Historic Events That Led to the First Clinical Implantation of a Total Artificial Heart. *Texas Heart Institute Journal*. 2013;40:117–9.

5. Altman L. The Feud. *New York Times*. 2007.

6. Maugh T. Denton Cooley, Texas Surgeon Who Performed First Successful Heart Transplant in U.S., Dies at 96. *Los Angeles Times*. 2016.

7. A Bitter Feud: Two Great Surgeons at War over the Human Heart. *Life*. April 1970.

8. Cooley. Some Thoughts About the Historic Events.

9. Altman L. The Feud.

10. Ibid.

11. Dr. Denton Cooley at 95: The Legend Speaks in a Video Interview. July 2016. www.houstonchronicle.com/local/prognosis/article/Cooley-at-95-Some-tidbits-from-an-interview-8387536.php.

12. Cooley D. *10,000 Hearts: A Surgeon's Memoir*. Austin: Briscoe Center for American History, University of Texas; 2012.

13. Dr. Denton Cooley at 95.

14. Maugh T. Denton Cooley, Texas Surgeon.

15. Miller LW, Rogers JG. Evolution of Left Ventricular Assist Device Therapy for Advanced Heart Failure: A Review. *JAMA Cardiology*. 2018;3:650–8.

16. Jakovljevic DG, Yacoub MH, Schueler S, et al. Left Ventricular Assist Device as a Bridge to Recovery for Patients with Advanced Heart Failure. *Journal of the American College of Cardiology.* 2017;69:1924–33.

17. McIlvennan CK, Wordingham SE, Allen LA, et al. Deactivation of Left Ventricular Assist Devices: Differing Perspectives of Cardiology and Hospice/Palliative Medicine Clinicians. *Journal of Cardiac Failure.* 2017;23:708–12.

18. Diop MS, Rudolph JL, Zimmerman KM, Richter MA, Skarf LM. Palliative Care Interventions for Patients with Heart Failure: A Systematic Review and Meta-Analysis. *Journal of Palliative Medicine.* 2017;20:84–92.

19. Warraich HJ, Hernandez AF, Allen LA. How Medicine Has Changed the End of Life for Patients with Cardiovascular Disease. *Journal of the American College of Cardiology.* 2017;70:1276–89.

20. Warraich HJ, Mentz RJ, Hernandez AF. Paving a Better Path for Patients Dying of Heart Disease. *Circulation.* 2018;137:1216–7.

21. Doctor Considers the Pitfalls of Extending Life and Prolonging Death. January 2017. www.npr.org/sections/health-shots/2017/01/30/512426568/doctor-considers-the-pitfalls-of-extending-life-and-prolonging-death.

22. Warraich, Hernandez, Allen. How Medicine Has Changed the End.

23. Goldstein NE, Mehta D, Siddiqui S, et al. "That's Like an Act of Suicide" Patients' Attitudes Toward Deactivation of Implantable Defibrillators. *Journal of General Internal Medicine.* 2008;23 Suppl 1:7–12.

24. Singh GK, Siahpush M, Azuine RE, Williams SD. Widening Socioeconomic and Racial Disparities in Cardiovascular Disease Mortality in the United States, 1969–2013. *International Journal of MCH and AIDS.* 2015;3:106–18.

25. Rosenson RS, Hegele RA, Fazio S, Cannon CP. The Evolving Future of PCSK9 Inhibitors. *Journal of the American College of Cardiology.* 2018;72:314–29.

26. Ray KK, Landmesser U, Leiter LA, et al. Inclisiran in Patients at High Cardiovascular Risk with Elevated LDL Cholesterol. *New England Journal of Medicine.* 2017;376:1430–40.

27. Singh, Siahpush, Azuine, Williams. Widening Socioeconomic and Racial Disparities.

Index